HEAT SHOCK PROTEINS AND THE CARDIOVASCULAR SYSTEM

Developments in Cardiovascular Medicine

M.LeWinter. H. Suga and M.W. Watkins (eds.): *Cardiac Energetics: From Emax to Pressure-volume Area*. 1995 ISBN 0-7923-3721-2

R.J. Siegel (ed.): *Ultrasound Angioplasty*. 1995   ISBN 0-7923-3722-0

D.M. Yellon and G.J. Gross (eds.): *Myocardial Protection and the Katp Channel*. 1995
ISBN 0-7923-3791-3
A.V.G. Bruschke. J.H.C. Reiber. K.I. Lie and H.J.J. Wellens (eds.): *Lipid Lowering Therapy and Progression of Coronary Atherosclerosis*. 1996 ISBN 0-7923-3807-3

A.S.A. Abd-Elfattah and A.S. Wechsler (eds.): *Purines and Myocardial Protection*. 1995
ISBN 0-7923-3831-6
M. Morad, S. Ebashi, W. Trautwein and Y. Kurachi (eds.): *Molecular Physiology and Pharmacology of Cardiac Ion Channels and Transporters*. 1996 ISBN 0-7923-3913-4

A.M. Oto (ed.): *Practice and Progress in Cardiac Pacing and Electrophysiology*. 1996
ISBN 0-7923-3950-9
W.H. Birkenhager (ed.): *Practical Management of Hypertension. Second Edition*. 1996
ISBN 0-7923-3952-5
J.C. Chatham, J.R. Forder and J.H. McNeill(eds.):*The Heart In Diabetes*. 1996
ISBN 0-7923-4052-3
M. Kroll, M. Lehmann (eds.): *Implantable Cardioverter Defibrillator Therapy: The Engineering-Clinical Interface*. 1996   ISBN 0-7923-4300-X

Lloyd Klein (ed.): *Coronary Stenosis Morphology: Analysis and Implication*.
1996   ISBN 0-7923-9867-X

Johan H.C. Reiber, Ernst E. Van der Wall (eds.): *Cardiovascular Imaging*.
ISBN 0-7923-4109-0
A.-M. Salmasi, A. Strano (eds.): *Angiology in Practice*. ISBN 0-7923-4143-0

Julio E. Perez, Roberto M. Lang, (eds.): *Echocardiography and Cardiovascular Function: Tools for the Next Decade*. 1996 ISBN 0-7923-9884-X

Keith L. March (ed.): *Gene Transfer in the Cardiovascular System: Experimental Approaches and Therapeutic Implications*. 1997 ISBN 0-7923-9859-9

Anne A. Knowlton (ed.): *Heat Shock Proteins and the Cardiovascular System*.
1997 ISBN 0-7923-9910-2

HEAT SHOCK PROTEINS AND THE CARDIOVASCULAR SYSTEM

edited by

A. A. Knowlton

Cardiology Section
Department of Medicine
V.A. Medical Center
and
Baylor College of Medicine
Houston, Texas, USA

KLUWER ACADEMIC PUBLISHERS

Boston / Dordrecht / London

Distributors for North America:
Kluwer Academic Publishers
101 Philip Drive
Assinippi Park
Norwell, Massachusetts 02061 USA

Distributors for all other countries:
Kluwer Academic Publishers Group
Distribution Centre
Post Office Box 322
NL-3300 AH Dordrecht, THE NETHERLANDS

Library of Congress Cataloging-in-Publication Data

A C.I.P. Catalogue record for this book is available
from the Library of Congress.

Contents

List of Contributors

Albert Amberger, Ph.D.
Institute for Biomedical Aging
Research
Austrian Academy of Sciences
6020 Innsbruck
Rennweg 10, Austria

R. William Currie, Ph.D.
Laboratory of Molecular Neurobiology
Department of Anatomy and
Neurobiology
Dalhousie University
Halifax, Canada B3H 4H7

Dipak K. Das, Ph.D.
Department of Surgery, Cardiovascular
Division
University of Connecticut
School of Medicine
Farmington, Ct. 06032

Wolfgang Dillmann, M.D.
Department of Medicine
University of California-
 San Diego
200 W. Arbor Drive
San Diego, Cal.92103-8412

Barney E. Dwyer, Ph.D.
Chief of Molecular Neurobiology
Laboratory
Veterans Affairs Hospital and
Dartmouth Medical School
Department of Medicine (Neurology)
Research Service 151
White River Junction, VT 05009

Timothy Fawcett, Ph.D.
Gene Expression/Aging
National Institutes on Aging
4940 Eastern Ave.
Baltimore, Md. 21224

Richard J. Heads, Ph.D.
Department of Cardiology
Guy's and St. Thomas Medical and
Dental Schools
The Rayne Institute
St. Thomas' Hospital
Lambeth Palace Rd,
London SE1 7EH
England, U.K.

Nikki Holbrook, Ph.D.
Gene Expression/Aging
National Institutes on Aging
4940 Eastern Ave.
Baltimore, Md. 21224

Shogen Isoyama, M.D.
First Department of Internal Medicine
Tohuku University School of Medicine
1-1 Seiryo-machi, Aobaku
Sendai 980, Japan

A.A.Knowlton, M.D.
Cardiology Section
V.A. Medical Center and
Baylor College of Medicine
2002 Holcombe
Houston, Tx. 77030

Douglas L. Mann, M.D.
Cardiology Section
V.A. Medical Center and
Baylor College of Medicine
2002 Holcombe
Houston, Tx. 77030

Nilanjana Maulik, Ph.D.
Department of Surgery, Cardiovascular
Division
University of Connecticut
School of Medicine
Farmington, Ct. 06032

Ruben Mestril, Ph.D.
Department of Medicine
University of California- San Diego
200 W. Arbor Drive
San Diego, Cal. 92103-8412

Bernhard Metzler, Ph.D.
Institute for Biomedical Aging
Research
Austrian Academy of Sciences
6020 Innsbruck
Rennweg 10, Austria

Dorothea Michaelis, Ph.D.
Institute for Biomedical Aging
Research
Austrian Academy of Sciences
6020 Innsbruck
Rennweg 10, Austria

Masayuki Nakano, M.D., Ph.D.
the Second Department of Internal
Medicine
Gunma University
School of Medicine 3-39-15
Showa-machi
Maebashi, Gunma
Japan 371

Robert N. Nishimura, M.D.
Molecular Neurobiology Laboratory
Veterans Affairs Hospital and UCLA
Dept. of Neurology, 111N-1
16111 Plummer St.
Sepulveda, Ca. 91343

J.-Christophe L. Plumier, Ph.D.
Department of Anatomy and
Neurobiology
Dalhousie University
Halifax, Nova Scotia,
Canada B3H 4H7

Maria Romen, Ph.D.
Institute for General and Experimental
Pathology
University of Innsbruck

6020 Innsbruck
Rennweg 10, Austria

Georg Schett, Ph.D.
Institute for Biomedical Aging
Research
Austrian Academy of Sciences
and Institute for General and
Experimental Pathology
University of Innsbruck
6020 Innsbruck
Rennweg 10, Austria

Hari S. Sharma, Ph.D.
Thorax Center
Erasmus University
3000 DR Rotterdam
The Netherlands

Dr. Joachim Stahl
Max-Delbrück-Center for Molecular
Medicine
Robert-Rössle-Str. 10
D-13122 Berlin-Buch
Germany

G.Wick, Ph.D.
Professor and Chairman
Institute for Biomedical Aging
Research
Austrian Academy of Sciences
and Institute for General and
Experimental Pathology
University of Innsbruck
6020 Innsbruck
Rennweg 10, Austria

Derek Yellon, Ph.D.
Division of Cardiology
Hatter Institute for Cardiovascular
Studies
London WC1E 6AU
England, U.K.

Robert Udelsman, M.D.
Department of Surgery
Johns Hopkins University

Baltimore, MD 21225

Qingbo Xu, Ph.D.
Institute for Biomedical Aging
Research
Austrian Academy of Sciences
6020 Innsbruck
Rennweg 10, Austria

Preface

Heat shock proteins (HSP) were originally described in heat-shocked drosophila by Ritossa in the early 1960's. In the last 5 years it has become apparent that these heat shock proteins have important functions both in the normal cell and in the stressed cell. These proteins constitute an endogenous protective system; mutations in the heat shock proteins can be lethal, and there are no known organisms without heat shock proteins. The first observations on heat shock proteins and the heart were made in the 1980's and interest in these proteins increased over the decade. In the last few years there has been an exponential growth in number of papers published on heat shock proteins and the heart. Heat shock proteins have been implicated in a number of cardiovascular research areas including ischemia, hypertrophy, aging, and atherosclerosis, and this list is growing.

The purpose of this volume is to give an overview of our current understanding of the heat shock proteins in the cardiovascular system, and to summarize the approaches to the study of heat shock proteins in the heart. This volume assembles results from a number of different cardiovascular fields. and provides a comprehensive review of heat shock proteins in the cardiovascular system.

The expression of the heat shock proteins in the heart is influenced by stimuli such as hypoxia and stretch. Our current understanding of regulation of HSP expression will be discussed. Most work has focused on HSP 70, the major inducible protein in the 70 kDa subfamily of heat shock proteins. Overexpression of HSP 70 can protect the heart from ischemic and hypoxic injury. There is ongoing debate about whether heat shock proteins have a role in either preconditioning or stunning. Both free radical scavengers and heat shock proteins have been shown to protect the heart from stress. What are the relative roles of these two systems and is one more important than the other? Might heat shock proteins have a role in cardioplegia and angioplasty? Could preinduction of the stress response before undertaking cardiac surgery or angioplasty, both of which are accompanied by brief periods of ischemia, protect the heart during the procedure? Cardiac hypertrophy is preceded by an early rise in HSP 70 accompanied by changes in the proto-oncogenes, c-myc and c-fos. Does this increase in HSP 70 reflect cardiac injury, or is it a growth response? Recently in my own laboratory in collaboration with Douglas Mann we have made some interesting observations on heat shock proteins, cytokines, and heart failure. Tumor necrosis factor, often elevated in advanced heart failure, induces expression of HSP 70 in isolated adult cardiocytes.

In the past few years it has become apparent that the aging organism has a decreased heat shock response. The aged heart has a blunted increase in HSP 70 in response to ischemia. This reduction in the heat shock response with age has implications for the ability of the elderly to withstand disease and to respond to the hemodynamic changes that accompany severe illness.

Less is known about the other eight to ten major heat shock proteins and their function(s) in the heart. HSP 60, a mitochondrial heat shock protein, increases with myocardial ischemia. HSP 27, which in response to stress undergoes phosphorylation, also increases in response to ischemia. HSP 27 overexpression has been reported to protect fibroblasts from injury. What are the roles of the heat shock proteins in the vasculature? Interesting observations have been made of changes in the expression in the vessel walls in response to varying types of stress. Again, age appears to blunt the heat shock response. More controversial is the theory that atherosclerosis is at least in part an immune response to HSP 65, a bacterial heat shock protein.

The heat shock proteins have become a burgeoning area of cardiovascular research because the heat shock proteins represent a vital group of proteins that potentially can be manipulated to have therapeutic benefit in the setting of myocardial ischemia and injury. The next decade is likely to bring even more interesting findings as investigators work to understand how these proteins protect the heart, and try to bring the beneficial effects of the heat shock proteins to the clinical setting.

A.A.Knowlton, M.D.
Cardiology Section
Department of Medicine
V.A. Medical Center
Baylor College of Medicine
Houston, TX, USA

1

AN OVERVIEW OF THE HEAT SHOCK PROTEINS, THEIR REGULATION, AND FUNCTION

A.A.Knowlton
Veterans Affairs Medical Center and Baylor College of Medicine, Houston, Tx.

This chapter is multifunctional, serving as an introduction to the heat shock proteins and as well as covering HSPs that have had limited or no study in the heart. The regulation of expression of the HSPs is reviewed here. Lastly, key research not included in the remainder of the volume, including the function of HSPs and nuclear localization, will be discussed.

The heat shock proteins, outlined in table I, can be subdivided into 5 groups: 1. the small HSPs, 20 to 30 kDa discussed in chapters 8 and 9; 2. the 50-60 kDa HSPs, also discussed in chapter 8; 3. the 70 kDa HSPs, discussed in chapters 2-6; 4. the 90 kDa HSPs, which have not been studied in any detail in the heart; and 5. the 100 kDa plus HSPs, which have not been studied in mammalian systems. The field of HSPs and ischemic injury in the brain has developed in parallel with studies on the heart, and Nishimura and Dwyer review this research in chapter 11. Interesting, new questions are being raised about heat shock proteins, and one of the most provocative is the potential role of HSP60 in autoimmune disease. In the cardiovascular field, an immune response to bacterial HSP65, the homolog of HSP60, may result in antibodies binding to human HSP60; this antibody response may have a role in atherogenesis. This area is reviewed in chapter 10 by Wick and his colleagues. Over the last few years it has become clear that the heat shock response diminishes with age, and this phenomena and its consequences are reviewed in Chapter 6.

The heat shock proteins were first identified by their induction by heat shock; hence the designation heat shock proteins for this ubiquitous group of proteins that constitute a diverse stress response. The heat shock proteins are characterized by their upregulation in response to stress, the presence of a weak ATPase, and a high degree

Table I - Summary of the Heat Shock Proteins

	ALTERNATE NAMES	LOCATION	CHARACTERISTICS
HSP10	GroES	MITOCHONDRIA	CHAPERONIN, WORKS IN CONJUNCTION WITH HSP60
HSP 25	HSP 27	CYTOPLASM / PERINUCLEAR MIGRATES TO NUCLEUS WITH STRESS	PHOSPHORYLATED OVEREXPRESSION PROTECTS AGAINST HEAT SHOCK
HSP40	DnaJ, hdj-1	CYTOPLASMIC; TO NUCLEUS WITH STRESS	WORKS WITH HSP70 AND HSC70 IN PROTEIN FOLDING
HSP 60	GroEL	MITOCHONDRIA SYNTHESIZED IN CYTOPLASM	CHAPERONIN; HELPS FOLD IMPORTED CYTOPLASMIC PROTEINS IN CONJUNCTION WITH HSP10
HSC 70	HSP73	CYTOPLASM, MIGRATES TO NUCLEUS WITH STRESS & CELL DIVISION	CONSTITUTIVE, ABUNDANT, ASSOCIATED WITH PROTEIN SYNTHESIS. CHAPERONE
HSP 70	HSP72, INDUCIBLE HSP70, DnaK	CYTOPLASM; MIGRATES TO NUCLEUS WITH STRESS & CELL DIVISION	INDUCIBLE, LITTLE TO NONE AT BASELINE; OVEREXPRESSION PROTECTS CELLS AGAINST HEAT STRESS AND HYPOXIA
HSP 75	GRP 75	MITOCHONDRIA	
GRP 78	BiP, HSP78	ENDOPLASMIC RETICULUM	EXPRESSION ALTERED BY GLUCOSE LEVELS; CHAPERONIN
HSP 90		CYTOPLASM; TO NUCLEUS WITH STRESS	2 PROTEINS, α & δ; CONSTITUTIVE, PHOSPHORYLATED BIND CYTOPLASMIC HORMONE RECEPTORS; ? REGULATE SRC & OTHER KINASES; ↑ SYNTHESIS WITH STRESS
HSP 104			ONLY IN YEAST TO DATE; CONVEYS THERMOTOLERANCE
HSP 110		CYTOPLASM & NUCLEOLI ? MIGRATES TO NUCLEUS WITH STRESS	CONSTITUTIVE ↑ SYNTHESIS WITH STRESS

of sequence homology among species. Mutation of the heat shock proteins can be lethal. Some of the proteins, such as HSP70, the inducible form of the 70 kDa HSP, are present in low amounts in normal mammalian tissue, in contrast to their absence in the unstressed lower organism. The initial heat shock protein research focused on Drosophila, yeast and Escherichia coli. This volume is testament to the importance of the most basic research and the foundation it forms for research on mammalian systems. The work in this volume is the prelude to application of heat shock protein to the clinical setting.

REGULATION OF EXPRESSION

A number of the heat shock proteins, HSC70, HSP27, HSP90, HSP60, and GRP78, are expressed at high levels in the normal, unstressed cell (Ciocca et al. 1993; Inaguma et al. 1993; Wilkinson & Pollard, 1993; Gutierrez & Guerriero,J,V, 1995; Quraishi et al. 1996). HSP70, the inducible protein, is present in normal mammalian heart and upregulated in response to stress (Gutierrez & Guerriero,V,Jr, 1991; Knowlton et al. 1991; Locke et al. 1996).. In contrast, in other organisms such as Drosophila melanogaster, HSP70 is absent from the unstressed cell and rapidly upregulated with increases of 100-fold in the protein in response to heat stress. Although in mammalian cells many of the heat shock proteins are present constitutively, all have been reported to increase in response to stresses such as heat or hypoxia/ischemia. The response varies by gene, by stress, and by cell type and organism; for example, GRP78 changes in response to changes in glucose concentration, and in the liver HSP70 expression is altered by insulin (Watowich & Morimoto, 1988; Ting et al. 1989).

A wide variety of stresses can induce the heat shock response. These include heat, hypoxia, amino acid analogues (which interfere with proper protein folding), ethanol, metabolic stress, and heavy metals. In the isolated, perfused heart stretch and altered shortening induce HSP70, while in isolated, neonatal cardiocytes stretch did not affect HSP70 expression (Sadoshima et al. 1992). These latter results suggest either that the microenvironment of the intact heart is important for the mechanical induction of HSP70 or that there is a difference between neonatal and adult cardiocytes. Interestingly, stretch has been reported to induce HSP70 in other tissues(Zhao et al. 1994).

Heat Shock Factors (HSF's)

The primary transcription factor involved in regulation of expression of heat shock proteins is HSF-1 (heat shock factor). There are at least three HSF's in mammalian cells, HSF-1 and HSF-2, and HSF-4 (Cotto et al. 1996). HSF-3 was cloned from the chicken (Nakai & Morimoto, 1993). HSF-2 has only been described to be activated by hemin-induced differentiation of a human erythroleukemia cell line (Sistonen et al. 1992). HSF-2 is not activated by stress and is not phosphorylated, unlike HSF-1. HSF-1 appears to be the transcription factor mediating the stress response regardless of the stress. Both heat and hypoxia activate HSF-1. HSF-1 is present in the cytoplasm in an

3

inactive form. With stress trimerization occurs as well as phosphorylation (Westwood & Wu, 1991). HSF-1 moves to the nucleus where it binds to the HSE (heat shock element), which is present in the promoter of the stress response genes. Recently it has been shown that serine phosphorylation occurs after DNA binding and before transcription occurs (Cotto et al. 1996). This inducible phosphorylation is necessary for transcription to occur. HSF-1 remains active for no more than a few hours; inactivation is thought to occur by dephosphorylation. Four highly conserved domains occur in HSF-1 and these consist of hydrophobic, heptad repeats, which form leucine zippers, one of the motifs for DNA binding proteins (Rabindran et al. 1993).

Although activation of HSF-1 is necessary for the stress response, it is not sufficient. Salicylate will activate binding of HSF-1 to HSE in HeLa cells, a human cell line derived from a cervical tumor (Jurivich et al. 1992; Giardina & Lis, 1995). However, despite binding of HSF-1, initiation of transcription does not occur. This is similar to what occurs in some less complex species, such as Drosophila melanogaster, where HSF is always bound to HSE. Salicylate activation of HSF-1 binding to HSE does not interfere with subsequent activation of the stress response by heat shock (Jurivich et al. 1995). The activation of HSF by nonsteroidal anti-inflammatory drugs results in a constitutive phosphorylation of the HSF, but does not trigger HSP transcription (Cotto et al. 1996). Cells pretreated with salicylate have a more rapid response to heat stress than controls. This is of particular interest given the widespread use of salicylates in cardiac patients and the protective benefits observed when treating unstable angina with salicylates. Perhaps this protective effect involves more than the anti-platelet properties of aspirin.

In muscle cells (C2C12 cell line), 20 min. of heat shock or two hours of hypoxia activated binding of HSF-1 (Benjamin et al. 1990). Cycloheximide did not block activation of HSF-1, demonstrating that inactive HSF-1 is present in the cytoplasm of nonstressed cells; thus, new synthesis of protein is not necessary to initiate HSP70 transcription. Inhibition of mitochondrial oxidative phosphorylation with rotenone resulted in activation of HSF-1 binding within 30 min. in C2C12 cells (Benjamin et al. 1992). In further experiments the investigators demonstrated that severe reduction in ATP levels (30% of control) was sufficient to activate HSF-1. In isolated neonatal rat heart cells, two hours of hypoxia activated HSF-1 (Iwaki et al. 1993). However, in these experiments steady-state levels of HSP70 mRNA increased before activation of HSF-1 was detected by gel-shift experiments. This was interpreted as insensitivity of the gel mobility shift assay, but it is also possible that hypoxia resulted in an increase in the stability of the HSP70 mRNA. A parallel for this was observed in HeLa cells where heat shock resulted in a marked increase in HSP70 mRNA half-life (Theodorakis & Morimoto, 1987).

Post-transcriptional regulation represents a second level of regulation of gene expression occurs in the cell. The initial steps still involve RNA, and include splicing to remove introns (noncoding regions of genes that are present within the coding region and must be removed before translation can occur), and the addition of a cap at the 5'end. Several of the heat shock proteins, particularly HSP70 contain no introns so that splicing is not needed before translation. Subsequent steps, including movement of the mRNA to the cytoplasm and assembly of the mRNA and ribosomal units, are regulated. The details of this regulation remains to be elucidated. A final factor governing expression is mRNA half-life. Some mRNA's, such as those encoding cytokines, contain sequences in their 3' region that marks them for rapid degradation, limiting the synthesis of the final protein product. Clearly HSPs are regulated transcriptionally, additional post-transcriptional regulation remains to be clarified.

Work on regulation of HSPs expression in the heart and in skeletal muscle has been limited. Hypoxia and ischemia induce HSP70 and other HSPs, but the underlying mechanisms controlling this induction have not been determined. It is likely that the many aspects of induction of the heat shock response are universal; thus, there will be many common features regulating induction of the heat shock response in heart, liver, and drosophila. However, there are likely other features that are specific for regulation of this response for different species and tissues.

HOW DO HEAT SHOCK PROTEINS FUNCTION IN THE CELL AND WHY ARE THEY PROTECTIVE?

Chaperones and Protein Folding

The heat shock proteins are chaperones, proteins that facilitate the folding of other proteins. Chaperons are not functional subunits of the proteins they interact with, rather they serve to modify the tertiary structure of the protein. There have been a number of excellent reviews on the subject of chaperones, many of which are not heat shock proteins and are not induced in response to stress (Gething & Sambrook, 1992; Hendrick & Hartl, 1995; Ellis, 1996; Hartl, 1996). Although it has been shown that a protein can achieve its correct tertiary structure when allowed to refold in a test tube under correct conditions, the cell represents a more complex environment. In the cell HSC70 facilitates the proper folding of newly formed peptides (Beckmann et al. 1990). HSC70 and possibly also HSP70 function in nuclear transport of proteins via the nuclear pore. Whether HSC functions by unfolding the protein to be transported, or whether it has other functions is not known. However, several studies have shown that nuclear transport of particular proteins requires HSC70 (Imamoto et al. 1992; Yang & DeFranco, 1994). It is thought, though not proven, that the requirement of HSC70 for nuclear transport may be a universal requirement for many if not all proteins. A more likely scenario is that HSC70 and/or HSP70 are needed to unfold select globular proteins before they can pass through the pore.

HSP 60 and the Mitochondria

HSP60 is also known as cpn60, or chaperonin 60. The chaperonins are a unique

5

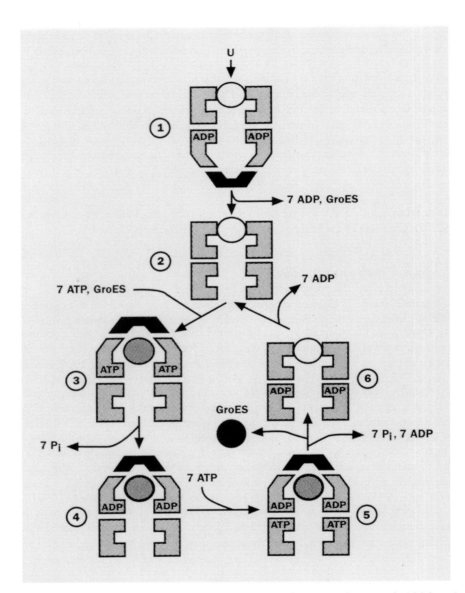

Figure 1 - Model of chaperonin-mediated folding from Mayhew et al. 1996. A vertical section of the complex shows a side view of the two rings with the dark GroES cap. The unfolded protein (U), shown as an open circle, enters at the top, darker shading of U indicates progression to its final folded form, and it is released. Refolding is accompanied by hydrolysis of ATP. Reprinted with permission from Nature 1996, MacMillan Magazines, Ltd.

subset of chaperons that possess sequence homology and were first described in chloroplasts. In mammalian cells HSP60 occurs predominantly in the mitochondria, though it is encoded by the nuclear and not the mitochondrial genome. HSP60 facilitates the proper folding of mitochondrial proteins (Cheng et al. 1989; Schröder et al. 1993). The TriC (TCP containing ring complex) family of proteins are thought to be the cytosolic counterparts of HSP60 for the chaperonin function. TCP-1 (t-complex polypeptide 1) facilitates the folding of actin and tubulin (Rommelaere et al. 1993). The folding mechanism of the bacterial homologues of HSP60 have been intensely studied. These proteins, GroEL(HSP60) and GroES (HSP10) form a barrel-like structure consisting of two stacked heptamerous rings of GroEL with GroES as a cap (figure 1). GroES also is an oligomer with seven 10 kDa subunits arranged in a ring. The unfolded protein enters the center of the barrel where the chaperonins interact with the exposed hydrophobic regions (Mayhew et al. 1996). Multiple ATP-dependent cycles of release and binding then occur, and these cycles result in refolding of the protein, which is then released. Recent observations suggest that GroES functions by aligning GroEL in the barrel, and then by binding at the opposite end of the barrel, facilitating the release of the folded polypeptide (Weissman et al. 1995). Interestingly, overexpression of GroEL and GroES in bacterial cells lacking the normal heat-shock response can protect them from heat-shock (1513); however, overexpression of GroEL alone is not protective. Thus the interaction between GroEL and GroES is integral to their protective function.

The HSP 70 family facilitates folding of proteins both under normal conditions and under stress. Although originally it had been thought that each HSP alone aided refolding, it is now apparent that often multiple HSPs act together in refolding denatured proteins (Gething & Sambrook, 1992; Langer et al. 1992; Frydman et al. 1994; Hartl, 1996). Under normal conditions in the cell, HSC 70, mitochondrial (mt) HSP70, and HSP 60 work in series to unfold and then refold proteins as they move from the cytosol to the interior of the mitochondria. Similar events occur in the cytoplasm where HSC70, HSP40, and TRiC act together to fold proteins as they are synthesized on the ribosome (Hendrick & Hartl, 1993; Freeman & Morimoto, 1996%). *In vitro* HSP70 (or HSC70), hdj-1 (HSP40), and either ATP or ADP can reactivate denatured ß-galactosidase (Freeman & Morimoto, 1996). The optimal stoichiometry for this reaction was a 24-fold molar excess of HSP70. HSP90 alone cannot reactivate the denatured enzyme, but can maintain the protein in a " folding-ready" state, preventing irreversible denaturation, until refolding by HSP70 and hdj-1 occurs (Freeman & Morimoto, 1996). This function of HSP90 parallels its interaction with the cytosolic hormone receptors discussed below.

The stoichiometry for optimal refolding by HSP70 has been shown by several laboratories to require a large excess of HSP70 (Skowyra et al. 1990; Freeman & Morimoto, 1996). This suggests that rather than indiscriminately interacting with all proteins that there may be selectivity in binding. Studies addressing this question have found that HSP70 binds to peptides containing a region with a minimal length of seven amino acids that are predominantly hydrophobic and basic(Fourie et al. 1994). Differences in affinity for a given protein also were observed among DnaK, BiP, and HSC. These observations support the concept of selective binding and selective renaturation.

Refolding and Stabilization of Macromolecular Structure During and After Stress

It is a natural extension from the chaperone and folding functions of the HSPs in the normal cell to the stabilization and refolding of macromolecules. Stress, such as heat or hypoxia, can result in denaturation of proteins (Lepock et al. 1993). The ability of the heat shock proteins to renature proteins was first demonstrated by Skowyra et al. who showed that DnaK, the Drosophila homologue of HSP70, could reactivate heat-inactivated RNA polymerase in an ATP dependent reaction (Skowyra et al. 1990). Preincubation of RNA polymerase with DnaK followed by heat shock prevented inactivation of the enzyme in an ATP independent process. Similarly, overexpression of HSP70 in a mammalian cell line protected the activity of co-expressed luciferase in cells subjected to metabolic poisoning (Williams et al. 1993). In contrast, Schroder et al. found that DnaK alone was insufficient to reactivate heat-inactivated luciferase, and that a combination of chaperons was needed for reactivation (Schröder et al. 1993). This result supports the concept that the interaction of multiple heat shock proteins is necessary for some of their functions, and that there is some specificity of action. All heat shock proteins cannot reactivate all proteins. The picture is complex with some proteins under some conditions being renatured by a single HSP, and other proteins requiring the coordinated action of several proteins in order to be refolded. It is clear that there are two groups of proteins involved in protein folding : 1) GroEL and GroES (HSP60 and HSP10) and 2) DnaK and DnaJ (HSP70 or HSC70 and HSP40). At least some of the time these two groups act sequentially as shown in figure 2. GroEL and GroES are mitochondrial proteins, but have cytoplasmic counterparts, the TRiC family of proteins.

Protection of Protein Synthesis

Following heat shock, HSP70 has been found associated with the ribosomal subunits, and is postulated to stabilize their structure (Beck & De Maio, 1994). Ribosomal RNA synthesis also has been shown to be protected by pretreating cells with brief heat shock before prolonged heat shock (Black & Subjeck, 1989). Protein synthesis post an inhibiting heat stress is proportional to the amount of HSP 70 present (Lindquist, 1981; Laszlo, 1988; Mizzen & Welch, 1988; Matts & Hurst, 1992; Matts et al. 1992). Likewise, there is a reduction in the amount of inhibition of protein synthesis in cells pretreated with brief heat shock before prolonged heat shock.

Data from studies on reticulocyte lysates suggests a role for HSP90, HSP70, and p56 in the regulation of heme regulated $eIF-2\alpha$ kinase (HRI) [Matts & Hurst, 1992]. Phosphorylation of $eIF-2\alpha$, a key initiation factor for protein synthesis, inhibits protein synthesis, and the phosphorylation state of $eIF-2\alpha$ is a primary regulator of protein synthesis (Chen,J-J & London, 1995). Studies of head-down tilt in rats, which results in decreased cardiac protein synthesis, demonstrated an increase in phosphorylation in $eIF-2\alpha$ and sequestration of HSC/HSP70 with the polysomes (Menon & Thomason,

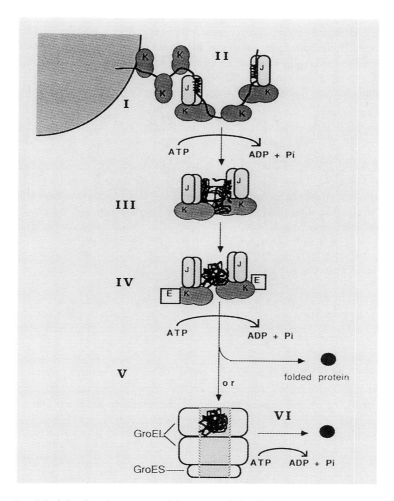

Figure 2 - Model showing sequential action of DnaK, DnaJ, GrpE, and GroEL/ES during folding of newly synthesized proteins. Similar events occur with mammalian homologs, HSC70, HSP40, and the TriC proteins. Reprinted with permission from the Annual Review of Biochemistry, vol. 62, c 1993, by Annual Reviews, Inc. (Hendrick and Hartl, 1993).

1995). In the absence of HSP70, HRI is free to phosphorylate eIF-2α, and inhibition of protein synthesis occurs.

In the normal cell HSC70 binds to newly formed peptides, as discussed above, and facilitates their correct folding. This is an important function, and some of the folding of new peptides is thought to occur in conjunction with the TriC family of proteins, similar to the coordination of HSC70, HSP60, and HSP10 in the eukaryotic mitochondria, and DnaK, GroEL, and GroES in bacteria (see figure 2).

Targeting Degradation

The heat shock proteins also direct irreversibly denatured proteins to degradation (Parsell & Lindquist, 1993; Hayes & Dice, 1996). Ubiquitin is a major component of one degradation pathway (Ciechanover & Schwartz, 1994, also see chapter 8). HSC70 can selectively target proteins to lysosomes for degradation, but regulation of this process is not completely understood.

OTHER HEAT SHOCK PROTEINS

Although 15 to 20 heat shock proteins have been identified, the vast majority of research in the heart has focused on HSP70. The lesser known heat shock proteins may have quite important functions in the heart, but these functions remain to be identified.

HSP 90

Most work on HSP90 has focused on its interaction with the cytoplasmic hormone receptors. HSP 90 binds the cytoplasmic hormone receptors, including receptors for glucocorticoid, dioxin, estrogen, and progesterone. HSP90 maintains the receptors in a conformation with a high affinity for the particular hormone. HSP 70 is needed for assembly of the receptor-HSP90 complex as are one or more smaller proteins including HSP56 and p23 (Hutchison et al. 1993, 1994, 1995; Johnson & Toft, 1995; Chen,S et al. 1996). Following binding of the hormone, HSP90 is released, and the receptor-hormone complex moves to the nucleus and activates expression of genes regulated by the particular hormone. While the glucocorticoid receptor is bound to HSP90, the nuclear localization signal (NLS) is concealed; with release of the receptor upon binding of glucocorticoid, the NLS is exposed, and nuclear translocation can occur (Scherrer et al. 1993).

A number of studies have demonstrated interaction between HSP90 and the tyrosine kinases pp60[v-src] (Xu & Lindquist, 1993; Aligue et al. 1994; Hartson & Matts, 1994; Whitesell et al. 1994; Mimnaugh et al. 1995; Nathan & Lindquist, 1995). More recently HSP 90 has been shown to interact with the tyrosine kinases Wee1 and p56[lck], and with two serine/threonine kinases, Raf and casein kinase II (Stancato et al. 1993; Aligue et al. 1994; Hartson & Matts, 1994; Miyata & Yahara, 1995). The studies on the interaction between HSP90 and pp60^{v-src} demonstrate that HSP 90 is necessary for stabilization and activation of the protein (Xu & Lindquist, 1993; Nathan & Lindquist, 1995). Others have shown that HSP90 folds two different basic helix-loop-helix proteins, E12 and MyoD, into their active conformations (Shue & Kohtx, 1994). All of these results suggest a role for HSP90 in regulating intracellular signalling, and more studies are needed to define further these interesting interactions.

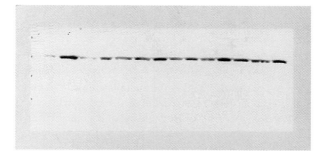

Figure 3 - Western blot demonstrating expression of HSP 90 in human heart. Samples are from normal donor hearts (first 2 lanes on left) and from explanted idiopathic cardiomyopathies(remaining lanes). Antibody to HSP 90 was the generous gift of Dr. Ann-Charlotte Wikström, Karolinska Institute, Novum, Sweden.

Our understanding of the function of HSP 90 beyond its role in regulating the effects of the cytoplasmic hormone receptors is limited. Interestingly, an elevation of HSP90 in peripheral lymphocytes precedes the development of lupus (Faulds et al. 1994; Latchman & Isenberg, 1994). HSP 90 is diffusely present in the brain (Izumoto & Herbert, 1993; Quraishi et al. 1996). Studies in the heart are finite. In our own laboratory we have examined levels of HSP90 in normal, human donor hearts. By adding a standard curve of purified HSP 90 to our western blots, we estimated levels of HSP 90 in normal donor hearts to be approximately 5.3 ± 0.9 ng/ug of cytosolic protein (figure 3, Knowlton,A.A. et al., unpublished data). Workers in Yellon's laboratory demonstrated that overexpression of HSP 90 in H9c2 cells (an embryonic, cardiac cell line) protected against heat shock, but not against 20 hrs. of substrate-free hypoxia (Heads et al. 1995). The many recent observations suggesting that frequently HSPs act in a coordinated fashion may explain these results; the increase of a single HSP may often be insufficient. Rather co-overexpression may be needed to achieve a protective effect. More work is needed to define the functions of HSP90 in the heart.

HSP40

The recently cloned HSP40 is the human homologue of bacterial DnaJ and functions in concert with HSP70/HSC70 (Ohtsuka, 1993). HSP40 co-immunoprecipitates with

HSP70 and HSC70; the addition of denatured protein increases the association between HSP40 and HSP70 (Sugito et al. 1995). The addition of HSP40 to HSC70 increased the hydrolysis of ATP by HSC70 seven-fold. Evidence to date indicates that HSP40, like the bacterial DnaJ, facilitates folding of proteins by HSP70 and HSC70. HSC70, HSP40, and ATP combined did not renature denature luciferase, but with the addition of rabbit reticulocyte lysate restoration of enzyme activity occurred (Sugito et al. 1995). These results suggest that at least some of the time HSC70 and HSP40 act in conjunction with other factors. This is consistent with the observations discussed above concerning the interaction of DnaK and DnaJ with GroEL/GroES and the interaction with HSP90.

GRP 78

GRP78, also known as BiP, is found in the endoplasmic reticulum in cells (Vogel et al. 1990; Nicchitta & Blobel, 1993; Heydari et al. 1995). Metabolic changes alter its expression. GRP78 is important for proper folding of proteins within the endoplasmic reticulum. Although this protein has been of great interest to immunologists, little is known about its possible role in cardiovascular tissue.

100 kDa Plus HSPs

There are at least two heat shock proteins over 100 kDa in size, HSP104 and HSP110. HSP104 was identified in yeast by Lindquist and her colleagues (Parsell et al. 1991). HSP104 overexpression confers thermotolerance on yeast cells (Sanchez & Lindquist, 1990; Parsell et al. 1993). A mammalian homologue remains to be identified. HSP110 is a cytoplasmic proteins that localizes to the nucleus with stress, only limited observations have been made on this protein, which was recently cloned (Subjeck et al. 1983; Shyy et al. 1986). Tissue distribution studies of HSP110 show the highest levels of the protein in the brain and then the liver, with low amounts in other tissues. HSP110 localizes to the cytoplasm and to the nucleoli. The functions of this protein are unknown, though it is presumed that HSP110 would have chaperone and refolding functions similar to other HSPs.

NUCLEAR LOCALIZATION WITH STRESS

Most nuclear proteins move to the nucleus once they are synthesized, but heat shock proteins belong to a subset of cellular proteins that selectively localize to the nucleus. HSP27, HSP70, and HSP 90 move to the nucleus with stress (Akner et al. 1992; Xia & Culp, 1995). The accumulation of HSC 70 in the nucleus is variable. Both HSC 70 and HSP 70 have important functions as chaperones for proteins entering the nucleus (Imamoto et al. 1992; Shi & Thomas, 1992; Yang & DeFranco, 1994). Nuclear localization is an integral part of the heat shock response; nuclear accumulation of HSPs starts within minutes of the heat stimulus, and peaks in a manner dependent on both the severity of the heating temperature and its duration (Welch & Feramisco, 1984; Ohtsuka & Laszlo, 1992). Once the heat insult is withdrawn, the protein starts moving out of the nucleus, but can still be detected in the nucleus up to sixteen hours later (Ohtsuka & Laszlo, 1992). The rate of nuclear accumulation of HSP70 was similar in both naive heat shocked cells and thermotolerant heat shocked cells, but for unknown reasons exit from the nucleus was faster during recovery period in thermotolerant cells (Ohtsuka & Laszlo, 1992).

Nuclear localization sequence (NLS), short stretches of four to 15 amino acids, characterized by the abundance of the basic amino acids lysine and arginine, are recognition signals for nuclear transport. A minority of NLSs vary from this pattern and have been identified by intensive mutational analysis (Siomi & Dreyfuss, 1995). These atypical sequences may bind to another protein, rather than to the nuclear pore, as the basic NLSs are thought to do (Imamoto-Sonobe et al. 1990; Adam,SA & Gerace, 1991; Adam,EJH & Adam, 1994; Imamoto et al. 1995). Recently, identification of one of the cytoplasmic receptors for the nuclear pore has been reported (Weis et al. 1995). Some proteins with NLS still need HSP 70 to move through the NPC, and this may reflect HSP 70's function as a chaperone; both SV40 large T antigen and nucleoplasmin contain NLS that are sufficient for nuclear localization, but both require HSP 70 for nuclear localization to occur (Shi & Thomas, 1992; Yang & DeFranco, 1994). NLSs may also be required for the for the efflux of proteins to the cytoplasm (Guiochon-Mantel et al. 1994). Proteins may have more than one NLS, though usually when redundant, one of the NLSs is relatively weak (Richter & Standiford, 1992). Myo D, the polyomavirus large-T antigen, p53, and the glucocorticoid receptor all contain more than one NLS.

Nuclear Localization of HSP 70

In our laboratory we have been interested in the role of nuclear localization of HSP70 in protection from ischemia. To date no definite known role for HSP70 in the nucleus is known, but this process is likely an important part of the cellular response to stress. The fact that HSP70 after heat shock associates with the periribosomal containing granular region of the nucleoli, and during recovery colocalizes with polyribosomes suggests that this localization into the nucleus may serve in preserving ribosomal assembly and function, and hence in the recovery of translation (Welch & Feramisco, 1984; Welch & Mizzen, 1988; Beck & De Maio, 1994).

Mutational Analysis of HSP 70

Several laboratories used large deletional mutations to try to identify the NLS for HSP 70 (Munro & Pelham, 1984; Milarski & Morimoto, 1989). A drawback of these studies is that some of the resulting proteins were small enough (less than 40 to 60 kDa) to move by passive diffusion to the nucleus. The single mutant that effected nuclear localization deleted 64 amino acids, reducing the molecular size to approximately 54 kDa, and not only prevented nuclear localization, but also prevented ATP binding. It was thought that this mutant had a significant conformational change, and that this change in conformation, rather than the deleted amino acids, was responsible for the decrease in nuclear localization.

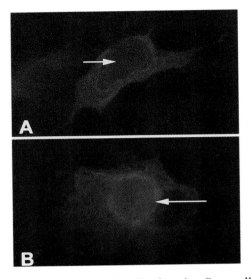

Figure 4 - Nuclear localization in Cos cells of transiently expressed human HSP70 containing an epitope tag at the carboxy terminus. A) Control cell. Tagged HSP70 localized in cytoplasm. B) Two hours of heat shock at 43° C result in nuclear localization of the protein. The arrow in both panels indicates the nucleus.

To more definitively explore nuclear localization of HSP 70, we have used site-directed mutagenesis to construct a series of mutants of human HSP 70 (Salfity & Knowlton, 1995). We identified the most likely nuclear localization sequences, based on primary sequence as discussed above. Nuclear localization sequence (NLS) 1, which overlapped with a sequence identified by others as able to function in a fusion protein as an NLS (Dang & Lee, 1989), and included amino acids 246 to 264, KRKHKKDISQNKRAVRRLR. Both deletional mutations and conservative mutations were done. In the latter alanines were substituted for lysines and arginines to minimize the effect of mutation on secondary structure. A unique epitope tag was inserted at the carboxy terminus to allow identification of the mutant protein (figure 4). When testing for nuclear localization of these mutants in transiently transfected Cos cells, it was apparent that mutation of KRKHKKDISQNKRAVRRLR altered, but did not totally abolish nuclear localization. This result suggests that there may be more than one NLSs for HSP70, and we are currently mutating several other likely sequences.

HSP70 accumulates in the nucleus only at certain times during the cell cycle (S phase), and at times of stress. Overexpression of HSP 70 will not result in nuclear translocation of the protein, suggesting that some other signal(s) is needed. This property distinguishes it from the majority of nuclear proteins, which accumulate in the nucleus at all times, and puts it in a class of proteins that are cytoplasmic until induced to enter the nucleus, such as the glucocorticoid receptor and certain transcription factors such as NFkB. The proteins with variable nuclear localization may be an important part of cell regulation, and understanding control of the translocation of these proteins will yield further understanding of cellular control mechanisms. Various regulatory processes have been described which regulate the intermittent nuclear localization of these proteins including: 1) Conformational change exposing an NLS as is thought to occur with binding of ligand to the glucocorticoid receptor (Simons, 1994), 2) Change in phosphorylation status as occurs with the NFkB inhibitor leading to its dissociation from the transcription factor with subsequent nuclear localization(Baeuerle & Baltimore, 1988), and as occurs with the Drosophila dorsal gene product, which is released from the cytoplasmic cactus protein resulting in nuclear localization (Whalen & Steward, 1993), and 3) cleavage of a part of the protein exposing a concealed NLS and resulting in nuclear localization. The mechanism(s) regulating nuclear localization of HSP70 have not been identified, and more work needs to be done in this area.

New Directions for Heat Shock Protein Research

Research in the heart has shown that a change in HSP70 with ischemia and that heat pretreatment to induce HSP70 can protect the heart from subsequent stress. Transgenic models as wells as transfected cell models have shown that overexpression of HSP70 prior to injury is protective. As heat shock induces many genes, interest has increased in alternative methods of inducing and suppressing HSP70 and other HSPs to aid in delineating their cellular functions. Of the many known agents influencing HSP70 expression, all are toxic. Herbimycin, a recently described agent that induces HSP70, is a tyrosine kinase inhibitor and can be expected to have a myriad of other effects besides the induction of HSP70. Herbimycin pretreatment to induce HSP70 can protect against injury at certain doses, and some investigators have not found it to be toxic (Hegde et al. 1995; Morris et al. 1996). Similarly, the flavanoids, such as quercetin, which has been described to inhibit HSP70 expression, have multiple effects. A brief review of the recent literature shows reports of quercetin effecting Na+/K+ ATPase, Ca+2/Mg+2 ATPase, mitochondrial respiration, inhibiting EF-1α, inhibiting platelet aggregation, inhibiting constitutive endothelial NO-synthase, "selectively" inhibiting phospholipase A2, and acting as a vasodilator (Lang & Racker, 1974; Beretz et al. 1978; Laughton et al. 1989; Duarte et al. 1993; Lindahl & Tagesson, 1993; Gu et al. 1994; Hodwick et al. 1994; Chiesi & Schwaller, 1995; Marcinkiewicz et al. 1995; Pace-Asciak et al. 1995). It is difficult to interpret experiments with quercetin because of its broad effects on the cell. The potential diverse effects of agents needs to be kept in mind when interpreting results. However, this is an important area because selective pharmacologic manipulation of the expression of the HSPs will be needed for clinical application.

To selectively alter HSP70 expression we have applied antisense treatment. Adult feline cardiac myocytes were treated with one of three 14 base phosphorothioate oligonucleotides: sense control, antisense, and antisense to MHCI (major histocompatibility complex 1) as a control for activation of RnaseH (Nakano et al. 1997). Treatment with antisense to HSP70 blocked the increase in HSP70 protein after hypoxia, and increased cellular injury. These experiments provide evidence of the importance of HSP70 in the endogenous stress response in cardiac myocytes. The same approach can be used to selectively impair expression of other HSPs, catalase, and superoxide dismutase. With careful controls, antisense experiments can shed light on the importance of the components of the stress response in protecting the cardiac myocyte against injury. Antisense experiments provide another method for elucidating the function of the HSPs in protecting the heart from injury.

SUMMARY

In the normal cell and tissue heat shock proteins function to: 1) Correctly fold newly synthesized proteins, 2) Act as chaperones unfolding and refolding proteins as they pass across membranes such as in the mitochondria and the nucleus, and 3) Maintain the cytoplasmic hormone receptors in proper conformation. With stress, heat shock proteins 1) Stabilize macromolecular structure, 2) Refold denatured proteins, possibly selectively refolding particular proteins, 3) Direct irreversibly denatured proteins to degradation, 4) Protect protein and ribosomal synthesis. Although under the optimal conditions proteins can assume their native conformation, it appears that in the complex environment of the cell that this does not occur spontaneously; rather, proteins are dependent on heat shock proteins and other chaperones to achieve correct conformation.

ACKNOWLEDGEMENTS

Supported in part by HL92510 (NHLBI).

REFERENCES

1.   Adam EJH, Adam SA. 1994. Identification of cytosolic factors required for nuclear location sequence-mediated binding to the nuclear envelope. J Cell Biol 125:547-555.

2.   Adam SA, Gerace L. 1991. Cytosolic proteins that specifically bind nuclear localization signals are receptors for nuclear import. Cell 66:837-847.

3.   Akner G, Mossberg K, Sundquist K-G, Gustafsson J-A, Wikstrom A-C. 1992. Evidence for reversible, non-microtubule and non-microfilament-dependent nuclear translocation of HSP 90 after heat shock in human fibroblasts. European Journal of Cell Biology 58:356-364.

4.   Aligue R, Akhavan-Niak H, Russell P. 1994. A role for HSP 90 in cell cycle control: Wee1 tyrosine kinase activity requires interaction with HSP 90. Embo 13:6099-6106.

5.   Baeuerle PA, Baltimore D. 1988. IkB: A specific inhibitor of the NF-kB transcription factor. Science 242:540-544.

6.   Beck SC, De Maio A. 1994. Stabilization of protein synthesis of thermotolerant cells during heat shock: Association of heat shock protein-72 with ribosomal subunits of polysomes. JBiolChem 269:21803-21811.

7.   Beckmann RP, Mizzen LA, Welch WJ. 1990. Interaction of HSP 70 with newly synthesized proteins: Implications for protein folding and assembly. Science 248:850-854.

8.   Benjamin IJ, Kroger B, Williams RS. 1990. Activation of the heat shock transcription factor by hypoxia in mammalian cells. ProcNatlAcadSci USA 87:6263-6267.

9.   Benjamin IJ, Horie S, Greenberg ML, Alpern RJ, Williams RS. 1992. Induction of stress proteins in cultured myogenic cells: Molecular signals for the activation of heat shock transcription factor during ischemia. JClinInvest 89:1685-1689.

10.   Beretz A, Anton R, Stoclet JC. 1978. Flavanoid compounds are potent inhibitors of cyclic AMP phosphodiesterase. Experientia 34:1054-1055.

11.   Black AR, Subjeck JR. 1989. Involvement of rRNA synthesis in the enhanced survival and recovery of protein synthesis seen in thermotolerance. JCellPhysiol 138:439-449.

12.   Chen J-J, London IM. 1995. Regulation of protein synthesis by heme-regulated eIF-2α kinase. TIBS 20:105-108.

13.   Chen S, Prapapanich V, Rimerman RA, Honoré B, Smith DF. 1996. Interactions of p60, a mediator of progesterone receptor assembly with heat shock proteins HSP90 and HSP70. MolEndocrin 10:682-693.

14.   Cheng MY, Hartl F-U, Martin J, et al. 1989. Mitochondrial heat-shock protein HSP60 is essentialfor assembly of proteins imported into yeast mitochondria. Nature 337:620-625.

15.   Chiesi M, Schwaller R. 1995. Inhibition of constitutive endothelial NO-synthase activity by tannin and quercetin. BiochemPharmacol 49:495-501.

16.   Ciechanover A, Schwartz AL. 1994. The ubiquitin-mediated proteolytic pathway: mechanisms of recognition of the proteolytic substrate and involvement in the degradation of native cellular proteins. FASEB J 8:182-191.

17.   Ciocca DR, Oesterreich S, Chamness GC, McGuire WL, Fuqua SAW. 1993. Biological and clinical implications of heat shock protein 27000 (Hsp27): a Review. JNatlCancer Inst 85:1558-1570.

18.   Cotto JJ, Kline M, Morimoto RI. 1996. Activation of heat shock factor 1 DNA binding precedes stress-induced serine phosphorylation. JBiolChem 271:3355-3358.

19.   Dang CV, Lee WMF. 1989. Nuclear and nucleolar targeting sequences of c-erb-A, c-myb, N-myc,

17

p53, HSP 70, and HIV tat proteins. JBiolChem 264:18019-18023.

20. Duarte J, Perez-Vizcaino F, Zarzuelo A, Jimenez J, Tamargo J. 1993. Vasodilator effects of quercetin in isolated rat vascular smooth muscle. European J Pharmacol 239:1-7.

21. Ellis RJ, ed. The Chaperonins. New York: Academic Press, 1996.

22. Faulds GB, Isenberg DA, Latchman DS. 1994. The tissue specific elevation in synthesis of the 90 kDa heat shock protein precedes the onset of disease in lupus prone MRL/lpr mice. JRheumatol 21:234-238.

23. Fourie AM, Sambrook JF, Gething M-JH. 1994. Common and divergent peptide binding specificities of HSP 70 molecular chaperones. JBiolChem 269:30470-30478.

24. Freeman BC, Morimoto RI. 1996. The human cytosolic molecular chaperones HSP90, HSP70 (HSC70) and HDJ-1 have distinct roles in recognition of a non-native protein and protein refolding. Embo 15:2969-2979.

25. Frydman J, Nimmesgern E, Ohtsuka K, Hartl FU. 1994. Folding of nascent polypeptide chains in a high molecular mass assembly with molecular chaperones. Nature 370:111-117.

26. Gething M, Sambrook J. 1992. Protein folding in the cell. Nature 235:33-45.

27. Giardina C, Lis JT. 1995. Sodium salicylate and yeast heat shock gene transcription. JBiolChem 270:10369-10372.

28. Gu ZL, Xiao D, Jin LQ, Fans PS, Qian ZN. 1994. Effects of quercetin on Na+/K+-exchanging ATPase and Ca+2/Mg+2 ATPase in rats. Chung-Kuo Yao Li Hsueh Pao - Acta Pharmacologica Sinica 15:414-416.

29. Guiochon-Mantel A, Delabre K, Lescop P, Milgrom E. 1994. Nuclear localization signals also mediate the outward movement of proteins from the nucleus. J Cell Biol 91:7179-7183.

30. Gutierrez JA, Guerriero J V. 1995. Relative abundance of bovine HSP 70 mRNA and protein. Biochimica et Biophysica Acta 1260:239-242.

31. Gutierrez JA, Guerriero V Jr. 1991. Quantitation of HSP 70 in tissues using a competitive enzyme-linked immunosorbent assay. Journal of Immunological Methods 143:81-88.

32. Hartl FU. 1996. Molecular chaperones in cellular protein folding. Nature 381:571-580.

33. Hartson SD, Matts RL. 1994. Association of HSP 90 with cellular Src-family kinases in a cell-free system correlates with altered kinase structure and function. Biochemistry 33:8912-8920.

34. Hayes SA, Dice JF. 1996. Roles of molecular chaperones in protein degradation. J Cell Biol 132:255-258.

35. Heads RJ, Yellon DM, Latchman DS. 1995. Differential cytoprotection against heat stress or hypoxia following expression of specific stress protein genes in myogenic cells. J Mol Cell Cardiol 27:1669-1678.

36. Hegde RS, Zuo J, Voellmy R, Welch WJ. 1995. Short circuiting stress protein expression via a tyrosine kinase inhibitor, Herbimycin A. JCellPhysiol 165:186-200.

37. Hendrick JP, Hartl FU. 1993. Molecular chaperone functions of heat shock proteins. AnnuRevBiochem 62:349-384.

38. Hendrick JP, Hartl F-U. 1995. The role of molecular chaperones in protein folding. FASEB J

9:1559-1569.

39.   Heydari AR, Conrad CC, Richardson A. 1995. Expression of heat shock genes in hepatocytes is affected by age and food restriction in rats. JNutr 125:410-418.

40.   Hodwick WF, Duval DL, Pardini RS. 1994. Inhibition of mitochondrial respiration and cyanide-stimulated generation of reactive oxygen species by selected flavanoids. BiochemPharmacol 47:573-580.

41.   Hutchison KA, Scherrer LC, Czar MJ, et al. 1993. Regulation of glucocorticoid receptor function through assembly of a receptor-heat shock protein complex. Ann NYAcadSci 684:35-48.

42.   Hutchison KA, Dittmar KD, Czar MJ, Pratt WB. 1994. Proof that HSP70 is required for assembly of the glucocorticoid receptor into a herocomplex with HSP90. JBiolChem 269:5043-5049.

43.   Hutchison KA, Stancato LF, Owens-Grillo JK, et al. 1995. The 23-kDa acidic protein in reticulocyte lysate is the weakly bound component of the HSP foldosome that is required for assembly of the glucocorticoid receptor into a functional heterocomplex with HSP90. JBiolChem 270:18841-18847.

44.   Imamoto N, Matsuoka Y, Kurihara T, et al. 1992. Antibodies against 70-kD heat shock cognate protein inhibit mediated nuclear import of karyophilic proteins. J Cell Biol 119:1047-1061.

45.   Imamoto N, Tachibana T, Matsubae M, Yoneda Y. 1995. A karyophilic protein forms a stable complex with cytoplasmic components prior to nuclear pore binding. JBiolChem 270:8559-8565.

46.   Imamoto-Sonobe N, Matsuoka Y, Semba T, Okada Y, Uchida T, Yoneda Y. 1990. A protein recognized by antibodies to Asp-Asp-Asp-Glu-Asp shows specific binding activity to heterogeneous nuclear transport signals. JBiolChem 265:16504-16508.

47.   Inaguma Y, Goto S, Shinohara H, Hasegawa K, Ohshima K, Kato K. 1993. Physiological and pathological changes in levels of the two small stress proteins, HSP 27 and αB crystallin, in rat hindlimb muscles. JBiochem 114:378-384.

48.   Iwaki K, Chi S, Dillmann WH, Mestril R. 1993. Induction of HSP 70 in cultured rat neonatal cardiomyocytes by hypoxia and metabolic stress. Circulation 87:2023-2032.

49.   Izumoto S, Herbert J. 1993. Widespread constitutive expression of HSP 90 messenger RNA in rat brain. Journal of Neuroscience Research 35:20-28.

50.   Johnson J, Toft DO. 1995. Binding of p23 and hsp 90 during assembly with the progesterone receptor. MolEndocrin 9:670-678.

51.   Jurivich DA, Sistonen L, Kroes RA, Morimoto RI. 1992. Effect of sodium salicylate on the human heat shock response. Science 255:1243-1245.

52.   Jurivich DA, Pachetti C, Qiu L, Welk JF. 1995. Salicylate triggers heat shock factor differently than heat. JBiolChem 270:24489-24495.

53.   Knowlton AA, Brecher P, Apstein CS. 1991. Rapid expression of heat shock protein in the rabbit after brief cardiac ischemia. JClinInvest 87:139-147.

54.   Lang DR, Racker E. 1974. Effects of quercetin and F1 inhibitor on mitochondrial ATPase and energy-linked reactions in submitochondrial particles. Biochimica et Biophysica Acta 333:180-186.

55.   Langer T, Lu C, Echols H, Flanagan J, Hayer MK, Hartl FU. 1992. Successive action of DnaK, DnaJ and GroEL along the pathway of chaperone-mediated protein folding. Nature 356:683-689.

56.   Laszlo A. 1988. The relationship of heat-shock proteins, thermotolerance, and protein synthesis. Exp Cell Res 178:401-414.

57.   Latchman DS, Isenberg DA. 1994. The role of HSP90 in SLE. Autoimmunity 19:211-218.

58.   Laughton MJ, Halliwell B, Evans PJ, Hoult JRS. 1989. Antioxidant and pro-oxidant actions of the plant phenolics quercetin, gossypol and myricetin. BiochemPharmacol 38:2859-2865.

59.   Lepock JR, Frey HE, Ritchie KP. 1993. Protein denaturation in intact hepatocytes and isolated cellular organelles during heat shock. J Cell Biol 122:1267-1276.

60.   Lindahl M, Tagesson C. 1993. Selective inhibition of group II phospholipase A2 by quercetin. Inflammation 17:573-582.

61.   Lindquist S. 1981. Regulation of protein synthesis during heat shock. Nature 293:311-314.

62.   Locke M, Tanguay RM, Ianuzzo CD. 1996. Constitutive expression of HSP 72 in swine heart. J Mol Cell Cardiol 28:467-474.

63.   Marcinkiewicz C, Galasinski W, Gindzienski A. 1995. EF-1α is a target site for an inhibitory effect of quercetin in the peptide elongation process. Acta Biochimica Polonica 42:347-350.

64.   Matts RL, Hurst R. 1992. The relationship between protein synthesis and heat shock protein levels in rabbit reticulocyte lysates. JBiolChem 267:18168-18174.

65.   Matts RL, Xu Z, Pal JK, Chen J. 1992. Interactions of the heme-regulated eIF-2α kinase with heat shock proteins in rabbit reticulocyte lysates. JBiolChem 267:18160-18167.

66.   Mayhew M, da Silva ACR, Martin J, Erdjument-Bromage H, Tempst P, Hartl FU. 1996. Protein folding in the central cavity of the GroEL-GroES chaperonin complex. Nature 329:420-426.

67.   Menon V, Thomason DB. 1995. Head-down tilt increases rat cardiac muscle eIF-2α phosphorylation. Am J Physiol 269:C802-C804.

68.   Milarski KL, Morimoto RI. 1989. Mutational analysis of the human HSP70 protein: Distinct domains for nucleolar localization and adenosine triphosphate binding. J Cell Biol 109:1947-1962.

69.   Mimnaugh EG, Worland PJ, Whitesell L, Neckers LM. 1995. Possible role for serine/threonine phosphorylation in the regulation of the heteroprotein complex between the HSP90 stress protein and the pp60vsrc tyrosine kinase. JBiolChem 270:28654-28659.

70.   Miyata Y, Yahara I. 1995. Interaction between casein kinase II and the 90-kDa stress protein, HSP 90. Biochemistry 34:8123-8129.

71.   Mizzen LA, Welch WJ. 1988. Characterization of the thermotolerant cell. I. Effects on protein synthesis activity and the regulation of heat-shock protein 70 expression. J Cell Biol 106:1105-1116.

72.   Morris SD, Cumming DVE, Latchman DS, Yellon DM. 1996. Specific induction of the 70-kD heat stress proteins by the tyrosine kinase inhibitor herbimycin-A protects rat neonatal cardiomyocytes. JClinInvest 97:706-712.

73.   Munro S, Pelham HRB. 1984. Use of peptide tagging to detect proteins expressed from cloned genes: deletion mapping functional domains of drosophila HSP 70. Embo 3:3087-3093.

74.   Nakai A, Morimoto RI. 1993. Characterization of a novel chicken heat shock transcription factor, heat shock factor 3, suggests a new regulatory pathway. MolCellBiol 13:1983-1997.

75.   Nakano M, Mann DL, Knowlton AA. 1997. Blocking the endogenous increase in HSP72 increases susceptibility to hypoxia and reoxygenation injury in isolated adult feline cardiocytes. Circulation, in press.

76.   Nathan DF, Lindquist S. 1995. Mutational analysis of HSP 90 function: Interactions with a steroid receptor and a protein kinase. MolCellBiol 15:3917-3925.

77.   Nicchitta CV, Blobel G. 1993. Lumenal proteins of the mammalian endoplasmic reticulum are required to complete protein translocation. Cell 73:989-998.

78.   Ohtsuka K. 1993. Cloning of a cDNA for heat-shock proein HSP 40, a human homologue of bacterial DnaJ. BiochemBiophysResCommun 197:235-240.

79.   Ohtsuka K, Laszlo A. 1992. The relationship between HSP 70 localization and heat resistance. Exp Cell Res 202:507-518.

80.   Pace-Asciak CR, Hahn S, Diamandis EP, Soleas G, Goldberg DM. 1995. The red wine phenolics trans-resveratrol and quercetin block human platelet aggregation and eicosanoid synthesis: implications for protection against coronary artery disease. Clinica Chimica Acta 235:207-219.

81.   Parsell DA, Lindquist S. 1993. The function of heat-shock proteins in stress tolerance: Degradation and reactivation of damaged proteins. AnnuRevGenet 27:437-496.

82.   Parsell DA, Sanchez Y, Stitzel JD, Lindquist S. 1991. HSP 104 is a highly conserved protein with two essential nucleotide-binding sites. Nature 353:270-273.

83.   Parsell DA, Taulien J, Lindquist S. 1993. The role of heat-shock proteins in thermotolerance. Philosophical Transactions of the Royal Society of London Series B - Biological Sciences 339:279-284.

84.   Quraishi H, Rush SJ, Brown IR. 1996. Expression of mRNA species encoding heat shock protein 90 (HSP90) in control and hyperthermic rat brain. Journal of Neuroscience Research 43:335-345.

85.   Rabindran SK, Haroun RI, Clos J, Wisniewski J, Wu C. 1993. Regulation of heat shock factor trimer formation: Role of a conserved leucine zipper. Science 259:230-234.

86.   Richter JD, Standiford D. Structure and regulation of nuclear localization signals. In: Feldherr CM, ed. Nuclear Trafficking. New York: Academic Press, 1992:90-121.

87.   Rommelaere H, Van Troys M, Gao Y, et al. 1993. Eukaryotic cytosolic chaperonin contains t-complex polypeptide 1 and seven related subunits. ProcNatlAcadSci USA 90:11975-11979.

88.   Sadoshima J, Jahn L, Takahashi T, Kulik TJ, Izumo S. 1992. Molecular characterization of the stretch-induced adaption of cultured cardiac cells. JBiolChem 267:10551-10560.

89.   Salfity MR, Knowlton AA. 1995. Site-directed mutagenesis of a highly conserved nuclear localization sequence in human HSP 72. J Cell Biochem 19B:204 (ABST.).

90.   Sanchez Y, Lindquist SL. 1990. HSP 104 required for induced thermotolerance. Science 248:1112-1115.

91.   Scherrer LC, Picard D, Massa E, et al. 1993. Evidence that the hormone binding domain of steroid receptors confers hormonal control on chirmeric proteins by determining their hormone-regulated binding to heat-shock protein 90. Biochemistry 32:5381-5386.

92.   Schröder H, Langer T, Hartl F, Bukau B. 1993. DnaK, DnaJ and GrpE form a cellular chaperone machinery capable of repairing heat-induced protein damage. Embo 12:4137-4144.

93.   Shi Y, Thomas JO. 1992. The transport of proteins into the nucleus requires the 70-kilodalton heat shock protein or its cytosolic cognate. MolCellBiol 12:2186-2192.

94.   Shue G, Kohtx DS. 1994. Structural and functional aspects of basic helix-loop-helix protein folding by heat-shock protein 90. JBiolChem 269:2707-2711.

95.   Shyy T-T, Subjeck JR, Heinaman R, Anderson G. 1986. Effect of growth state and heat shock on nucleolar localization of the 110,000 Da heat shock protein in mouse embryo fibroblasts. Cancer Research 46:4738-4745.

96.   Simons SS Jr. 1994. Function/activity of specific amino acids in glucocorticoid receptors. Vitamins and Hormones 49:49-130.

97.   Siomi H, Dreyfuss G. 1995. A nuclear localization domain in the hnRNP A1 protein. J Cell Biol 129:551-560.

98.   Sistonen L, Sarge KD, Philips B, Abravaya K, Morimoto RI. 1992. Activation of heat shock factor 2 (HSF2) during hemin-induced differentiation of human erythroleukemia cells. MolCellBiol 12:4104-4111.

99.   Skowyra D, Georgopoulos C, Zylicz M. 1990. The E. coli dnaK gene product, the HSP70 homolog, can reactivate heat-inactivated RNA polymerase in an ATP hydrolysis-dependent manner. Cell 62:939-944.

100.   Stancato LF, Chow Y, Hutchison KA, Perdew GH, Jove R, Pratt WB. 1993. Raf exists in a native heterocomplex with HSP 90 and p50 that can be reconstituted in a cell-free system. JBiolChem 268:21711-21716.

101.   Subjeck JR, Shyy T, Shen J, Johnson RJ. 1983. Association between the mammalian 110,000-dalton heat-shock proein and nucleoli. J Cell Biol 97:1389-1395.

102.   Sugito K, Yamane M, Hattori H, et al. 1995. Interaction between HSP 70 and HSP 40, eukaryotic homologues of DnaK and DnaJ, in human cells expressing mutant-type p53. FEBS Letters 358:161-164.

103.   Theodorakis NG, Morimoto RI. 1987. Posttranscriptional regulation of HSP 70 expression in human cells: Effects of heat shock, inhibition of protein synthesis, and adenovirus infection on translation and mRNA stability. MolCellBiol 7:4357-4368.

104.   Ting L-P, Tu C-L, Chou C-K. 1989. Insulin induced expression of human heat-shock protein gene HSP 70. JBiolChem 264:3404-3408.

105.   Vogel JP, Misra LM, Rose MD. 1990. Loss of BiP/GRP78 function blocks translocation of secretory proteins in yeast. J Cell Biol 110:1885-1895.

106.   Watowich SS, Morimoto RI. 1988. Complex regulation of heat shock- and glucose-responsive genes in human cells. MolCellBiol 8:393-405.

107.   Weis K, Mattaj IW, Lamond AI. 1995. Identification of hSRP1α as a functional receptor for nuclear localization sequences. Science 268:1049-1053.

108.   Weissman JS, Hohl CM, Kovalenko O, et al. 1995. Mechanism of GroEL action: Productive release of polypeptide from a sequestered position under GroES. Cell 83:577-587.

109.   Welch WJ, Feramisco JR. 1984. Nuclear and nucleolar localization of the 72,000-dalton heat shock protein in heat-shocked mammalian cells. JBiolChem 259:4501-4513.

110.   Welch WJ, Mizzen LA. 1988. Characterization of the thermotolerant cell. II. Effects on the

intracellular distribution of heat-shock protein 70, intermediate filaments, and small nuclear ribonucleoprotein complexes. J Cell Biol 106:1117-1130.

111.   Westwood JT, Wu C. 1991. Stress-induced oligomerization and chromosomal relocalization of heat-shock factor. Nature 353:822-827.

112.   Whalen AM, Steward R. 1993. Dissociation of the dorsal-cactus complex and phosphorylation of the dorsal protein correlate with the nuclear localization of dorsal. J Cell Biol 123:423-534.

113.   Whitesell L, Mimnaugh EG, De Costa B, Myers CE, Neckers LM. 1994. Inhibition of heat shock protein HSP90-pp60v-serc heteroprotein complex formation by benzoquinone ansamycins: Essential role for stress proteins in oncogenic transformation. ProcNatlAcadSci USA 91:8324-8328.

114.   Wilkinson JM, Pollard I. 1993. Immunohistochemical localisation of the 25 kDa heat shock protein in unstressed rats. AnatRec 237:453-457.

115.   Williams RS, Thomas JA, Fina M, German Z, Benjamin IJ. 1993. Human heat shock protein 70 (HSP 70) protects murine cells from injury during metabolic stress. JClinInvest 92:503-508.

116.   Xia P, Culp LA. 1995. Adhesion activity in fibronectin's alternatively spliced domain EDa(EIIIA): Complementatiry to plasma fibronectin functions. Exp Cell Res 217:517-527.

117.   Xu Y, Lindquist S. 1993. Heat-shock protein HSP 90 governs the activity of pp60v-src kinase. ProcNatlAcadSci USA 90:7074-7078.

118.   Yang J, DeFranco DB. 1994. Differential roles of heat shock protein 70 in the in vitro nuclear import of glucocorticoid receptor and Simian virus 40 large tumor antigen. MolCellBiol 14:5088-5098.

119.   Zhao Y, Chacko S, Levin RM. 1994. Expression of stress proteins (HSP-70 and HSP-90) in the rabbit urinary bladder subjected to partial outlet obstruction. MolCellBiochem 130:49-55.

2

ISCHEMIA, INFARCTION AND HSP70

Wolfgang H. Dillmann and Ruben Mestril
Department of Medicine, Division of Endocrinology and Metabolism
University of California, San Diego, La Jolla, CA 92093-0618.

INTRODUCTION

Acute myocardial infarction remains one of the major causes of death among men in the Western World. The most common cause of acute myocardial infarction is thrombosis or occlusion of the coronary arteries that feed the left ventricle of the heart. The lack of blood flow to the cardiac muscle can result in severe cellular damage that eventually may compromise the muscle's ability to contract. Coronary thrombosis is a direct consequence of coronary artery disease or more specifically atherosclerosis. Recent research aimed at identifying the cause of atherosclerosis and efforts to prevent it have contributed to a decreased incidence of myocardial infarction in the past decade. However, in spite of this recent improvement, the incidence of myocardial infarction leading to subsequent severe cardiac failure still remains a significant medical problem. Therefore, the salvage of additional myocardium following an infarction is a highly desirable aim. Recent evidence indicates that endogenous protective mechanisms are readily activated in cardiomyocytes during an ischemic event, thus a better understanding of these endogenous protective mechanisms will most likely lead to additional myocardial salvage in the reperfused myocardium.

Myocardial infarction and the resulting ischemia produce a number of intracellular changes within the cardiomyocyte. These changes include among others increased cellular calcium levels, altered osmotic control, membrane damage, free radical production, decreased intracellular pH, depressed ATP levels, oxygen depletion, and decreased intracellular glucose levels, etc, (Bonventre, 1988). These events represent a form of stress which is known to result in protein denaturation within the cell. An increase in denatured proteins in the cell has previously been reported to trigger the heat shock response which increases the synthesis of the so-called heat shock proteins (HSPs) (Ananthan et al., 1986). This heat shock response produces a transient rearrangement of cellular activities in order to cope with the stress period by protecting essential components within the cell, so as, to permit it to resume normal activity during recovery from the stress (Lindquist, 1986). This ability of the cell for self-preservation has attracted the attention of several investigators in the field of cardiovascular research. The present chapter will attempt to cover what is known about these heat shock proteins, in particular the HSP70, and the recent studies related to their expression and involvement in myocardial protection against ischemic damage.

MYOCARDIAL ISCHEMIA AND ISCHEMIC INJURY

Myocardial ischemia and acute myocardial infarcts result from an imbalance between the supply of oxygenated blood and the oxygen requirement. Ischemia is best defined in relative rather than in absolute terms (Braunwald and Sobel, 1992; Reimer and Jennings, 1986). Complete and sudden occlusion of a large epicardial artery results in a wave front of myocardial necrosis starting at the subendocardial region and extending towards the epicardial part of the myocardium (Reimer et al., 1977). In experimental animals such as dogs after 20 minutes of coronary occlusion, increasing numbers of myocytes become irreversibly damaged in the subendocardial zone and by 40 minutes the majority of the myocytes are destined to necrose (Jennings et al., 1960). In small rodents (mice and rats), infarct size is primarily determined by the size of the occluded vessel because no significant collateral vessels exist (Fishbein et al., 1978). It is important to note that ischemic myocytes do not die within a few minutes after the onset of complete ischemia. Not all myocytes die simultaneously and islands of viable myocytes remain in ischemic regions for a long time or indefinitely (Reimer et al., 1977; Reimer and Jennings, 1979). In addition, it appears that myocytes exposed to milder ischemia can survive for longer times (Reimer, 1980). These are then important considerations to keep in mind when setting strategies aimed at protecting the ischemic myocardium.

Complete ischemia, at the cellular level, leads within 8 to 10 seconds to a cessation of oxidative phosphorylation and a switch to anaerobic glycolysis (Kubler and Spieckermann, 1970; Neely and Morgan, 1974). Anaerobic glycolysis results in much less efficient production of high energy phosphates and the demand for high energy phosphates quickly outpaces supply. Reduction of ATP concentrations below 20% of normal levels leads to the cells inability to regenerate high energy phosphates, maintain ion gradients, and to control their volume (Jennings et al., 1978). Metabolic products, especially lactate, accumulate contributing to pH lowering and increasing the osmotic load to the cell (Rovetto et al., 1975). Loss of volume control, increasing osmotic load, and intracellular volume expansion stretches the fragile sarcolemma which together with mechanical forces provided by myocardial contraction leads to disruption of the sarcolemma (Jennings et al., 1986). The ruptured sarcolemma presents a hallmark of irreversible myocardial damage resulting in cell death (Jennings et al., 1986; Jennings et al., 1990a). Rupture of the sarcolemma is evidenced by the release of cytosolic proteins including creatine phosphokinase (CPK) and lactate dehydrogenase (LDH). Severe ischemia markedly depresses protein synthesis due to decreased translational initiation and elongation (Schreiber et al., 1975; Kao et al., 1976; Williams et al., 1981). This leads to the synthesis of incomplete polypeptides which cannot fold properly and form complexes of denatured proteins. The acidic pH, abnormal ionic milieu, and formation of oxygen radicals during reperfusion will further contribute to protein malfolding and denaturation. The presence of denatured proteins in myocytes presents probably one of the major triggering mechanisms for the induction of HSP70 gene

26

expression. Renaturation of malfolded proteins, removal of irreversibly denatured proteins, and the resumption of protein synthesis present important cell functions especially in myocytes recovering from ischemic injury after reperfusion. Brief episodes of severe ischemia can lead to prolonged contractile dysfunction in the absence of severe myocyte damage as determined by histological changes. This condition has been termed myocardial stunning (Heyndrickx et al., 1975). Its cellular basis is currently only incompletely explored, but a recent report has shown that HSP70 may also play a protective role during this condition (Sun et al., 1995). In addition, severe chronic ischemia can lead to myocardial dysfunction which can be ameliorated by the relief of ischemia and has been termed myocardial hibernation (Rahimtoola, 1989). An interesting phenomenon known as preconditioning which refers to the exposure of the myocardium to brief episodes of ischemia appears to exert a protective effect for several hours against subsequent more prolonged ischemia (Murry et al., 1986). This effect may be mediated by adenosine and its receptors (Lasley et al., 1990). A protective effect occurring 24 hours after the initial ischemic preconditioning episode has recently postulated to be due to HSP70 (see chapter 4).

MYOCARDIAL REPERFUSION

Early in the course of severe ischemia a large number of jeopardized but not irreversibly injured myocytes exist, especially at the border of the wave front progressing from the subendocardial to the epicardial portion of the myocardium. These myocytes can be salvaged by timely reperfusion (Jennings et al., 1990b; Ellis et al., 1983). Early recanalization of an occluded coronary artery by pharmacological or mechanical means has led to a significant improvement in short- and long-term outcomes of acute myocardial infarcts (Lavie et al., 1990). Reperfusion leads to myocardial salvage, but can also result in damage (Braunwald and Kloner, 1985). The timing of reperfusion appears to make the crucial difference for the development and the extent of reperfusion injury. In reversibly injured myocytes, reperfusion leads only to temporary changes like cell swelling (Jennings et al., 1985). In contrast, in irreversibly injured myocytes, reperfusion leads to explosive cell swelling and accelerated cell death (Jennings and Reimer, 1981). In isolated myocytes, reoxygenation leads also to cell death which may result from oxygen radicals and calcium influx (Josephson et al., 1991; Quaife et al., 1991; Hohl et al., 1982). The findings summarized above indicate the importance of salvage of the myocardium by early reperfusion. It has been hypothesized that increased levels of HSP70 in cardiomyocytes contribute to a protective effect and accelerate recovery from ischemic damage by promoting normal protein folding. The normal folding state of proteins is a crucial requirement for proper cell function. Definitive evidence that HSP70 can fulfill this protective role has recently been shown (Marber et al., 1995; Plumier et al., 1995) and may eventually lead to future treatment strategies which will further enhance myocardial tissue salvaged after severe ischemia.

THE MAMMALIAN HEAT SHOCK PROTEINS

HSP70 is a member of the mammalian heat shock proteins. These proteins can be grouped in three subgroups according to their molecular mass. The high molecular mass HSPs include three major members namely HSP110, HSP90-α and HSP90-β. The last two HSPs have attracted much interest due to their ability to bind to steroid receptors and are presumably involved in the regulation of these molecules with their ligands (Pratt, 1993). The HSP70 family is the most abundant and complex of the HSPs. This subgroup includes the HSP70 and HSP60 proteins. The HSP70 group is made up of at least three to four members in mammalian cells (Lowe and Moran, 1986; Harrison et al., 1987). One of the HSP70s is expressed constitutively in all cells and is slightly increased in expression by a heat shock or other oxidative stresses. The other three HSP70 members are inducible isoforms which are expressed exclusively when the cell is under stress, exception in primate cells which constitutively express a considerable amount of these inducible forms of HSP70 under normal conditions (Welch et al., 1983). HSP60 is nuclearly encoded, but resides in the mitochondria where it is believed to be involved in the assembly of macromolecular complexes (Ostermann et al., 1989). The small molecular mass HSPs are HSP47, HSP40, HSP27, αB-crystallin (20kD), heme oxygenase (32kD) and ubiquitin (8kD). HSP47 is an endoplasmic reticulum resident protein which has a high binding affinity for collagen (Nagata et al., 1991) and recently has been postulated to serve as a molecular chaperone (Sauk et al., 1994). HSP40 has recently been found to be in close association with HSP70 and is believed to be involved in the same processes as HSP70 (Hattori et al., 1993; Frydman et al., 1994). HSP27 has been shown to also be involved in the development of the thermotolerant phenotype in the cell (Kampinga et al., 1994). Interestingly, HSP27 is the target of phosphorylation in response to mitogens and tumor promoters (Welch, 1985). The αB-crystallin is highly homologous to the small heat shock proteins (Ingolia and Craig, 1982; Southgate et al., 1983) and has recently been reported to be induced by heat shock (Klemenz et al., 1991). In addition, αB-crystallin has been found to be an abundant protein in cardiac muscle cells (Bennardini et al., 1992). The heme oxygenase besides being induced by several of the common stressors (heat shock in rodents, hypoxia, hydrogen peroxide, cadmium) as other HSPs is also induced by hemin as are other stress proteins (Sistonen et al., 1992). Ubiquitin, the smallest member in this subgroup, is induced by similar stresses as the major HSPs (heat shock, amino acid analogues, denatured proteins) and plays a vital role in the process of protein degradation (Mayer et al., 1991).

The most abundant HSPs are the members of the HSP70 group. The constitutively expressed HSP70 (apparent molecular weight 73 kd) is found in the cytoplasm under non-stress conditions, while the inducible HSP70 (apparent molecular weight 72 kD) is found in the nucleus and more precisely in the nucleolus during a heat shock. Heat shock proteins besides having the common feature of being induced by stress have been found to bind denatured or nascent polypeptides in the different compartments of the cell. This characteristic of heat shock proteins has made them a good candidate to be involved in a cellular defense mechanism.

The protective nature of heat shock proteins has been documented mainly by the observation that a mild heat shock (42°C) confers resistance to the cell against a subsequent lethal heat shock (45°C) (Li and Werb, 1982). This phenomenon usually

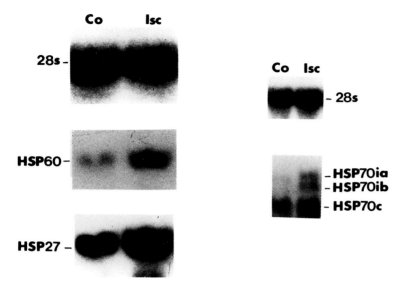

FIGURE 1: Northern blot analysis of total RNA from control rat hearts (Co) and rat hearts submitted to *in vivo* occlusion of the left descending coronary artery for 30 minutes (Isc). Northern blot was sequentially probed with the human HSP70, HSP60 and HSP27 cDNAs, as well as a probe specific for the ribosomal 28s RNA so as to assess loading differences.

referred to as thermotolerance is a transient resistance to the cytotoxic effects of a subsequent lethal hyperthermic treatment which is induced by a non-lethal heat treatment. The synthesis and degradation of heat shock proteins directly correlates with the development and decay of thermotolerance (Li and Mak, 1985). This fact has been taken as evidence that these proteins are involved in the acquisition, maintenance and decay of thermotolerance.

HSP70 has been recently found to be an "unfoldases" which functions to facilitate the transport of proteins through the membranes of the endoplasmic reticulum (ER) and mitochondria (Deshaies et al. 1988; Chirico et al., 1988). Due to this property of facilitating the translocation of other proteins through the membranes of the different intracellular compartments, HSP70 has been classified as a molecular chaperone. Other investigators have found that the mammalian constitutive HSP70 (73 kd) is involved in a mechanism that targets intracellular proteins for lysosomal degradation during periods of serum withdrawal. According to their findings, HSP70 recognizes and binds a short peptide sequence found in certain intracellular proteins which are preferentially degraded when cells are deprived of serum (Chiang et al., 1989). These findings suggest that HSPs have a vital function within the cell even under non-stress conditions.

The increased synthesis of HSPs during cellular stress may reflect the need for these proteins to protect different structures within the diverse cellular compartments. Evidence that seems to support this hypothesis comes from two reports that show when HSP70 is depleted in cells either by micro-injection of antibodies specific to HSP70 (Riabowal et al., 1988) or by reducing the expression of HSP70 by genetic means (promoter competition) [Johnston and Kucey, 1988] cells are rendered sensitive to a subsequent heat shock. Although the most convincing evidence for the protective role of HSP70 against heat stress has been recently reported in two parallel studies. In these studies, the constitutive expression of a stably transfected HSP70 gene either in a rat fibroblast cell line (Li et al., 1991) or in simian CV cells (Angelidis et al., 1991) resulted in a higher resistance to thermal stress. It would then seem that HSP70s are involved in vital functions within the cell and that its presence is of crucial importance for cell survival during a heat shock. In addition, numerous studies have shown that increased levels of HSPs by a heat shock will also protect against others stresses and vice versa (Mizzen and Welch, 1988; Hahn and Li, 1990; Polla et al., 1991). This phenomenon of cross-protection or cross-tolerance has attracted the attention of many investigators, especially those attempting to find new means of protecting cardiac myocytes against ischemia-induced injury.

THE CARDIAC CELL AND HSP70

In the last fifteen years, several studies have shown that heat shock proteins are readily synthesized in cardiac cells during tissue trauma (Currie and White, 1981), aortic banding and hyperthermia (Hammond et al., 1982). Further studies have shown that HSP70 is induced to high levels of expression following conditions similar to those encountered during myocardial ischemia. Ligation of the left anterior descending coronary artery in the heart of experimental animals for several hours produces acute myocardial ischemia which was found to increase expression of the HSP70 inducible gene (Dillmann et al., 1986; Mehta et al., 1988). Although HSP70 is the main HSP exhibiting increased expression following *in vivo* experimental ischemia, other HSPs are also induced by the ischemic event. Figure 1 shows a representative Northern blot containing total RNA from rat hearts that were submitted to 30 minutes of *in vivo* ischemia as well as control hearts. As can be observed, the two inducible isoforms of HSP70, as previously defined (Mestril et al., 1994a), as well as HSP60 and HSP27 were all induced by the ischemic stress. Obviously, the level of expression of HSP70 is greater due to the low basal level of expression of the inducible isoforms of HSP70 in rodent cells. This is markedly evident in the case of the isolated perfused rat heart model, as can be seen in Figure 2, and as shown by other investigators (Currie, 1988a). Figure 2A shows a representative Northern blot analysis of total RNA from isolatedperfused rat hearts while control hearts express negligible amounts of the inducible HSP70. Hearts submitted to heat stress (42°C for 30 minutes) or global

30

A

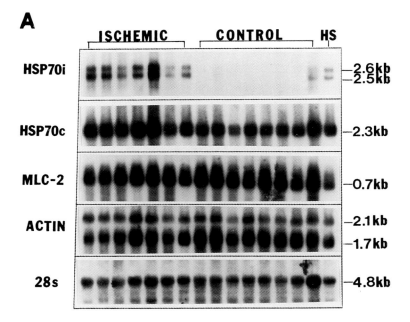

FIGURE 2A: Northern blot analysis of total RNA from isolated perfused rat hearts that were either submitted to global ischemia for 30 minutes followed by 90 minutes of reperfusion, heat shock (42°C for 30 minutes) or left untreated. Northern blot was sequentially probed with the inducible human HSP70 (HSP70i), constitutive rat HSP70 (HSP70c), rat myosin light chain-2 (MLC-2), rat β-actin (ACTIN) cDNAs and a ribosomal RNA 28s probe.

ischemia (no perfusion for 30 minutes) expressed significant amounts of HSP70 mRNA as can be seen in Figure 2B.

Hypoxia decompression which produces hypoxic hypoxia, a form of oxygen depletion, was also found to increase the synthesis of HSP70 *in vivo* in rodent cardiac tissue (Howard and Geoghegan, 1986). We have also found that the expression of HSP70 is induced in cultured rat neonatal myocytes during stresses similar to those encountered in ischemia. Neonatal rat myocytes exposed to ATP depletion using metabolic inhibitors or oxygen depletion exhibit high levels of HSP70 mRNA and protein (Iwaki et al., 1993). The rapid induction of HSP70 in cardiac tissue during oxidative stress has prompted interest in investigating the possible protective role that it may play in the heart during myocardial ischemia. It has shown that a whole animal pre-heat shock treatment of rats confers enhanced post-ischemic recovery in an isolated reperfused rat heart model system (Currie et al., 1988b). Currie and co-workers found that isolated

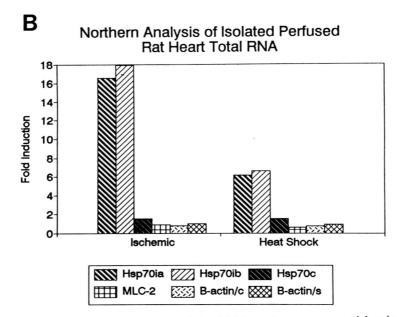

FIGURE 2B: Graphic representation of the fold induction over control levels of the normalized values obtained for the expression of the different mRNAs HSP70ia (2.6kb), HSP70ib (2.5kb), HSP70c (2.3kb), MLC-2 (0.7kb), cardiac β-actin/c (1.7kb), cellular β-actin/s (2.1kb) during ischemic stress (n=7) and heat stress (n=3).

perfused hearts from rats which had received a 15 minute heat treatment at 42°C, 24 hours previously, exhibited an improved contractile recovery after a 30 minute period of low-flow ischemia followed by reperfusion as compared to hearts from non-heat treated animals. In addition, these investigators found that the pre-heat treatment of animals produced less ultrastructure disruption of the mitochondria and a decrease in creatine kinase release in rat heart tissue following ischemia/reperfusion injury. Upon examination of the changes in the rat heart after the heat treatment, they found increased levels of HSP70 protein and an increase in enzymatic activity for the anti-oxidative enzyme catalase. The increase in catalase activity following whole-body heat stress

remains unclear and subsequent studies have shown that it does not involve any changes in transcription activation of the gene coding for catalase (Currie and Tanguay, 1991). In addition, it has been suggested that the heat induced increase in catalase activity may be secondary to a direct heat shock protein interaction which modulates the activity of the enzyme (Kukreja and Hess, 1992). Although, recent studies indicate that catalase may not play a role in the myocardial protection conferred by a whole body heat stress, either in isolated perfused rat hearts (Wall et al., 1993) or *in vivo* rat hearts (Auyeung et al., 1995). In addition, other studies have confirmed that a hyperthermic treatment of experimental animals can result in a significantly improved myocardial salvage following coronary occlusion and reperfusion *in vivo* (Donnelly et al., 1992; Currie et al., 1993) as well as in an isolated perfused heart model (Walker et al., 1993). A more recent study has shown that the sympathomimetic drug, amphetamine, is capable of producing a whole body stress in pigs at a concentration of 3 mg/kg. This dose of amphetamine was found to induce the expression of several of HSPs: HSP70, HSP27 and HSP90, as well as, two antioxidant enzymes (superoxide dismutase and catalase) in the heart, lung, liver, brain, kidney and intestine of pigs. The hearts of these amphetamine-treated animals were found to exhibit improved post-ischemic left ventricular global as well as regional contractile functions and reduced myocardial cellular injury after left arterial descending coronary artery occlusion and hypothermic cardioplegic arrest (Maulik et al, 1995).

Obviously, all studies have not shown a correlation between an increase in heat shock proteins and resistance to myocardial ischemic injury. Although one must bear in mind that the majority of these studies have used periods of coronary occlusion or ischemia that reach the late irreversible phase of injury (Jennings and Reimer, 1981). Therefore, if the ischemic episode persists for a long period of time where the majority of the cardiomyocytes have suffered irreversible ischemic injury, there is little that the increased presence of HSP70 or any other protective agent can do to protect the integrity of the myocyte. A good example of this point is the work of Donnelly and co-workers (Donnelly et al, 1992) who demonstrated that in the *in situ* rat heart, a whole body heat stress can result in a significant reduction in infarct size after a 35 minute, but not after a 45 minute coronary occlusion. A similar study in an *in vivo* rabbit heart model by Marber and co-workers (Marber et al, 1993) showed that heat stress is protective against a 30 minute period of coronary occlusion and reperfusion, while the same group of investigators had previously failed to find any protective effects of a heat stress followed by a 45 minute period of occlusion in the same model (Yellon et al, 1992).

It is obvious that a whole-body heat stress results in many cellular changes in an organism besides an increase in the expression of heat shock proteins which could be responsible for the observed protection against myocardial ischemia. Nonetheless, several studies have shown that HSPs and, in particular, the amount of HSP70 present following a whole-body heat shock is directly related to the degree of myocardial protection obtained (Hutter et al., 1994; Marber et al., 1994). Further direct evidence that HSP70 is able to cross-protect against ischemic injury has recently been obtained using myogenic cell lines. It was found that when myogenic cells that had previously received a mild heat shock were submitted to conditions mimicking ischemia *in vitro* (hypoxia, glucose deprivation, hypotonicity, restricted intercellular volume) or simulated ischemia, these cells were then able to survive significantly better than cells that had not been pre-heat shocked (Mestril et al., 1994b). Similar results were obtained when a stably transfected human HSP70 was over-expressed in myogenic cells. Overexpression of the human HSP70 in rodent myogenic cell lines either by transient or stable transfection has shown to confer a protective effect against metabolic stress (Williams et al., 1993) and simulated ischemia (Mestril et al., 1994b). Interestingly, this myogenic stably transfected cell line overexpressing HSP70 has recently been found to also be resistant to endotoxemia (Chi et al., 1996).

These results indicate that HSP70, if not solely responsible, must play an important role in the myocardial protection obtained following a whole body heat stress. Conclusive evidence that HSP70 plays this protective role *in vitro* has been shown using neonatal rat cardiomyocytes where the delivery of exogenous copies of HSP70 using recombinant adenoviral vectors (e.g. human adenovirus 5) results in a marked tolerance of the cardiomyocyte to simulated ischemic conditions (Mestril et al., 1996). In addition, transgenic mice that overexpress HSP70 in cardiac muscle have now been shown using an isolated perfused heart preparation. The hearts of these mice have a significantly marked recovery in contractile function as well as a reduction in infarct size and creatine release after ischemia and reperfusion (Marber et al., 1995). Similar results using an independently generated transgenic mouse strain was found by other investigators (Plumier et al., 1995). These results have been further confirmed by the finding that the hearts of these transgenic mice overexpressing the HSP70 gene show a marked reduction in infarct size in an *in vivo* model of ischemia and reperfusion (Hutter et al., 1996).

The amount of evidence presently available indicate that HSP70 plays an important role in myocardial protection against ischemic and reperfusion injury. The future challenges will be to fully understand the precise mechanism in which HSP70 confers myocardial protection and in finding pharmacological means of increasing the amount of HSP70 in the heart of patients undergoing cardiopulmonary by-pass, thrombolytic or coronary angioplastic therapies.

REFERENCES

Angelidis CE, Lazaridis I, Pagoulatos GN. Constitutive expression of heat shock protein 70 in mammalian cells confers thermoresistance. Eur J Biochem 1991;199:35-39.

Ananthan J, Goldberg AL, Voellmy R. Abnormal proteins serve as eukaryotic stress signals and trigger the activation of heat shock genes. Science 1986;232:522-524.

Auyeung Y, Sievers RE, Weng D, Barbosa V, Wolfe CL. Catalase inhibition with 3-amino-1,2,4-triazole does not abolish infarct size reduction in heat-shocked rats. Circulation 1995;92:3318-3322.

Bennardini F, Wrzosek A, Chiesi M. αB-crystallin in cardiac tissue, association with actin and desmin filaments. Circ Res 1992;71:288-294.

Bonventre JV. Mediators of ischemic renal injury. Ann Rev Med 1988;39:531-544.

Braunwald E, Kloner RA. Myocardial reperfusion: a double-edged sword? J Clin Invest 1985;76:1713-1719.

Braunwald E, Sobel BE. "Coronary blood flow and myocardial ischemia." In *Heart Disease*, Braunwald E, ed. Philadelphia, PA: W.B. Saunders Co., 1992.

Chi SH, Mestril R. Stable expression of a human hsp70 gene in a rat myogenic cell line confers protection against endotoxin. Amer J Physiol (in press)

Chiang HL, Terlecky SR, Plant CP, Dice JF. A role for a 70 kilodalton heat shock protein in lysosomal degradation of intracellular proteins. Science 1989;246:382-385.

Chirico WJ, Walters MG, Blobel G. 70 K heat shock related proteins stimulate protein translocation into microsomes. Nature 1988;332:805-810.

Currie RW, White FP. Trauma induced protein in rat tissues: a physiological role for a "heat shock" protein? Science 1981;214:72-73.

Currie RW. Protein synthesis in perfused rat hearts after in vivo hyperthermia and in vitro cold ischemia. Biochem Cell Biol 1988a;66:13-19.

Currie RW, Karmazyn M, Kloc M, Mailer K. Heat shock response is associated with enhanced post-ischemic ventricular recovery. Circ Res 1988b;63:543-549.

Currie RW, Tanguay RM. Analysis of RNA for transcripts for catalase and SP71 in rat hearts after in vivo hyperthermia. Biochem Cell Biol 1991;69:375-382.

Currie RW, Tanguay RM, Kingma Jr JG. Heat shock response and limitation of tissue necrosis during occlusion/reperfusion in rabbit hearts. Circulation 1993;87:963-971.

Deshaies RJ, Koch BD, Werner-Washburne M, Craig EA, Schekman R. A subfamily of stress proteins facilitates translocation of secretory and mitochondrial precursor polypeptides. Nature 1988;332:800-805.

Dillmann WH, Mehta HB, Barrieux A, Guth BD, Neeley WE, Ross J. Ischemia of the dog heart induces the appearance of a cardiac mRNA coding for a protein with migration characteristics similar to heat shock/stress protein 71. Circ Res 1986;59:110-114.

Donnelly TJ, Sievers RE, Vissern FLJ, Welch WJ, Wolfe CL. Heat shock protein induction in rat hearts. Circulation 1992;85:769-778.

Ellis SG, Henschke CI, Sandor T, Wynne J, Braunwald E, Kloner RA. Time course of functional and biochemical recovery of myocardium salvaged by reperfusion. J Am Coll Cardiol 1983;1:1047-1055.

Fishbein MC, Maclean DM, Maroko PR. Experimental myocardial infarction in the rat: qualitative and quantitative changes during pathologic evaluation. Am J Pathol 1978;90:57-70.

Frydman J, Nimmesgern E, Ohtsuka K, Hartl FU. Folding of nascent polypeptide chains in a high molecular mass assembly with molecular chaperones. Nature 1994;370:111-117.

Hahn GM, Li GC. "Thermotolerance, thermoresistance and thermosensitization." In Stress Proteins in Biology and Medicine, Morimoto RI, Tissieres A, Georgopoulos C, eds. Cold Spring Harbor, NY: Cold Spring Harbor Laboratory Press, 1990.

Hammond GL, Lai YK, Markert CL. Diverse forms of stress lead to new patterns of gene expression through a common and essential metabolic pathway. Proc Natl Acad Sci USA 1982;79:3485-3488.

Harrison GS, Drabkin HA, Kao FT, Hartz J, Hart IM, Chu EHY, Wu BJ, Morimoto RI. Chromosomal location of human genes encoding major heat shock protein HSP70. Som Cell Mol Gen 1987;13:119-130.

Hattori H, Kaneda T, Lokeshwar B, Laszlo A, Ohtsuka K. A stress-inducible 40 kDa protein (hsp40): purification by modified two-dimensional gel electrophoresis and co-localization with hsc70 (p73) in heat-shocked Hela cells. J Cell Sci 1993;104:629-638.

Heyndrickx GR, Millard RW, McRitchie RJ, Maroko PR, Vatner SF. Regional myocardial functional and electrophysiological alterations after brief coronary artery occlusion in conscious dogs. J Clin Invest 1975;56:978-985.

Hohl C, Ansel A, Altshuld R, Brierley GP. Contracture of isolated rat heart cells on anaerobic to aerobic transition. Am J Physiol 1982;242:H1022-H1030.

Howard G, Geoghegan TE. Altered cardiac tissue gene expression during acute hypoxic expression. Mol Cell Biochem 1986;69:155-160.

Hutter MM, Sievers RE, Barbosa V, Wolfe CL. Heat shock protein induction in rat hearts: a direct correlation between the amount of heat shock protein induced and the degree of myocardial protection. Circulation 1994;89:355-360.

Hutter JJ, Mestril R, Tam EKW, Sievers RE, Dillmann WH, Wolfe CL. Overexpression of inducible heat shock protein (HSP)72 in transgenic mice decreases infarct size. J Amer Coll Cardiol 1996;27:33A

Ingolia TD, Craig EA. Four small Drosophila heat shock proteins are related to each other and to mammalian α-crystallin. Proc Natl Acad Sci USA 1982;79:2360-2364.

Iwaki K, Chi SH, Dillmann WH, Mestril R. Induction of HSP70 in cultured rat neonatal cardiomyocytes by hypoxia and metabolic stress. Circulation 1993;87:2023-2032.

Jennings RB, Sommers HM, Smyth GA, Flack HA, Linn H. Myocardial necrosis induced by temporary occlusion of a coronary artery in the dog. Arch Pathol 1960;70:68-78.

Jennings RB, Hawkins HK, Lowe JE, Hill ML, Klotman S, Reimer KA. Relation between high energy phosphate and lethal injury in myocardial ischemia in the dog. Am J Pathol 1978;92:187-214.

Jennings RB, Reimer KA. Lethal myocardial ischemic injury. Am J Pathol 1981;102:241-255.

Jennings RB, Schaper J, Hill ML, Steenbergen C, Jr, Reimer KA. Effect of reperfusion late in the phase of reversible ischemic injury. Changes in cell volume, electrolytes, metabolites and ultrastructure. Circ Res 1985;56:262-278.

Jennings RB, Reimer KA, Steenbergen C, Jr. Myocardial ischemia revisited. The osmolar load, membrane damage and reperfusion. J Mol Cell Cardiol 1986;18:769-780.

Jennings RB, Murry CE, Steenbergen C,Jr, Reimer KA. Development of cell injury in sustained acute ischemia. Circulation 1990a;82(Suppl.3):II2-II12.

Jennings RB, Murry CE, Reimer KA. Myocardial effects of brief periods of ischemia followed by reperfusion. Adv Cardiol 1990b;37:7-31.

Johnston RN, Kucey BL. Competitive inhibition of HSP70 gene expression causes thermosensitivity. Science 1988;242:1551-1554.

Josephson RA, Silverman HS, Lakatta EG, Stern MD, Zweier JL. Study of the mechanisms of hydrogen peroxide and hydroxyl free radical-induced cellular injury and calcium overload in cardiac myocytes. J Biol Chem 1991;266:2354-2361.

Kampinga HH, Brunsting JF, Stege GJ, Konings AW, Landry J. Cells overexpressing hsp27 show accelerated recovery from heat-induced nuclear protein aggregation. Biochem Biophy Res Comm 1994;204:1170-1177.

Kao R, Rannels DE, Morgan HE. Effects of anoxia and ischemia on protein synthesis in perfused rat hearts. Circ Res 1976;38:I125-I130.

Klemenz R, Frohli E, Steiger RH, Schafer R, Aoyama A. Alpha B-crystallin is a small heat shock protein. Proc Natl Acad Sci USA 1991;88:3652-3656.

Kubler W, Spieckermann PG. Regulation of glycolysis in the ischemic and the anoxic myocardium. J Mol Cell Cardiol 1970;1:351-377.

36

Kukreja RC, Hess ML. The oxygen free radical system: from equations through membrane protein interactions to cardiovascular injury and protection. Cardiovasc Res 1992;26:641-655.

Lasley RD, Rhee JW, Van Wylen DGL, Mentzer RM, Jr. Adenosine A1 receptor mediated protection of the globally ischemic isolated rat heart. J Mol Cell Cardiol 1990;22:39-47.

Lavie CJ, Gersh BJ, Chesebro JH. Reperfusion in acute myocardial infarction Mayo Clin Proc 1990;65:549-564.

Li GC, Werb Z. Correlation between synthesis of heat shock proteins and development of thermotolerance in Chinese hamster fibroblasts. Proc Natl Acad Sci USA 1982;79:3218-3222.

Li GC, Mak JY. Induction of heat shock protein synthesis in murine tumors during the development of thermotolerance. Cancer Res 1985;45:3816-3824.

Li GC, Li L, Liu YK, Mak JY, Chen L, Lee WMF. Thermal response of rat fibroblasts stably transfected with the human 70 kD heat shock protein encoding gene. Proc Natl Acad Sci USA 1991;88:1681-1685.

Lindquist S. The heat shock response. Ann Rev Biochem 1986;55:1151-1191.

Lowe DG, Moran LA. Molecular cloning and analysis of DNA complementary to three mouse Mr=68,000 heat shock protein mRNAs. J Biol Chem 1986;261:2102-2112.

Marber MS, Latchman DS, Walker JM, Yellon DM: Cardiac stress protein elevation 24 hours after brief ischemia or heat stress is associated with resistance to myocardial infarction. Circulation 1993;88:1264-1272.

Marber MS, Walker JM, Latchman DS, Yellon DM. Myocardial protection after whole body heat stress in the rabbit is dependent on metabolic substrate and is related to the amount of the inducible 70kD heat stress protein. J Clin Invest 1994;93:1087-1094

Marber MS, Mestril R, Chi SH, Sayen MR, Yellon DM, Dillmann WH. Overexpression of the rat inducible 70-kD heat stress protein in a transgenic mouse increases the resistance of the heart to ischemic injury. J Clin Invest 1995;95:1446-1456

Maulik N, Engelman RM, Wei Z, Liu X, Rousou JA, Flack JE, Deaton DW, Das DK: Drug-induced heat-shock preconditioning improves postischemic ventricular recovery after cardiopulmonary bypass. Circulation 1995;92(II):II-381-II388.

Mayer RJ, Lowe J, Landon M, McDermott H, Tuckwell J, Doherty F, Laszlo L. "Ubiquitin and the lysosomal system: molecular pathological and experimental findings." In *Heat Shock*, Maresca B and Lindquist S, eds. Berlin, Germany: Springer-Verlag, 1991.

Mehta HB, Popovich BK, Dillmann WH. Ischemia induces changes in the level of mRNAs coding for stress protein 71 and creatine kinase M. Circ Res 1988;63:512-517.

Mestril R, Chi SH, Sayen MR, Dillmann WH. Isolation of a novel inducible rat heat shock protein (HSP70) gene and its expression during ischemia-hypoxia and heat shock. Biochem J 1994a;298:561-569.

Mestril R, Chi SH, Sayen MR, O'Reilly K, Dillmann WH. Expression of inducible stress protein 70 in rat heart myogenic cells confers protection against simulated ischemia induced injury. J Clin Invest 1994b;93:759-767.

Mestril R, Giordano FJ, Conde AG, Dillmann WH. Adenovirus mediated gene transfer of a heat shock protein 70 (hsp70i) protects against simulated ischemia. J Mol Cell Cardiol (in press)

Mizzen LA, Welch WJ. Characterization of the thermotolerant cell. I. Effects on protein synthesis activity and the regulation of heat shock protein 70 expression. J Cell Biol 1988;106:1105-1116.

Murry CE, Jennings RB, Reimer KA. Preconditioning with ischemia: a delay of lethal cell injury in ischemic myocardium. Circulation 1986;74:1124-1136.

Nagata K, Nakai A, Hosokawa N, Kudo M, Takechi H, Sato M, Hirayoshi K. "Interaction of HSP47 with newly synthesized procollagen and regulation of HSP expression." In *Heat Shock*, Maresca B, Lindquist S, eds. Berlin, Germany: Springer-Verlag, 1991.

Neely JR, Morgan HE. Relation between carbohydrate and lipid metabolism and the energy balance of heart muscle. Ann Rev Physiol 1974;36:413-459.

Ostermann J, Horwich AL, Neupert W, Hartl FV. Protein folding in mitochondria requires complex formation with hsp60 and ATP hydrolysis. Nature 1989;341:125-130.

Polla BS, Mili N, Kantengwa S, 1991. "Heat shock and oxidative injury in human cells." In *Heat Shock*, Maresca B, Lindquist S, eds. Berlin: Springer-Verlag, 1991.

Pratt WB. The role of heat shock proteins in regulating the function, folding, and trafficking of the glucocorticoid receptor. J Biol Chem 1993;268:21455-21458.

Plumier JC, Ross BM, Currie RW, Angelidis CE, Kazlaris H, Kollias G, Pagoulatos GN. Transgenic mice expressing the human heat shock protein 70 have improved post-ischemic myocardial recovery. J Clin Invest 1995;95:1854-1860.

Quaife RA, Kohmoto O, Barry WH. Mechanisms of reoxygenation injury in cultured ventricular myocytes. Circulation 1991;83:566-577.

Rahimtoola SH. The hibernating myocardium. Am Heart J 1989;117:211-221.

Reimer KA, Lowe JE, Rasmussen MM, Jennings RB. Myocardial infarct size vs. duration of coronary occlusion in dogs. Circulation 1977;56:786-794.

Reimer KA, Jennings RB. Transmural progression of necrosis within the framework of ischemic bed size (myocardium at risk) and collateral flow. Lab Invest 1979;40:633-644.

Reimer KA. Myocardial infarct size. Measurements and predictions. Arch Pathol Lab Med 1980;104:225-230.

Reimer KA, Jennings RB. "Myocardial ischemia, hypoxia and infarction." In *The Heart and Cardiovascular System*, Fozzard HA, Jennings RB, Haber E, Katz AM, Morgan HE, eds. New York, NY: Raven Press, 1986.

Riabowol KT, Mizzen LA, Welch WJ. Heat shock is lethal to fibroblasts microinjected with antibodies against HSP70. Science 1988;242:433-436.

Rovetto MJ, Lamberton WF, Neely JR. Mechanisms of glycolytic inhibition in ischemic rat hearts. Circ Res 1975;37:742-751.

Sauk JJ, Smith T, Norris K, Ferreira L. HSP47 and the translation-translocation machinery cooperate in the production of alpha1(I) chains of type I procollagen. J Biol Chem 1994;269:3941-3946.

Schreiber SS, Rothschild MA, Evans C, Reff F, Oratz M. The effect of pressure or flow stress on right ventricular protein synthesis in the face of constant and restricted coronary perfusion. J Clin Invest 1975;55:1-11.

Sistonen L, Sarge KD, Phillips B, Abravaya K, Morimoto RI. Activation of heat shock factor 2 during hemin induced differentiation of human erythroleukemia cells. Mol Cell Biol 1992;12:4104-4111.

Southgate R, Ayme A, Voellmy RW. Nucleotide sequence analysis of the Drosophila small heat shock gene cluster at locus 67B. J Mol Biol 1983;165:35-57.

Sun JZ, Tang XL, Knowlton AA, Park SW, Qiu Y, Bolli R. Late preconditioning against myocardial stunning. An endogenous protective mechanism that confers resistance to postischemic dysfunction 24 h after brief ischemia in conscious pigs. J Clin Invest 1995;95:388-403.

Walker DM, Pasini E, Kucukoglu S, Marber MS, Iliodromitis E, Ferrari R, Yellon DM. Heat stress limits infarct size in the isolated perfused rabbit heart. Cardiovasc Res 1993;27:962-967.

Wall SR, Fliss H, Korecky B. Role of catalase in myocardial protection against ischemia in heat shocked rats. Mol Cell Biochem 1993;129:187-194.

Welch WJ, Garrels JI, Thomas GP, Lin JJC, Feramisco JR. Biochemical characterization of the mammalian stress proteins and identification of two stress proteins as glucose and calcium ionophore regulated proteins. J Biol Chem 1983;258:7102-7111.

Welch WJ. Phorbol ester, calcium ionophore, or serum added to quiescent rat fibroblast cells all result in the elevated phosphorylation of two 28,000 dalton mammalian stress proteins. J Biol Chem 1985;260:3058-3062.

Williams EH, Kao RL, Morgan HE. Protein degradation and synthesis during recovery from myocardial ischemia. Am J Physiol 1981;240:E268-E273.

Williams RS, Thomas JA, Fina M, German Z, Benjamin IJ. Human heat shock protein 70 (HSP704) protects murine cells from injury during metabolic stress. J Clin Invest 1993;92:503-508.

Yellon DM, Iliodromitis E, Latchman DS, Van Winkle DM, Downey JM, Williams FM, Williams TJ: Whole body heat stress fails to limit infarct size in the reperfused rabbit heart. Cardiovasc Res 1992;26:342-346.

39

3

DO HEAT SHOCK PROTEINS PLAY A ROLE IN MYOCARDIAL PRECONDITIONING?

Richard J. Heads
Department of Cardiology, Guys' and St. Thomas' Medical and Dental Schools, Rayne Institute, St. Thomas' Hospital, Lambeth Palace Road, London SE1 7EH.

Derek M. Yellon
The Hatter Institute, Department of Academic and Clinical Cardiology, University College London Medical School and Hospitals, Grafton Way, London, WC1E 6DB.

Abbreviations.

HSP	Heat shock protein
HSP70	Inducible 70 kDa heat shock protein (also synonymous with 72 kDa HSP; HSP70i; HSP71 or HSP72)
HSC70	Constitutive 70 kDa HSP (also synonymous with HSP73; 73 kDa HSP)
HSP60	60 kDa heat shock protein
HSP27	27 kDa heat shock protein
PKC	Protein kinase C
CPK	Creatine phosphokinase
TTC	Triphenyl tetrazolium chloride
SOD	Superoxide dismutase
SPT	8-sulphophenyl theophylline
2-DOG	2-deoxyglucose
H9c2	Embryonal rat heart derived myoblast cell line
CCPA	2-chlorocyclopentyl-N_6-adenosine
4xPC	Preconditioning with 4x5 minute coronary occlusions separated by10 minute reperfusions
HSF	Heat shock (transcription) factor
SDS-PAGE	Sodium dodecyl sulphate polyacrylamide gel electrophoresis
LVEDP	Left ventricular end diastolic pressure
IL-1	Interleukin 1
TNF	Tumour necrosis factor
NFkB	Nuclear factor kappa B

INTRODUCTION

This area of investigation has evolved from the idea that an adaptive response to stress in the heart could be harnessed in order to delay or prevent the onset of tissue necrosis following a prolonged episode of myocardial ischaemia. The observation by Curries' group that sub-lethal, whole-body heat stress could protect the isolated, Langendorff perfused heart against ischaemia [Currie et al, 1988] initially focussed attention on the heat shock (or stress) proteins (HSPs) and anti-oxidant enzymes such as catalase [Karmazyn et al, 1990] as having a potential prominent role in this form of adaptation. The 70 kDa heat shock protein (HSP70) was then shown to be elevated by brief, intermittent ischaemia and reperfusion of the kind that is likely to cause 'preconditioning' [Knowlton et al, 1991]. Subsequently, the discovery of a delayed, 'second window' of protection 24-72 hours following sublethal ischaemia [Marber et al, 1993; Kuzuya et al, 1993; Baxter et al, 1993] has extended the therapeutic potential of the now well known ischaemic preconditioning phenomenon. In this respect, attention has focussed primarily on the inducible isoform of HSP70, rather than the constitutive HSC70, as having a major protective role, based on the assumption that it is the major inducible stress protein in myocardium. However, more recently other potential mediators of delayed preconditioning such as antioxidant enzymes have received considerable attention.

It is the purpose of this chapter to review the data with regard to the potential role of HSP70 and other HSPs in protection following 'preconditioning', or delayed adaptation to sublethal ischaemia. Despite the now moderate numbers of studies documenting elevation of HSP70 following ischaemia, surprisingly the question of whether HSP70 is directly involved in this phenomenon, or is an epiphenomenon, is still an area of controversy. The persistence of this controversy is largely due to the fact that the majority of studies on HSP70 expression following ischaemia are merely correlative, ie. showing an *association* between HSP70 elevation and the degree of protection. Whilst HSP70 is clearly induced by ischaemia and reperfusion, there is little direct *in vivo* evidence for HSP70 being causative in reducing or delaying the degree of infarction following its induction by ischaemia, or its being involved in the normal tissue response to ischaemic preconditioning. Information regarding a direct protective role for HSP70 comes only from over-expression of HSP70 in transfected cell lines or transgenic mouse models. There are few studies in the heart literature which are designed to determine the mechanisms of HSP70 gene expression and whether these are the same mechanisms as occur during delayed preconditioning. In fact, these types of studies are difficult, if not impossible to carry out *in vivo*.

Delayed ischaemic preconditioning, in common with acute ('classical') preconditioning has now been shown by work from our own laboratory to be both adenosine receptor [Baxter et al, 1994] and protein kinase C (PKC) [Baxter et al, 1995] dependent. Therefore, if these are important pathways leading to adaptation to stress (ischaemia) and the expression of certain classes of genes, it is not unreasonable to assume that evidence should exist that these same pathways lead to HSP expression if HSPs are to have a direct protecive role in precondtioning. So where is this evidence ? Whilst HSPs clearly play an important a role in adaptation following thermal preconditioning, the response to myocardial ischaemia is seemingly very complex in that anti-oxidant genes, immediate-early genes encoding transcriptional regulators,

43

genes for enzymes of intermediary metabolism and angiogenic growth factors and so on, are all transcriptionally activated following ischaemia. It is therefore, likely that not only HSPs, but also many other classes of genes will play an important role in the 'second window'.

HEAT STRESS AND DELAYED ADAPTATION TO ISCHAEMIA

Heat Stress and Myocardial Protection

Currie et al, (1988) demonstrated that hearts from rats which had been given whole-body heat stress at 42°C for 15 minutes, 24 hours prior to removal and perfusion in Langendorff mode, had improved return of contractile function, reduced creatine phosphokinase (CPK) release and less ultrastructural damage following 30 minutes of global ischaemia. These hearts had elevated levels of HSP70 at 24 hours following heat stress, which may have been associated with the protection. This would, then appear to be an example of the well described phenomenon of adaptive thermotolerance. Protection was also associated with elevation of activity of the anti-oxidant enzyme catalase. A subsequent study by Karmazyn et al, (1990) demonstrated that the peak of protection occurred at 48 hours post-heat stress and that catalase activity was elevated from 24 to 96 hours post-heat stress and was maximal at 48 hours. HSP70 elevation also appeared maximal between 24 to 48 hours. We have demonstrated significant preservation of mitochondrial function 24 hours following *in vivo* heat stress in rabbits when hearts were subjected to coronary artery occlusion *in situ* [Yellon et al, 1992]. Currie et al (1993) subsequently demonstrated that whole-body heat stress protected the *in situ* rabbit heart against tissue necrosis following a 30 minute coronary artery occlusion and 3 hour reperfusion at 24 hours but not 40 hours post-heat stress as determined by triphenyltetrazolium chloride (TTC) staining. Again, HSP70 was detected by immuno (Western) blotting at 48 hours post-heat stress. In addition, elevation of HSP70 mRNA was detected by Northern blotting at 1.5 to 3 hours post-heat stress.

Donnelly et al, (1992) showed that hyperthermic pretreatment of rats (42°C; 20 minutes) 24 hours prior to 35 minutes left coronary artery occlusion and 120 minutes reperfusion improved myocardial salvage (TTC staining) compared to controls. This protection was associated with significantly increased levels of HSP70. Following this, Hutter et al, (1994) determined that 24 hours following heat stress the degree of protection against ischaemic injury produced by a 35 minute coronary artery occlusion and 2 hours reperfusion in the rat heart appeared proportional to the severity of the preconditioning heat stress. Again, infarct size was determined by TTC staining and was inversely proportional to the accumulation of HSP70. As one would expect, the degree of HSP70 accumulation was proportional to the severity of the preconditioning heat stress, as presumably, would be other factors such as catalase activity or other HSPs, which were not measured. Marber et al, (1994) demonstrated that whole body heat stress with 24 hours recovery improved functional recovery in isolated ventricular papillary muscles subjected to hypoxic superfusion with pyruvate as substrate. There was no protection when the muscles were superfused with glucose as substrate. The degree of recovery was also proportional to the content of HSP70 in the contralateral papillary muscle from the same hearts. Therefore, whilst these studies are again suggestive of HSP70 (as elevated by heat stress) protecting against ischaemia, the HSP70 expression cannot be causatively or mechanistically linked to protection.

In attempts to develop clinically relevant models to test the protective effects of heat stress, two studies come to mind. Firstly, Lui et al, (1992) used 15 minutes of warm blood cardiolpegia at 42°C in the pig heart on cardiopulmonary bypass in an attempt to improve functional recovery following 2 hours of hypothermic, hyperkalaemic arrest. They found that functional recovery was improved in the heat shock group and this difference reached significance after 60 minutes of normothermic reperfusion. There was also a marginal reduction in CPK release. HSP70 and SOD activity were also increased in the heat shock group-again this was only significant after 60 minutes of reperfusion.

Secondly, in an interesting study by McCully et al, (1996) retrograde hyperthermic perfusion was used for 15 minutes, 5 minutes prior to global ischaemia in the isolated, perfused rat heart. This caused a significantly enhanced dP/dT and peak developed pressure and a reduction in end diastolic pressure follwing 15 minutes of global ischaemia when compared to control normothermically perfused hearts. These authors also demonstrated a 9-fold increase in HSP70 mRNA levels by 30 minutes of normothermic reperfusion and a 1.7-fold increase in HSP70 protein at the same time. Whilst this procedure clearly led to an enhanced functional recovery of the hearts, the protection occurred prior to, or at least co-incident with, the elevation in HSP70 message/protein. Therefore, these authors appear to observe an acute 'preconditioning' type phenomenon which may be due to release of catecholamines or other mediators during hyperthermic perfusion. This protection is, therefore, probably independent of the observed small increase in HSP70, given that other workers have observed that (i) the peak in HSP70 mRNA occurs at 1.5-2 hours post-stress [Knowlton et al, 1991; Currie et al, 1993]; (ii) in cells exposed to heat shock or simulated ischaemia the maximal levels of HSP70 induction reach up to 100-fold [Heads et al, 1994]; (iii) the peak in protection normally associated with HSP elevation occurs 24 to 48 hours post-heat stress [Currie et al, 1988; Karmazyn et al, 1990].

In conclusion, the ability of thermal preconditioning to improve myocardial salvage is a robust phenomenon which is associated with and, at the very least partially dependent upon, expression of 72 kDa heat shock protein in the 24 to 48 hour time frame (see table 1 for a summary of protocols).

Delayed Ischaemic Preconditioning and Myocardial Protection

In its classical form, ischaemic preconditioning is an *acute* protective phenomenon which is charactersied by a short, or series of short, periods of ischaemia (coronary artery occlusion) seperated by brief periods of reperfusion. The myocardium is transiently protected against a subsequent ischaemic episode severe enough to cause infarction in control animals and is characterised by a slower rate of ATP depletion during the subsequent ischaemia and a reduction, or delay in the degree of tissue necrosis [see Murry et al, 1991]. This acute phase of protection has rapid onset (present within 1-2 minutes of reperfusion) and is transient, lasting for between 60 to 120 minutes. It is also dependent on adenosine receptor activation in the rabbit and dog [see

Author	Date	Species	PC Protocol	Recovery	Improved Parameters
Currie et al.	1988	Rat	Whole Body HS 42°C/15 min.	24h	Contractile function, CPK release, Ultrastructure; HSP70(wb);catalase
Yellon et al.	1992	Rabbit	Whole Body HS 42°C/15 min.	24h	Mitochondrial respiration
Donnelly et al.	1992	Rat	Whole Body HS	24h	Infarct size
Lui et al.	1992	Pig	Cardioplegia 1h 42°C		Contractile function, CPK release; HSP70(wb), SOD
Currie et al.	1993	Rabbit	Whole Body HS 42°C/15 min.	24-40h	Infarct size@24h, not 40h; HSP70(wb)
Marber et al.	1993	Rabbit	Whole Body HS 42°C/15 min.	24h	Isolated papillary muscle function (pyruvate not glucose) HSP70 (wb)
Hutter et al.	1994	Rat	Whole Body HS	24h	Infarct size; HSP70 (wb)
McCully et al.	1996	Rat	Retrograde perfusion 42°C/15 min.		Contractile function; End diastolic pressure; HSP70(wb)
Kuzuya et al.	1993	Dog	4x5 min CAO	0-24h	Infarct size@0 and 24 h, not 3 and 12h
Marber et al.	1993	Rabbit	4x5 min CAO 10 min Repn	24h	Infarct size; HSP70 (wb)
Baxter et al.	1994	Rabbit	4x5 min CAO 10 min Repn	24h	Infarct size; ADO-R-dependent
Tanaka et al.	1994	Rabbit	4x5 min CAO 5 min Repn	24h	No change in infarct size; HSP70 (ihc)
Sun et al.	1995	Pig	10x2 min CAO 2 min Repn x 3 days		Systolic wall thickening; HSP 70 (ihc)
Baxter et al.	1996	Rabbit	4x5 min CAO 10 min Repn	24-96h	Infarct size @24-72h; No change in HSP70(wb)

Table 1: Summary of published Heat Shock and Delayed Preconditioning Protocols and their principal findings. Key: HS-Heat shock, CAO-Coronary artery occlusion, Repn-Reperfusion, SOD-Superoxide dismutase, ADO-R-Adenosine receptor, (wb)-Western blot, (ihc)-Immunohistochemistry.

Murry et al, 1991; Walker and Yellon, 1992; Baxter and Yellon, 1994] and has been linked to subsequent activation of protein kinase C (PKC) in the rabbit [Speechley-Dick et al, 1994] and rat heart [Mitchell et al, 1995]. Ischaemic preconditioning has also been shown to lead to a delayed protective adaptation of the myocardium, again characterised by a reduction or delay in the degree of tissue necrosis (infarct size) and therefore, the protection appears to be biphasic. The 'second window of protection', 'delayed' or 'late' preconditioning, as it has been variously termed, is also adenosine receptor dependent [Baxter et al, 1994] and has, at least in some cases, been associated with increased myocardial HSP70 within the risk zone [Marber et al, 1993] and increased activity of the superoxide dismutase enzyme [Yamashita et al, 1994].

Liu et al , (1991) have shown non-selective adenosine receptor antagonists (ie.with mixed A_1 and A_2 effects) to abolish the effects of *acute* preconditioning in the rabbit heart. Selective A_1 receptor agonists have also been shown to be effective as preconditioning agents in limiting infarct size. The *acute* phase of preconditioning also appears to be dependent on G-protein coupling (G_i) since preconditioning is blocked by pre-treatment with pertusis toxin. As described above it has recently been shown by work from our own laboratory that the *delayed* phase of protection is also both adenosine receptor- and PKC-dependent [Baxter et al, 1994; Baxter et al, 1995]. Evidence from several groups indicate that activation of PKC may be a crucial signal transduction event in acute ischaemic preconditioning. However, it is not known at present which target protein(s) are phosphorylated by PKC and therefore, which is the final effector pathway for protective adaptation. One suggested candidate is the ATP-dependent potassium channel (see [Walker and Yellon, 1992] and references within). Both stress protein and anti-oxidant genes may be activated in a PKC-dependent manner during delayed adaptation (see below).

Bolli and colleagues have described a late preconditioning against myocardial stunning, rather than against infarction. Conscious pigs underwent 10x2 minute coronary occlusions separated by 2 minutes reperfusion on 3 consecutive days. Recovery of systolic wall thickening was substantially improved on days 2 and 3 of the protocol. Blockade of adenosine receptors with 8-sulphophenyl theophylline (SPT) did not block the preconditioning against stunning. Therefore, this result appears to differ from the adenosine A_1-receptor-dependent protection against infarction. HSP70 mRNA was reported to be elevated 2 hours following preconditioning and increased immunohistochemical staining of HSP70 in the nucleus was observed. Maximal protection was observed at 24-48 hours after preconditioning, at which time HSP70 was also elevated as determined by Western blotting [Sun et al, 1995]. It would be interesting to determine whether this protocol is also able to protect against infarction in the pig heart. However, again HSP70 elevation is *associated* with protection 24-48 hours after brief, repetitive ischaemia (see table 1 for a summary of protocols).

An important goal has been to establish cell-based models for both acute and delayed preconditioning. In such systems it may be possible to more closely dissect the mechanisms of preconditioning at the levels of the signal transduction events and end-effector molecules. Several recent studies have described a preconditioning-like phenomenon in isolated primary cardiomyocytes. For instance, Ikonomidis et al, (1994) recently described acute preconditioning of a population of cells derived and cultured from adult human ventricular myocytes with low volume anoxia. Decreased trypan blue uptake; fall in intracellular pH and lactate dehydrogenase release were observed.

However, the phenotype of these cells is such that they are substantially de-differentiated, despite expressing some myocyte-specific markers (Li et al, 1996). In another study Armstrong *et al*, (1994) described acute preconditioning of adult rabbit ventricular myocytes with a combination of hypotonic buffer followed by ischaemic pelletting of the cells. The observed acute protection appeared to be both adenosine and PKC-dependent. Yamashita *et al*, (1994) have described *delayed* preconditioning 24 hours after hypoxic treatment of neonatal rat ventricular cardiocytes which was associated with elevation of Mn-SOD mRNA and activity. Interestingly and perhaps, importantly, we have also been able to induce delayed preconditioning, not only in neonatal cardiocytes, but also in the embryonal rat heart-derived cell line H9c2 following differentiation into myotubes by low serum (R.J. Heads, unpublished data). This seems to be consistent with an idea that ischaemic tolerance can be induced in terminally differentiated but not dividing cells put forward by Osborne et al (1994). They described the development of ischaemic tolerance in rat small intestinal mucosa which appeared to be due to adaptational changes in the differentiated lamina propria, but not the rapidly dividing epithelium. Molecular adaptation of vascular endothelial cells to oxidative stress has also been described, which involved elevation of both HSP70 and various anti-oxidant enzymes (see Lu et al, 1993). It will be interesting to determine to what extent these effects are related to delayed preconditioning rather than another form of adaptation and whether delayed preconditioning is itself muscle cell specific.

We have developed a delayed preconditioning model in neonatal rat cardiocytes in which they can be preconditioned with simulated ischaemia consisiting of treatment with the glycolytic inhibitor 2-deoxyglucose (2-DOG) and lactate, pH6.5. 24 hours later, the cells are resistant to a more severe form of simulated ischaemia consisting of 2-DOG, lactate, KCl and an oxygen scavenger (dithionite). Interestingly, preliminary data suggests that this form of delayed preconditioning can be inhibited by both a PKC inhibitor and by an adensoine A_1 receptor antagonist and so appears to be consistent with the mechanisms of *in vivo* delayed preconditioning (Cumming et al, 1996 and R.J. Heads unpublished results).

HSP70 Expression During Delayed Preconditioning

Coronary artery occlusions have been reported to result in rapid transcription of the HSP70 gene and transient accumulation of HSP70 mRNA [Knowlton et al, 1991]. It has also recently been shown that induction of HSP70, HSP27, c-*myc*, *jun*-B and ubiquitin occur at the mRNA level following brief ischaemia [Das et al, 1993]. The changes in hsp 70 may be due to both changes in the stability of HSP70 mRNA as well as an increase in transcriptional activity. In the study of Knowlton et al, (1991) accumulation of HSP70 protein following ischaemia was detectable at 2 hours and was maximal at approximately 24-48 hours and therefore, this time-course seems to be similar to that observed following *in vivo* heat shock (see above).

The degree of the infarct-size-limiting effect observed in myocardium [Marber et al, 1994; Currie and Tanguay, 1991] or cytoprotection in myogenic cells [Heads et al, 1995 (1); Mestril et al, 1994] following mild heat stress correlates approximately with levels of induced HSP70. Although the *acute* phase of preconditioning has been

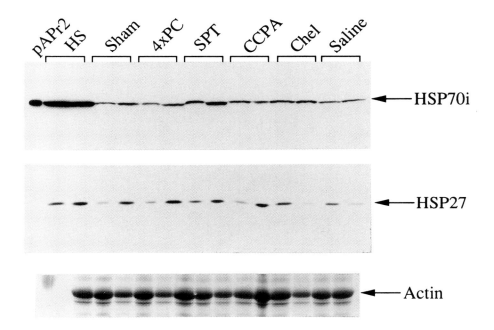

Figure 1a. HSP70 and HSP27 were analysed by SDS-PAGE and Western blotting. An approximately 2.5-fold elevation of HSP70i was apparent 24 hours following heat stress (HS) but no elevation ws observed following 4xPC or treatment with the A_1-specific adenosine receptor agonist 2-chlorocyclopentyl-N^6-adeosine (CCPA)[see 1b below]. No overall change in HSP27 levels were observed on one dimensional gels. pAPr2: Neuronal cells stably transfected with HSP70. Figure taken from Heads et al, (1995(3)).

shown to limit infarct size, this does not appear to correlate with changes in HSP70 [Heads et al, 1995 (2)]. However, the re-appearance of protection 24 hours following brief coronary artery occlusion has been reported in some cases to be associated with both elevation of HSP70 [Marber et al, 1993] and increased anti-oxidant enzyme activity [Yamashita et al, 1994]. Elevation of HSP70 has also been observed in two other studies following brief myocardial ischaemia, but in the absence of any induced protection [Donnelly et al, 1992; Tanaka et al, 1994]. The lack of protection in these

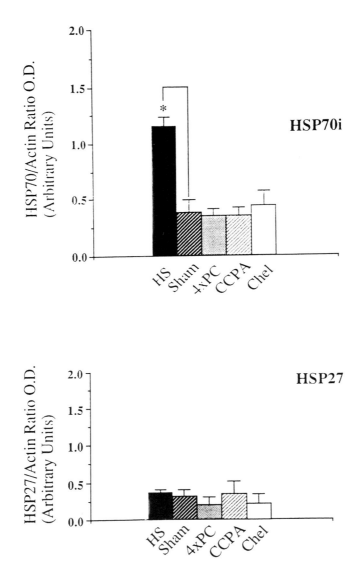

Figure 1b .HSP70 and HSP27 were analysed by densitometry. An approximately 2.5-fold elevation of HSP70i was apparent 24 hours following heat stress (HS) but no elevation was observed following 4xPC or treatment with the A_1-specific adenosine receptor agonist 2-chlorocyclopentyl-N6-adeosine (CCPA). No overall change in HSP27 levels were observed on one dimensional gels. pAPr2: Neuronal cells stably transfected with HSP70. Figure taken from Heads et al, (1995(3)).

studies was attributed by the authors to levels of induced HSP70 being below a hypothetical 'threshold' for protection.

HSP70 mRNA and/or protein expression following four, five-minute coronary occlusions separated by ten minute reperfusions (4xPC) has been demonstrated in a number of studies [Knowlton et al, 1991; Marber et al, 1993; Das et al, 1993]. We are currently analysing stress protein and anti-oxidant mRNA and protein expression 24 hours following 4xPC with and without SPT and the PKC inhibitor chelerythrine and following pre-treatment with the adenosine A_1 receptor specific agonist 2-chlorocyclopentyl-N_6-adenosine (CCPA). Baxter et al, (1994; 1995) have described an infarct-limiting effect following both 4xPC and CCPA pre-treatments in this model which was inhibited by both SPT and chelerythrine. Again, we have found that adenosine receptor-dependent protection appears to occur in the absence of HSP70 elevation (see figure 1) in contrast to the results of Knowlton et al, (1991) and our earlier study (Marber et al, 1993).

In the present study, the sham-operated hearts had a relatively high basal level of HSP70 which was not further modulated by any treatment, at least as determined by Western blotting compared to approximately four-fold induction by heat shock. However, the sensitivity of current methods is such that, for instance, a change of 20% would be at the limit of detection. Also, the physiological relevance of changes of less than one- to two-fold would be questionable. In the study of Marber et al, 1993 the sham operated hearts appeared to have only very low levels of HSP70. The reason for this difference in basal HSP70 levels between the two studies is not known, but may be due to one or a combination of the following: (i) that a silk ligature was placed under the artery in the sham-operated rabbits in the present study (but not occluded), leading to a difference in the level of surgically-induced stress to the myocardium (in the study of Knowlton et al, 1991 the authors reported that sham-operated controls were performed both with and without placing the silk ligature in the myocardium. Although they state that no difference in HSP70 mRNA levels between the two was observed, the Northern blots show that some of the sham-operated hearts expressed levels of HSP70 mRNA only slightly lower than that observed following occlusion); (ii) it is possible that the stress of recovery of the animals over a 24 hour period, albeit with antibiotic and analgesic cover, leads to appreciable expression of myocardial HSP70; (iii) it was apparent that naive (non-sham operated) rabbits from the same batch also had relatively high basal levels of HSP70 (R.J. Heads, unpublished observation), therefore, it is likely that a genuine shift in the baseline occurred in the rabbits supplied prior to any experimentation. Never-the-less, despite relatively high basal levels of HSP70 observed in the sham operated animals, protection (ie. infarct size limitation) was not observed in these hearts. Therefore, preconditioning would have to induce some other, subsequent effect such as translocation of the HSP70 in order to elicit protection.

Since the optimal protection following 4xPC is seen at 48-72 hours and not 24 hours, we have also analysed data with respect to the expression of HSP70 mRNA and protein at time points other than at 24 hours following 4xPC. The time-course of HSP70 protein expression at 24, 48, 72 and 96 hours following 4xPC has been determined and again appears to show no difference in HSP70 levels (G.F. Baxter, submitted). We found that HSP70 mRNA was elevated only inconsistently two hours following 4xPC compared to strong induction by heat stress or bacterial endotoxin pretreatment. Again HSP70 mRNA was not induced by CCPA pretreatment (see figure 2). However, we

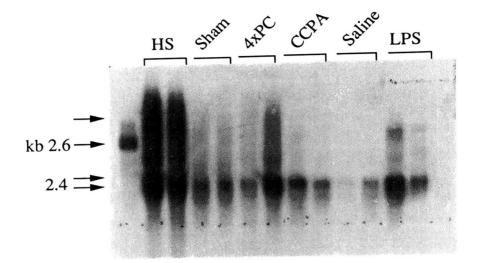

Figure 2. HSP70 mRNAs were analysed by Northern blotting 90 minutes after treatment with heat stress (HS), 4xPC, CCPA, saline or bacterial lipopolysaccharide (LPS). Strong induction of two inducible mRNAs (2.4/2.6 kb) was observed following HS as well as induction of constutive HSP70 mRNAs (2.2/2.3 kb). HSP70 mRNAs were also induced, although inconsistently, by 4xPC. Induction by LPS occurred to a lesser extent than HS (R.J. Heads, G.F. Baxter and D.M. Yellon, unpublished observations).

have also demonstrated that elevation of both Mn- and Cu/Zn-superoxide dismutase (SOD) activities were observed 24 hours after 4xPC (R.J. Heads, unpublished observation) indicating a possible role for these antioxidants in delayed protection.

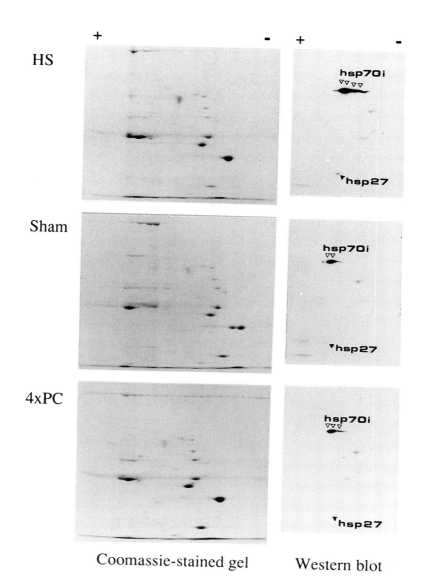

Coomassie-stained gel   Western blot

Figure 3.HSP70 and HSP27 were analysed by 2D-PAGE and Western blotting. In sham-operated hearts there were two major isoforms of HSP70i expressed constitutively. 24 hours following heat stress both the levels and heterogeneity of HSP70i was increased, constituted by a shift to more basic isoforms. A similar but much smaller shift was observed in some samples following 4xPC. Two isoforms of HSP27 were oberved in sham hearts, which increased in amount following heat stress but not 4xPC. This data has appeared in Heads et al, (1995(3)).

Knowlton et al, (1991) observed that the induction of HSP70 following 4xPC appeared to involve a shift in the isoform pattern to a more basic pI as determined by two-dimensional isoelectric focussing/SDS-PAGE. However, they did not quantitate the level of HSP70 induction in this study and only a comparison with normal left ventricle tissue was shown. Since a sham-operated control taken after 24 hours recovery was not shown for comparison, it is possible that the stress associated with the recovery process could have contributed to the induction of HSP70 in these animals. Notwithstanding this, we surmised that whilst we were not able to observe any overall increase in HSP70 compared to shams at 24 hours as determined by one-dimensional Western blots, there may be a change in the isoform distribution following preconditioning. Therefore, we ran two-dimensional gels of various pre-treatments. As can be seen from figure 3 control hearts expressed two HSP70 isoforms as detected by a specific monoclonal antibody recognising inducible HSP70. These two isoforms were induced by both heat stress and bacterial endotoxin pre-treatment 24 hours previously by approximately the same extent. In addition, heat stress induced a third isoform. Preconditioning did not induce the two control isoforms to higher level nor did it strongly induce the third isoform, although in some 4xPC samples there was a slight shift of the HSP70 to a more basic position. This latter data appears to confirm our data from one dimensional blots that, in our hands, there is no consistent gross induction of HSP70 by 4xPC. The changes that were detected were very subtle.

Since we found that control surgical sham hearts after 24 hours expressed detectable levels of HSP70 we thought it necessary to determined whether the protective interventions ie. 4xPC and CCPA pre-treatment were able to induce translocation of HSP70 to different subcellular compartments where it may exert some protective effect. A crude subcellular fractionation based on differential centrifugation revealed that both heat stress and 4xPC appeared to cause a redistribution of HSP70 from the soluble fraction (cytosol) to the low speed (cytoskeleton/nuclear) fraction and also to the high speed (membrane) fraction (see figure 4). CCPA also appeared to cause a similar redistribution. Therefore, the protective interventions appear to involve a translocation of HSP70 which may indicate that post-translational mechanisms involved in the regulation of HSP70, where it is already expressed, are important in the protection afforded by delayed preconditioning.

Therefore, the involvement of HSP70 in protection is a two-step process: (i) induction of HSP70 expression at the transcriptional level and (ii) translocation to a functional compartment. If, as in our study, HSP70 is already expressed at relatively high levels prior to preconditioning, the preconditioning stimulus only needs to cause the translocation in order to elicit the protection. It is also worth bearing in mind that high basal expression of HSP70 may exert a negative feed back effect on further expression, therefore, one would not necessarily expect further expression unless basal levels were low initially. However, the post translational events leading to translocation are essential for protection in both scenarios.

54

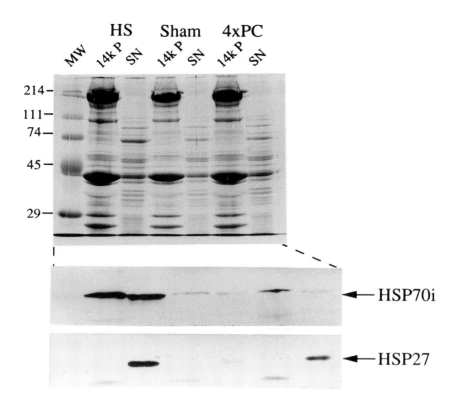

Figure 4. Analysis of the compartmentalisation of HSP70 and HSP27 into cytoskeletal/myofibrillar and membrane/cytosolic fractions by differential centrifugation, SDS-PAGE and Western blotting. Following heat stress (HS) an increase in HSP70 was apparent in both low speed cytoskeletal fractions (14 kP-this fraction also contains nuclei) and the membrane-associated cytoskeletal and soluble fraction (SN), indicating translocation of newly synthesised HSP70 to the cytoskeletal/myofirillar and/or nuclear compartments. A small increase in HSP70 in this fraction was also observed following 4xPC, although this appeared to involve a redistribution rather than net synthesis. An increase in HSP27 was observed following HS and although not apparent from this figure, involves a shift from the membrane-associated fraction to the soluble fraction. A similar shift was observed following 4xPC. This data has appeared in Heads et al, (1995(3)).

IS HSP70 A PROTECTIVE PROTEIN DURING ISCHAEMIA ?

To determine the ability of HSP70 to protect cells against heat stress or simulated ischaemia, we and others have transfected the clonal rat myogenic cell line H9c2 [Heads et al, 1995 (1); Mestril et al, 1994] or mouse 10T1/2 cells [Williams et al, 1993] with a cDNA encoding human HSP70. Cells expressing high levels of HSP70 relative to cells transfected with the control vector (containing no HSP70 but expressing only the antibiotic resistance marker) were significantly protected against both lethal heat stress and simulated ischaemia. This demonstrates that although the *in vivo* response to stress is very complex, resulting in the elevated expression of several genes, a single stress-related gene product can protect cells against more than one stress, including simulated ischaemia when expressed at high levels. This indicates that HSP70 may play a role in protection of myocytes against ischaemia and that the ability of HSP70 to protect against more than one stress is consistent with the idea of cross-tolerance.

The use of cultured neonatal rat primary cardiac myocytes for similar studies comparing the cytoprotective potential of the same HSP70 construct in transient transfection experiments yielded the same protection against heat stress and simulated ischaemia as that described above for H9c2 cells [Cumming et al, 1996]. The H9c2 cells express a predominantly skeletal myoblast phenotype, therefore it was important to repeat this experiment in cardiac cells. However, the H9c2 cells do appear to be a suitable cell line for screening the function of these HSPs. This is probably due to the highly conserved nature of stress protein function in different cell types, rather than the phenotypic nature of H9 cells being truely representative of cardiocytes. In addition, the H9c2 cells have the advantage of being clonal and therefore, stably transfected cell lines can be established, something which cannot be achieved in primary cells at present.

Nakano et al, (1996) have used an antisense oligonucleotide approach to determine the role of HSP70 in protection within the physiological range of its endogenous expression in response to mild (8 hours) or severe (12 hours) hypoxia in isolated adult feline cardiocytes. Cells transfected with antisense cDNAs to HSP70 showed a 40% decrease in HSP70 levels and increased susceptibility to hypoxic injury. These results appear to indicate a physiological role for HSP70 in protection against hypoxic injury. This is an important example of the type of approach needed to determine specifically the role of HSP70 within the physiological context of delayed preconditioning.

An important experimental goal is to specifically determine the involvement of HSP70 in ischaemic tolerance *in vivo*. In the last year there have been three separate reports of transgenic mouse models which over-express HSP70 and these have been used to test the ability of HSP70 to protect the heart against ischaemia *in vivo* [Plumier et al, 1995; Radford et al, 1994; Marber et al, 1995]. These studies have all used a similar strategy to introduce copies of either human or rat HSP70 genes into the mouse genome. In the study of Marber *et al*, (1995), transgenic mice were generated using a chimaeric transgene consisting of a rat inducible HSP70 (rHSP70-[Mestril et al, 1994]) inserted into the vector pCAGGS. This placed the rHSP70 gene under the control of the cytomegalovirus immediate-early enhancer (hCMV-IE) and chicken β-actin promoter. The chimaeric transgene was then excised from the vector and injected into the male pro-nuclei of fertilised eggs from hyper-ovulated B6xSJL mice. The injected eggs were

A: Hsp 60

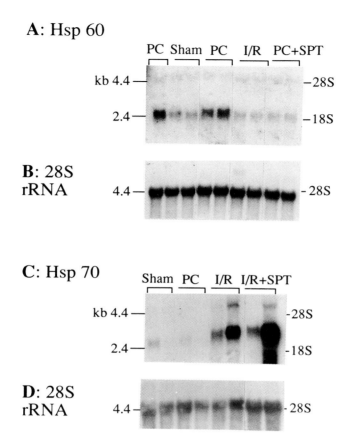

B: 28S
rRNA

C: Hsp 70

D: 28S
rRNA

Figure 5. Northern blotting of left ventricle ischaemic zone samples from two representative hearts each from: sham-operated (sham); preconditioned hearts [5 minutes ischaemia+10 minutes reperfusion (PC)]; hearts subjected to PC+30 mins ischaemia+2 hours reperfusion (I/R) and following treatment with the non-selective adenosine recptor antagonist 8-sulphophenyl theophyline (SPT:7.5 mg kg⁻¹). Northern blots were probed for HSP60 and HSP70 mRNAs. Panel (A): sham-operated (Sham); Preconditioning [5 minutes ischaemia+10 minutes reperfusion (PC)]; PC+30 mins ischaemia+2 hours reperfusion (I/R); SPT treatment followed by preconditioning (PC+SPT). Panel (C): groups were as for panel (A), except that SPT treatment followed by PC+I+R is shown (I/R+SPT). Blots were probed for: (A): hsp60 transcripts; (C): hsp70 transcripts; (B) and (D): 28S rRNA as a comparison for total RNA loading. Filters were sequentially stripped and re-probed in that order. The position of RNA size markers are shown on the left for comparison and positions of 28S and 18S rRNA on the right. Hsp60 probe (λ22a) hybridised to a single band at approximately 2.4 kb. Hsp70 probe (DP8) hybridised to bands at approximately 2.4 and 2.6 kb. Figure taken from reference [Heads et al, 1995(2)].

then implanted into pseudo-pregnant CD1 mice. Genomic DNA from tail clips from three week old mice were then analysed by Southern blotting with a probe specific for the chimaeric transgene to detect the presence of the transgene.

Transgene-positive heterozygous mice showed a high level of HSP70 expression in the un-stressed condition compared to transgene-negative mice, without apparent detriment. Hearts from the transgene positive and negative mice were subjected to 20 minutes of zero-flow ischaemia at 37°C followed by 120 minutes of reperfusion in Langendorff mode. The transgene-positive hearts showed a 40% reduction in infarct size, as determined by TTC staining; a doubling of contractile recovery and a 50% decrease in CPK release. There was no difference in endogenous catalase activity between transgene positive and transgene-negative mice. Similar positive results were obtained in the studies of Plumier *et al*, (1995) and Radford *et al*, (1994). In the latter study, metabolic determinants such as ATP/P_i and PCr/P_i ratios were improved as determined by phosphorous-31 nuclear magnetic resonance spectroscopy, despite only a modest elevation in HSP70 levels.

Together, these important studies represent a direct demonstration of the ability of HSP70, elevated in unstressed hearts, to protect the isolated heart against ischaemia/reperfusion damage in the absence of other contemporaneous factors and confirm the results obtained by transfection of isolated/cultured cells with the HSP70 gene.

MECHANISMS OF HSP70 INDUCTION: DOES HSP70 EXPRESSION CORRELATE WITH ADENOSINE RECEPTOR OR PROTEIN KINASE C ACTIVATION ?

In order to establish a role for HSP70 in delayed preconditioning it is important to determine which mechanisms are involved in the expression of HSP70 during ischaemia and reperfusion and whether these correspond to those pathways activated by preconditioning. We examined changes in HSP gene expression during a typical *acute* preconditioning protocol using Northern blotting to determine changes in HSP mRNA. This showed that mRNA for HSP60 was induced within 15 mins of a 5 min coronary occlusion. However, HSP70 mRNA had a different pattern of expression since it was only induced during the 30 min ischaemic episode and two-hour reperfusion that succeeded the preconditioning (see figure 5). Therefore, HSP expression is not co-ordinately regulated in response to ischaemia. The increase in HSP70 mRNA involved the induction of a new transcript (2.6 kb) which accumulated to high levels during reperfusion [Heads et al, 1995 (2)] similar to an inducible transcript described by others [Currie et al, 1991; Mestril et al, 1994].

Since *acute* preconditioning is dependent on adenosine receptor activation [Lui et al, 1991] and we have also recently demonstrated the dependence of the delayed phase of preconditioning on adenosine receptor activation [Baxter et al, 1994], to conclude a role for HSP70 in acute or delayed preconditioning it is, therefore, important to determine whether HSP mRNA expression could be modulated by adenosine receptor activation during ischaemia. Administration of the adenosine receptor antagonist SPT, 5 mins prior to coronary artery occlusion, abolished the elevation of HSP60 mRNA seen after the 5 min occlusion and a following 10 min reperfusion (PC), but had no effect on

HSP70 mRNA expression either after PC or following a subsequent 30 min occlusion and two hours reperfusion. Substitution of preconditioning with the selective adenosine A_1 receptor agonist, CCPA, had no appreciable effect on either HSP60 or HSP70 mRNA expression after 15 mins ([Heads et al, 1995 (2)] and see figure 5). Adenosine receptor modulation therefore, appeared to regulate HSP60 mRNA expression, but not HSP70 mRNA. The differential effect of SPT and CCPA on HSP60 expression may indicate involvement of the A_2 or A_3-receptor subtypes, which are not activated by CCPA due to its specificity for the A_1-receptor. Strong activation of HSP70 gene expression only appears to occur during more prolonged ischaemia and particularly reperfusion, indicating that multiple, parallel responses may occur during adaptation and that reperfusion may play an important role in HSP70 induction. HSP70 mRNA expression did not appear to be directly due to adenosine receptor activation and therefore may occur in parallel to adenosine-dependent preconditioning rather than being directly downstream of it. These data also suggest that the thresholds for preconditioning and HSP70 expression may be different.

In addition to the above studies, we and others have established that similar differences in HSP60 and HSP70 expression occur in cardiac myocytes or myogenic cells following exposure to various metabolic inhibitors, free-radical generating agents and hypoxia. Using combinations of these agents to simulate ischaemia and reperfusion injury it may be possible to model the different phases of ischaemia and reperfusion and therefore to deduce which factors are involved in the initiation and maintainence of the preconditioning/adaptation response and may be important for determining the nature and sites of the metabolic lesions which lead to HSP expression during adaptation.

Benjamin et al, (1990) demonstrated that whilst hypoxic treatment of mouse myogenic cells leads to activation of heat shock transcription factor (HSF) which is temporally related to HSP70 gene promoter activity and transcription, this occurs after a delay of approximately two hours, in contrast to the rapid activation seen following heat stress. Iwaki et al, (1993) found that DNA binding of HSF was observed between two to four hours of continuous hypoxia in primary neonatal rat cardiocytes. However, in this case, HSP70 mRNA accumulation was observed prior to this, indicating that HSF-independent mechanisms of HSP70 promoter activation may occur following hypoxia. These two studies indicate that complex regulation of HSP70 gene expression may occur under different circumstances and that other regulatory factors acting on elements within the HSP70 promoter distinct from the heat shock element (HSE), such as those described during growth, differentiation and development, may be involved (see Welch, 1990).

It has been proposed that the fall in $[ATP]_i$ may be a trigger for HSP70 synthesis following oxidative/metabolic stress. Iwaki et al, (1993) demonstrated that HSP70 was induced by both hypoxia/re-oxygenation and metabolic stress (2-deoxyglucose and sodium cyanide). However, in the case of hypoxia but not metabolic stress, the HSP70 elevation *preceded* the fall in intracellular ATP. In a similar study, Benjamin et al, (1992) showed that HSP70 was induced by glucose deprivation and treatment with the mitochondrial inhibitor rotenone, conditions of metabolic stress which incurred severe intracellular acidosis and ATP-depletion.

In our preconditioning model described above in primary neonatal rat cardiocytes, the preconditioning simulated ischaemia (2-DOG; lactate, pH6.8) was

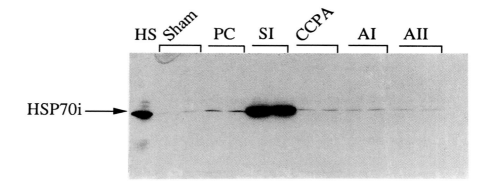

Figure 6. SDS-PAGE and Western blotting of samples from cultured neonatal rat cardiocytes 24 hours following pre-treatment with mild (preconditioning) simulated ischaemia (2-deoxyglucose, lactate, pH 6.8: PC); simulated ischaemia (2-deoxyglucose; lactate; KCl; dithionite; pH 6.8:SI); the adenosine A_1 receptor agonist 2-chlorocyclopentyl-N^6-adenosine (CCPA) or angiotensins I (AI) and II (AII). Slight induction of HSP70 was observed following PC and strong induction following SI. The PC pre-treatment was able to precondition the cells against CPK release and cell viability in an adenosine A_1 and PKC-dependent manner (see text). CCPA caused no induction of HSP70. Lane one contains protein from heat stressed rabbit heart for comparison (A. Punn, unpublished observations).

associated with only a very slight HSP70 elevation (approx.2-3-fold) as compared to an approximately 100-fold elevation by heat stress or a more severe simulated ischaemia (2-DOG; lactate; KCl; dithionite). However, a modest decrease in pH from 6.8 to 6.5 or 6.3 produced a marked increase in HSP70 expression (A. Punn, unpublished). These data also suggest that glycolytic inhibition and high (extracellular) lactate alone are insufficient to induce HSP70. It is apparent that a potent stimulus for HSP70 induction may be inhibition (uncoupling) of mitochondrial respiration and/or free radical generation, which may explain the pH effect on HSP70 expression. These of course, could have a significant reperfusion/reoxia-dependent component, as suggested above. In addition 5 μM CCPA did not elevate HSP70 (see figure 6). Therefore, in keeping with our *in vivo* data, we were again able to demonstrate a PKC and adenosine-dependent preconditioning effect in the absence of significant HSP70i elevation under conditions of mild metabolic inhibition.

HSP70 mRNA induction has been observed following the oxidative stress induced by xanthine/xanthine oxidase in rat myocardium [Kukreja et al, 1994]. This may indicate that there is a significant reperfusion-dependent component to HSP70 mRNA induction, as suggested above. This would also support the observation that HSP70 mRNA does not appear to be induced directly by adenosine receptor activation, but accumulates to high levels during reperfusion.

HSP70 mRNA induction has been observed in rat myocardium concomitantly with c-*myc* and c-*fos* mRNA expression following systemic treatment with phenylephrine and vasopressin or in rat aorta following angiotensin II (AII) treatment [Moalic et al, 1989]. This suggests that α1, vasopressin or AII receptor-dependent expression of HSP70 may occur in myocardium. Interestingly, these receptors are coupled to the phosphoinositide pathway and PKC. However, induction of HSP70 following AII treatment appears to be secondary to arterial hypertension. This observation is, none-the-less, intriguing considering that these substances may be released in relatively large quantities during myocardial ischaemia and it is possible that such a neurohumoral axis, at least in part, may contribute to the elevation of stress proteins. In isolated neonatal rat cardiocytes we have found no direct activation of HSP70i expression following petreatment with AI or AII (see figure 6). It has also been suggested that c-*myc* may itself regulate HSP70 expression as does AP-1 (*fos/jun*) [Morimoto and Milarski, 1990]. This may highlight possible involvement in delayed preconditioning of receptors other than the adenosine receptor, particularly in HSP70 elevation. Therefore, adenosine receptor activation may mediate effects contributing to delayed preconditioning of the myocardium which are, never-the-less, separate from HSP70 elevation.

In a study designed to shed light on the mechanisms of HSP70 elevation, Knowlton et al, (1991(2)) showed that brief myocardial stretch strongly induced HSP70 mRNA expression. The presence of an intraventricular balloon inflated to give a left ventricular end diastolic pressure (LVEDP) of 10 mmHg was sufficient to cause a 3-fold elevation of HSP70 mRNA within 30 minutes and 7-fold within 2 to 4 hours. Also, a single myocardial stretch induced by a 7 second aortic cross-clamp *in situ* or initial ballon inflation caused rapid induction of HSP70 message. Interestingly, isovolumic hearts with an LVEDP of 10 mmHg subjected to global ischaemia for varying times up to 2 hours showed no additional HSP70 mRNA induction, indicating that it was probably already maximal. It is therefore, possible that the dyskinesis, reduced systolic shortening and increased diastolic segment length which occur during ischaemia may contribute to the rapid expression of HSP70 mRNA after coronary occlusion.

As described above, delayed preconditioning has been shown to be PKC-dependent, since the infarct limitation seen 24 hours following 4xPC is abolished by chelerythrine. Since this is an important mechanism in preconditioning, it follows that HSP70 expression may also be PKC-dependent if it is directly related to the preconditioning mechanism. In the study of Knowlton et al (1991(2)) described above, the PKC inhibitor H7 was unable to block the stretch-induced elevation in HSP70 mRNA. In our own study, since we were unable to demonstrate elevation of HSP70 protein 24 hours following 4xPC or CCPA pretreatment, we were unable to demonstrate any effect of chelerythrine on HSP70 protein expression (see figure 1). In addition, chelerythrine did not appear to block the translocation of HSP70 to the low speed cytoskeletal and membrane fractions following 4xPC.

However, following heat shock, we have been able to show that the highly selective PKC inhibitor Ro31, 8220 is able to block both HSP70 and HP60 induction by approximately 50% following heat shock in H9c2 myogenic cells. Therefore, PKC appears to play some role in regulating HSP70 expression under certain conditions. However, the role of PKC in regulating HSP70 expression following ischaemia requires further clarification. The HSP70 gene promoter contains a phorbol ester responsive element (ie, activated via PKC) [Morimoto and Milarski, 1990] and it is likely that there may be some interaction between this element and the HSE under certain conditions (such as heat shock). We have also shown using the fluorescent PKC probe FIM-1 that PKC is activated by heat stress in H9 cells (R.J. Heads, unpublished observations). However, it is possible that the HSP70 gene is activated via a mechanism not involving binding of HSF to the HSE as suggested above for HSP70 activation following hypoxia [Benjamin et al, 1990], or that individual components of ischaemia and reperfusion activate different elements within the HSP70 promoter.

As mentioned above, α1-adrenergic mechanisms have been implicated in the expression of HSP70 under certain conditions [Moalic et al, 1989]. Banerjee and co-workers [Mitchell et al, 1995] have determined that α1 stimulation may be an important mechanism involved in acute preconditioning in the isolated rat heart against the mechanical dysfunction induced by global ischaemia and reperfusion. α1-receptors are coupled to PKC via phopspholipase C which releases the PKC activator-second messenger diacylglycerol (DAG) from membrane phospholipid. Transient ischaemia, the α1 agonist phenylephrine and a DAG analogue were all able to induce functional preconditioning. These were in turn blocked by the non-selective PKC antagonist staurosporine at a dose which did not have a negative inotropic effect or affect left ventricular developed pressure. These experiments when repeated with the selective PKC antagonist chelerythrine gave similar results.

Indirect immunofluorescence microscopy using antibodies directed against different PKC isoforms demonstrated that the Ca^{++}-independent (novel) nPKC isoforms PKCδ and ϵ were translocated with transient ischaemia. PKCδ translocated to the sarcolemma, whereas PKCϵ translocated to the nucleus. However, direct α1 stimulation did not translocate PKCδ to the nucleus, but caused sporadic translocation of another nPKC isoform, PKCζ to myocyte nuclei [Mitchell et al, 1995]. This translocation of different PKC isoforms to sarcolemma and nuclei of cardiomyocytes could mediate different aspects of acute and delayed preconditioning, respectively. Nuclear translocation could be involved in certain gene activation pathways. This is an interesting area which has yet to be investigated, particularly with respect to stress protein (in particular HSP70) expression.

A delayed form of preconditioning has been reported in several studies following activation of pro-inflammatory pathways *in vivo* by cytokines such as interleukin-1 (IL-1) [Maulik et al, 1993] and by bacterial endotoxin [Brown et al, 1989, Baxter et al, 1996]. Heat shock is also known to stimulte the release of arachidonic acid metabolites such as prostaglandins and leukotrienes in mammalian cells [Calderwood et al, 1989] and prostaglandins have been shown to induce HSP [Santoro et al, 1989]. Whilst these treatments and also tumour necrosis factor alpha (TNFα)] increase the activity of antioxidants such as catalase [Brown et al, 1989], they also may lead to HSP70 expression and phosphorylation of HSP27 [see Heads et al, (1996) for review]. Therefore, activation of these mediators *in vivo*, possibly following myocardial

62

ischaemia, could contribute to the preconditioning effect and/or the induction of HSP70.

We and others have shown pharmacological induction of HSP70 following treatment of cardiocytes [Morris et al, 1996] or non-cardiac cells [Hedge et al, 1995] with the benzoquinone ansamycin antibiotic herbimycin. This agent was also reported to induce a preconditioned state against lethal heat stress or simulated ischaemia 24 hours following treatment [Morris et al, 1996]. Although herbimycin has been reported to inhibit the tyrosine kinase activity of pp-60^{v-src}, another tyrosine kinase inhibitor, genistein had no protective effect nor any induction of HSP70. The mechanism of HSP70 induction and protection was, therefore, apparently not due to tyrosine kinase inhibition, directly. Since benzoquinones are strong reducing agents, they could potentially induce some intracellular stress by reducing disulphide bridges in proteins. In fact, this has been reported as being one mechanism by which herbimycin may inactivate the transcription factor NFκB and modify tyrosine kinases. Interestingly, sodium salicylate potentiates the stress response by increasing HSF binding to DNA and also inhibits NFκB activity [see Morris et al, (1996) and references within]. In the paper by Welch and co-workers [Hedge et al, 1995], there does appear to be some stress to the cells following herbimycin pretreatment as determined by the level of protein denaturation, although this was mild compared to heat stress. Therefore, whilst a pharmacologocal route to the elevation of HSP70 is an important and desirable goal, only dissection of the signal transduction pathways involved will lead to the discovery of specific agents which work in the absence of 'stress'.

5) EVIDENCE FOR THE INVOLVEMENT OF OTHER HSPS IN PRECONDITIONING

As discussed above, other genes such as HSP27, c-*myc* and *jun*-B are induced by ischaemia in the myocardium and could have a potential role in delayed preconditioning. We have also found that HSP60 mRNA expression is rapidly induced following a single, 5 minute coronary occlusion in the rabbit heart in a partially adenosine receptor dependent fashion. This is an intriguing result considering that HSP60 is located within the mitochondrial matrix and may protect against mitochondrial protein denaturation. The mitochondrion may be an important site of early ischaemia/reperfusion lesions and, as also suggested above, perturbations in mitochondrial function may play a role in the induction of stress proteins at the transcriptional level.

In an extension of the transfection approach to determine the cytoprotective potential of individual stress proteins, cells were transfected with HSP constructs other than HSP70. Transfected cell lines (H9c2) over-expressing HSP90 showed enhanced survival against lethal heat stress but no increased survival against simulated ischaemia. In contrast, transfected HSP60 was unable to protect against either heat stress or simulated ischaemia [Heads et al, 1995(1)]. This indicates possible functional differences between different stress proteins in their ability to protect against diverse stresses. However, there are possible explanations as to the inability of HSP60 to protect in the experiment described above. These are that the H9c2 cell line has fewer mitochondria than cardiac myocytes and therefore, some of the over-expressed HSP60 may not reach a functional intracellular compartment. The counter argument to this is that endogenous HSP60 is upregulated to relatively high levels following heat stress in H9c2 cells and therefore, presumably represents a functional response. An alternative explanation is that HSP60 functions *in vivo* in co-operation with other factors, including mHSP70 and the 10 kDa chaperonin (cpn10) and that the endogenous expression of these may be too low in the absence of a preconditioning stress to confer function to the additional transfected HSP60. An intriguing experiment would be to co-express HSP60 with cpn10, for instance. Similar results were also obtained using cultured neonatal rat primary cardiac myocytes [Cumming et al, 1996].

In an interesting and important experiment by Martin *et al*, (1995), replication-deficient adenoviral vectors were used to transfect neonatal cardiocytes with sense, anti-sense and non-phosphorylatable mutants of HSP27. They found that whilst increasing the levels of the already abundant HSP27 was not protective in itself, anti-sense and the mutant HSP27s rendered the cells more susceptible to simulated ischaemia. This indicates an important constitutive role for HSP27 and that phosphorylation of HSP27 is important in regulating its protective effects. The gene transfection approach will yield vital data on the cytoprotective potential of various proteins and can be extended to compare other HSPs and anti-oxidant genes such as Mn-SOD. We are currently examining the role of HSP27 and Mn-SOD in delayed preconditioning in rabbit heart and neonatal rat cardiocytes and also hope to assess the importance of post-translational phosphorylation in regulating the activity of HSP27 [Heads et al, 1995(3)].

In summary, although little work has been done on the role of other HSPs such as HSP60 and HSP27 in preconditioning, it is likely that they may also have important functions in protecting the mitochondria and the cytoskeleton, respectively, from ischaemia/reperfusion damage. Since these proteins are constitutively expressed in the myocyte, there may be an important role for post translational modification, particularly phosphorylation, in regulating their protective functions at the organelle level.

CONCLUSIONS

The evidence is clear that HSP70 is an important cytoprotective protein in the cardiac myocyte, protecting against both heat stress and ischaemia/reperfusion injury when expressed at high levels. It is also clear that HSP70 mRNA and protein are induced by ischaemia in cardiac myocytes. However, what is less clear is the severity of the ischaemia that is required to induce HSP70 at the transcriptional level and whether this corresponds to the mild stimulus required to precondition cardiac myocytes. At the present time, this remains equivocal. It is our feeling that the evidence suggests that the thresholds for preconditioning and HSP70 induction are, infact different. This is highlighted by the fact that induction in HSP70 at the protein level has not been reproducibly shown in all studies of delayed preconditioning. However, the phenomenon of the infarct-limiting effect of preconditioning is extremely robust and reproducible.

The threshold of ischaemia required for HSP70 induction is probably slightly higher than that required to precondition. This would explain the variable levels of HSP70 mRNA obtained in 4xPC hearts in our own laboratory. These studies are also confounded by the fact that variable constitutive basal levels of HSP70 protein are found in different species and institutions. One thing that is quite clear, is that HSP70 is not induced at the transcriptional level in an adenosine receptor-dependent fashion. Therefore, since both acute and delayed preconditioning are adenosine receptor dependent phenomena, at least in the rabbit and dog, any elevation in HSP70 probably occurs *in parallel* to preconditioning rather than directly downstream of adenosine receptor activation. In addition, the events associated with reperfusion such as oxygen-derived free radical generation and mitochondrial uncoupling appear to be stronger stimuli for HSP70 induction *in vivo* than brief ischaemia itself. Again, the strength of this stimulus depends on the severity of the preceeding ischaemia. In our hands at least, 10-30 minutes of continuous ischaemia is required for significant induction of the HSP70 message in rabbit heart and the subsequent reperfusion is required for accumulation to high levels. This length of ischaemia is therefore, likely to lead to at least some patchy necrosis.

In conclusion, although HSP70 is clearly protective, there is little compelling evidence that significant HSP70 induction at the trancriptional level is *directly* involved in the preconditioning mechanism as classically defined by its adenosine receptor dependence. However, there is evidence for an increase in HSP70 in specific subcellular compartments which may occur in parallel and contribute to the delayed preconditioning mechanism. This appears to be adenosine receptor-dependent and may involve a post-translational mechanism which results in translocation of HSP70. Therefore, it is at this point that we should think about our approach to manipulating HSP70 levels *in vivo* and maybe regard the mechanisms of HSP70 induction in their own right as being possibly separate from the phenomenon of preconditioning. There is clearly much potential in the therapeutic manipulation of this important cytoprotective protein, either pharmacoligically or via the use of appropriate gene transfer vectors. However, future studies should be designed in such a way as provide *mechanisitic* information on HSP70 expression, rather than merely *correlating* elevated HSP70 with protection. We look forward to an exciting future!

ACKNOWLEDGEMENTS

The authors would like to express their gratitude to Dr Gary F. Baxter for preparing myocardial tissue for the molecular studies of delayed preconditioning. Our own work described herein was carried out on a progam grant funded by the British Heart Foundation.

REFERENCES

Armstrong, S., Downey, J.M. and Ganote, C.E. 1994. Preconditioning of isolated rabbit cardiomyocytes: Induction by metabolic stress and blockade by the adenosine antagonist SPT and calphostin C, a protein kinase C inhibitor. Cardiovasc. Res.; **28**: 72-77.

Baxter, G.F., Marber, M.S., Patel, V.C. and Yellon, D.M. 1993. A 'second window of protection' 24 hours after ischaemic preconditioning may be dependent on adenosine receptor activation. Circulation; **88** (suppl.I):

I-101 (abstract).

Baxter, G.F., Marber, M.S., Patel, V.C. and Yellon, D.M. 1994. Adenosine receptor involvement in a delayed phase of myocardial protection 24 hours after ischemic preconditioning. Circulation; **90**: 2993-3000.

Baxter, G.F. and Yellon, D.M. 1994. Ischaemic preconditioning of myocardium: a new paradigm for clinical cardioprotection? Br.J. Clin. Pharmacol.; **38**: 381-387.

Baxter, G.F., Goma, F.M and Yellon, D.M. 1995. Involvement of protein kinase C in the delayed cytoprotection following sublethal ischaemia in rabbit myocardium. Br. J. Pharmacol.; **114**: in press.

Baxter, G.F., Goodwin, R.W., Wright, M.J. *et al.* 1996. Myocardial protection after monophosphoryl lipid A: studies of delayed anti-ischaemic properties in rabbit heart. Br.J.Pharmacol., **117**:*in press.*

Benjamin, I.J., Kroger, B. and Williams, R.S. 1990. Activation of heat shock transcription factor by hypoxia in mammalian cells. Proc.Natl.Acad.Sci.USA.; **87**: 6263-6267.

Benjamin, I.J., Horie, S., Greenberg, M.L. et al. Induction of stress proteins in cultured myogenic cells.: Molecular signals for the activation of heat shock transcription factor during ischemia. J. Clin. Invest., 1992; **89**: 1658-1689.

Brown, J.M., Grosso, M.A., Terada, L.S. *et al.* 1989. Endotoxin pretreatment increases endogenous myocardial catalase activity and decreases ischemia-reperfusion injury of isolated rat hearts. Proc.Natl.Acad.Sci.USA, **86**: 2516-2520.

Calderwood, S.K., Bornstein, B., Farnum, E.K. and Stevenson, M.A., 1989. Heat shock stimulates the release of arachidonic acid and the synthesis of prostaglandins and leukotriene B_4 in mammalian cells. J.Cell.Physiol., **141**:325-333.

Cumming, D.V.E., Heads, R.J., Brand, N.J. *et al.* 1996. The ability of heat stress and metabolic preconditioning to protect primary rat cardiac myocytes. Basic Res.Cardiol., **91**: 79-85.

Cumming, D.V.E., Heads, R.J., Watson, A. *et al.* 1996. Differential protection of primary rat cardiocytes by transfection of specific heat stress proteins. J.Mol.Cell.Cardiol., **28**: *in press.*

Currie, R.W., Karmazyn, M., Kloc, M. and Mailer, K. 1988. Heat shock response is associated with enhanced postischemic ventricular recovery. Circ. Res.; **63**: 543-549.

Currie, R.W. and Tanguay, R.M. 1991. Analysis of RNA for transcripts for catalase and SP71 in rat hearts after *in vivo* hyperthermia. Biochem. Cell Biol.; **69**: 375-382.

Currie, R.W., Tanguay, R.M. amd Kingma, J.G. 1993. Heat-shock response and limitation of tissue necrosis during occlusion/reperfusion in rabbit hearts. Circulation; **87**: 963-971.

Das, D.K., Engelman, R.M. and Kimura, Y. 1993. Molecular adaptation of cellular defences following preconditioning of the heart by repeated ischaemia. Cardiovascular Res.; **27**: 578-584.

Donnely, T.J., Seivers, R.E., Vissern, F.L.J., *et al.* 1992. Heat shock protein induction in rat hearts: A role for improved myocardial salvage after ischemia and reperfusion ? Circulation, 1992; **85**: 769-778.

Heads, R.J., Latchman, D.S. and Yellon, D.M. 1994. Stable high level expression of a transfected human hsp70 gene protects a heart-derived muscle cell line against thermal stress. J. Mol. Cell. Cardiol.; **26**: 695-699.

Heads, R.J., Yellon, D.M. and Latchman, D.S. 1995(1). Differential cytoprotection against heat stress or hypoxia following expression of specific stress protein genes in myogenic cells. J. Mol. Cell. Cardiol.; **27**: 1669-1678.

Heads, R.J., Latchman, D.S. and Yellon, D.M. 1995(2). Differential stress protein mRNA expression during early ischaemic preconditioning and its relationship to adenosine receptor function. J.Mol.Cell Cardiol.; **27**: 2133-2148.

Heads, R.J., Baxter, G.F., Latchman, D.S. and Yellon, D.M., 1995(3). Delayed protection in rabbit heart following ischaemic preconditioning is associated with modulation of HSP27 and superoxide dismutase at 24 hours. J.Mol.Cell.Cardiol., **27**: A163 (abstract).

Heads, R.J., Latchman, D.S. and Yellon, D.M. 1996. Molecular Basis of adaptation to ischemia in the heart: The role of stress proteins and anti-oxidants in the ischemic and reperfused heart. In: Karmazyn, M., Editor. Myocardial Ischemia: Mechanisms, Reperfusion, Protection. Birkhauser Verlag, Switzerland: *in press.*

Hedge, R.S., Zuo, J., Voellmy, R. and Welch, W.J., 1995. Short-circuiting stress protein expression via a tyrosine kinase inhibitor, herbimycin-A. J.Cell.Physiol., **165**: 186-200.

Hutter, M.M., Sievers, R.E., Barbosa, V. and Wolfe, C.L. 1994. Heat shock protein induction in rat hearts: A direct correlation between the amount of heat shock protein induced and the degree of myocardial protection. Circulation; **89**: 355-360.

Ikonomidis, J.S., Tumiati, L.C., Weisel, R.D. *et al.* 1994. Preconditioning human ventricular cardiomyocytes with brief periods of simulated ischaemia. Cardiovascular Res.; **28**: 1285-1291.

Iwaki, K., Chi, S-H., Dillman, W.H. and Mestril R. 1993. Induction of HSP70 in cultured rat neonatal cardiomyocytes by hypoxia and metabolic stress. Circulation; **87**: 2023-2032.

Karmazyn, M., Mailer, K. and Currie, R.W. 1990. Aquisition and decay of heat-shock-enhanced postischemic ventricular recovery. Am. J. Physiol.; **259** Heart Circ. Physiol.): H424-H431.

Knowlton, A.A., Brecher, P. and Apstein, C.S. 1991. Rapid expression of heat shock protein in the rabbit after brief cardiac ischemia. J.Clin.Invest.; **87**: 139-147.

Knowlton, A.A., Eberli, F.R., Brecher, P. *et al.* 1991. A single myocardial stretch or decreased systolic fiber shortening stimulates the expression of heat shock protein 70 in the isolated, erythrocyte-perfused rabbit heart. J.Clin.Invest., **88**: 2018-2025.

Kukreja, R.C., Kontos, M.C., Loesser, K.E., *et al.* 1994. Oxidant stress increases heat shock protein 70 mRNA in isolated perfused rat heart. Am. J. Physiol.; **267** (6 pt 2): H2213-H2219.

Kuzuya, T., Hoshida, S., Yamashita, N., et al. 1993. Delayed effects of sublethal ischemia on the aquisition of tolerance to ischemia. Circ. Res.; **72**: 1293-1299.

Li, R-K., Mickle, D.A.G.,Weisel, R.D. *et al.* 1996.Human pedeatric and adult ventricular cardiomyocytes in culture: assessment of phenotypic changes with passaging. Cardiovascular Res. 323.

Lu, D., Maulik, N., Moraru, I.I *et al.* 1993. Molecular adaptation of vascular endothelial cells to oxidative stress. Am.J.Physiol., **264**: C715-C722.

Lui, G.S., Thornton, J., Van Winkle, D.M. *et al.* 1991. Protection against infarction afforded by preconditioning is mediated by adenosine A1 receptors in rabbit heart. Circulation; **84**: 350-356.

Lui, X., Engelman, R.M., Moraru, I.I *et al.* 1992. Heat shock: A new approach for myocardial preservation in cardiac surgery. Circulation, **86** (suppl II): II-358-363.

Marber, M., Latchman, D.S., Walker, J.M. and Yellon, D.M. 1993. Cardiac stress protein elevation 24 hours following brief ischemia or heat stress is associated with resisitance to myocardial infarction. Circulation; **88**: 1264-1272.

Marber, M.S., Walker, J.M., Latchman, D.S. and Yellon, D.M. 1994. Myocardial protection after whole body heat stress in the rabbit is dependent on metabolic substrate and is related to the amount of inducible 70 kD heat stress protein. J.Clin.Invest., **93**:1087-1094.

Marber, M.S., Mestril, R., Chi, S-H., Sayen, M.R. *et al.* 1995. Overexpression of the rat inducible 70 kDa heat stress protein in a transgenic mouse increases the resistance of the heart to ischemic injury. J. Clin. Invest.; **95**: 1446-1456.

Martin, J.L., Mestril, R., Hickey, E. *et al.* 1995. HSP27 and protection against ischemic damage. J. Mol. Cell. Cardiol.; **27** (5) (suppl): A20 (abstract).

Maulik, N., Engelman, R.M., Wei, Z. *et al.* 1993. Interleukin-1α preconditioning reduces myocardial ischemia reperfusion injury. Circulation **88** (Suppl.II): II-387-394.

McCully, J.D., Lotz, M.M., Krukenkamp, I.B. and Levitsky, S. 1996. J.Mol.Cell.Cardiol., **28**:231-241.

Mestril, R., Chi, S-H., Sayen, R. *et al.* 1994. Expression of inducible stress protein 70 in rat heart myogenic cells confers protection against simulated ischemia-induced injury. J. Clin. Invest.; **93**: 759-767.

Mestril, R., Chi, S-H., Sayen, M.R. and Dillman, W.H. 1994. Isolation of a novel inducible rat heat-shock protein (HSP70) gene and its expression during ischaemia/hypoxia and heat shock. Biochem. J.; **298**: 561-569.

Mitchell, M.B., Meng, X., Ao, L. *et al.* 1995. Preconditioning of isolated rat heart is mediated by protein kinase C. Circ. Res.; **76**: 73-81.

Moalic, J.M., Bauters, C., Himbert, D. *et al.* 1989. Phenylephrine, vasopressin and angiotensin II as determinants of proto-oncogene and heat shock protein gene expression in adult rat heart and aorta. J. hypertension; 7: 195-201.

Morimoto, R. and Milarski, K.L. 1990. Expression and function of vertebrate hsp70 genes. In: Morimoto, R.I., Tissieres, A. and Georgopoulos, C., Editors. Stress proteins in biology and medicine, Cold Spring Harbour Laboratory Press: 223-278.

Morris, S., Cumming, D.V.E., Latchman, D.S. and Yellon, D.M., 1996. Specific induction of the 70 kD heat stress proteins by the tyrosine kinase inhibitor herbimycin-A protects rat neonatal cardiomyocytes. J.Clin.Invest., **97**: 706-712.

Murry, C.E., Jennings, R.B. and Reimer, K.A. 1991. New insights into potential mechanisms of ischemic preconditioning. Circulation; **84**(1): 442-445.

Nakano, M, Mann, D.L. and Knowlton, A.A. 1996. Blocking the endogenous increase in HSP 72 increases susceptibility to hypoxia and reoxygenation in isolated adult feline cardiocytes. J.Am.Coll. Cardiol. 27:294A (abst.).

Osborne, D.L., Aw, T.Y., Cepinskas, G. *et al.* 1994. Development of ischemia/reperfusion tolerance in the rat small intestine: an epithelium-dependent event. J. Clin. Invest.; **94**: 1910-1918.

Plumier, J-C. L., Ross, B.M., Currie, R.W., *et al.* 1995. Transgenic mice expressing the human heat shock protein 70 have improved post-ischemic myocardial recovery. J. Clin. Invest.; **95**: 1854-1860.

Radford, N., Fina, M., Benjamin, I.J. *et al.* 1994. Enhanced functional and metabolic recovery following ischemia in intact hearts from *hsp*70 transgenic mice. Circulation; **90** (4 part 2): I-G (abstract).

Santoro, M.G., Garaci, E. and Amici, C., 1989. Prostaglandins with antiproliferative activity induce the synthesis of a heat shock protein in human cells. Proc.Natl.Acad.Sci.USA., **86**: 8407-8411.

Speechley-Dick,M.E., Mocanu, M.M. and Yellon, D.M. 1994. Protein kinase C: It's role in ischaemic preconditioning. Circ. Res. **75**: 586-590.

Sun, J.Z., Tang, X.L., Knowlton, A.A. *et al.* 1995. Late preconditioning against myocardial stunning: An endogenous protective mechanism that confers resistance to postischemic dysfunction 24h after brief ischemia in conscious pigs. J. Clin. Invest. **95** (1): 388-403.

Tanaka, M., Fujiwara, H., Yamasaki, K. *et al.* 1994. Ischemic preconditioning elevates cardiac stress protein but does not limit infarct size 24 or 48 h later in rabbits. Am. J. Physiol.; **267**: H1476-H1482.

Walker, D.M. and Yellon, D.M. 1992. Ischaemic preconditioning: from mechanisms to exploitation. Cardiovasc. Res.; **26**: 734-739.

Welch, W.J. 1990. The mammalian stress response: cell physiology and biochemistry of stress proteins. In: Morimoto, R.I., Tissieres, A. and Georgopoulos, C., Editors. Stress proteins in biology and medicine, Cold Spring Harbour Laboratory Press: 223-278.

Williams, R.S., Thomas, J.A., Fina, M. *et al.* 1993. Human heat shock protein 70 (hsp70) protects murine cells from injury during metabolic stress. J. Clin. Invest.; **92**: 503-508.

Yamashita, N., Nishida, M., Hoshida, S. *et al*, 1994. Induction of mangenese superoxide dismutase in rat cardiac myocytes increases tolerance to hypoxia 24 hours after preconditioning. J. Clin. Invest., 1994; **94**: 2193-2199.

Yellon, D.M., Pasini, E., Cargnoni, A., Marber, M.S., Latchman, D.S. and Ferrari, R. 1992. The protective role of heat stress in the ischaemic and reperfused rabbit myocardium. J.Mol.Cell Cardiol.; **24**: 895-907.

4

HEAT SHOCK PROTEINS AND ANTIOXIDATIVE ENZYMES IN MYOCARDIAL PROTECTION

R. William Currie and J.-Christophe L. Plumier
Department of Anatomy and Neurobiology
Dalhousie University
Halifax, Nova Scotia, Canada B3H 4H7
Telephone 902 494 3343
Fax 902 494 8008

The heart is composed primarily of post-mitotic cells. This means that if the cardiomyocytes are injured and die, there is no replacement. Thus prevention of cell loss after metabolic injury, such as brief ischemia, is paramount to myocardial functional recovery. While various pharmacological treatments have been shown to be of some benefit, interest has also developed on endogenous cellular mechanisms which can increase cellular protection and functional recovery of injured myocardial cells. It seems reasonable that post-mitotic cells should have multiple strategies for changing their metabolism to adapt to changes (and stressors) in their local environment. In this chapter we discuss the evidence for antioxidants and heat shock proteins for protecting the heart from ischemia and reperfusion injury.

HEAT SHOCK PROTEINS IN THE HEART

Heat shock proteins were first identified in the heart in 1981. In the preceeding years, Hsps had been detected in *Drosophila melanogaster* (Mirault et al., 1978; Mitchell et al., 1979), in culture mammalian cells (Hightower, 1980), and in incubated rat brain slices (White, 1980). Heat shock proteins were first demonstrated in rats following hyperthermia or following ischemic injury (Currie and White, 1981). In this early study, the core body temperature of the rats was elevated to 42° - 42.5°C for 15 minutes. Proteins were metabolically labeled with [^{35}S]-methionine during a 2 hour recovery period. Examination of [^{35}S]-methionine labeled proteins revealed that 1 or 2 proteins were synthesized at a high level and that overall protein synthesis was suppressed. The highly induced protein was referred to as SP71 (Stress-induced protein of 71 kDa molecular mass; now Hsp70) and the other moderately induced protein was referred to a P73 (protein of 73 kDa molecular mass; now Hsc70).

ISCHEMIC INJURY INDUCES A HEAT SHOCK RESPONSE

Expression of Hsps in hearts during various pathophysiological conditions continues to be of interest. In the heart, a potent inducer of the heat shock reponse is ischemic injury. Ischemic injury caused by occluding the common carotid arteries in rats (Currie and White, 1981) induces the expression of Hsp70 in the brain, liver and kidney, but not in the heart. Occlusion of a coronary artery in dog hearts induced the expression of Hsp70 in the ischemic area (Dillmann et al., 1986; Mehta et al., 1988). Even in isolated rat hearts, Hsp70 was expressed after ischemic injury (Currie, 1987, 1988). In rabbits, coronary artery occlusion for only 5 minutes induced Hsp70 mRNA accumulation in the ischemic area during a 1 hour reflow period as revealed by Northern analysis (Knowlton et al., 1991). It seems clear that brief ischemia injures myocytes and one of their responses is to express Hsps. At the other extreme, ischemia of long duration, with no reflow causes cell death and necrosis in a large part of the ischemic area. Only in the transition zone between the ischemic area and the non-ischemic area are heat shock proteins synthesized. We have recently demonstrated using *in situ* hybridization in rat hearts exposed to 30 min of coronary artery occlusion that the distribution of *hsp70* mRNA was restricted to the area surrounding the necrotic zone (Plumier et al., 1996). Some have suggested that the regions expressing Hsp70 protein will survive the ischemic insult (Kinouchi et al., 1993). We believe that after ischemic injury cells expressing elevated levels of Hsp70 are clearly injured, and whether the cells survive depends on the severity (duration) of the injury, i.e., whether the cells are reversibly or irreversibly injured.

Exercise has been shown to induce heat shock transcription factors and Hsps in rat hearts (Locke et al., 1995). As most long distance and marathon runners know, exercise elevates body temperature. In fact, rats that are run to exhaustion on a tread mill, have an elevated body temperaure of approximately 42°C. These rats showed a progressive increase in the amount of at least 4 heat shock proteins in spleen, skeletal muscle and lymphocytes correlated with the duration of exercise and body temperature (Locke et al., 1990).

HEAT SHOCK PROTEINS AND ENDOGENOUS CELLULAR PROTECTION IN HEART

Heat shock treatment of rats has been shown to in induce a significant level of myocardial protection to ischemic injury (Currie et al., 1988; Karmazyn et al., 1990; Currie and Karmazyn, 1990). In these experiments, the rat's body temperature was raised to 42°C for 15 minutes. After a 24 hour recovery period, control and heat shocked hearts were isolated, perfused at a rate of 10 ml/min and electrically paced at 300 beats per minute. Hearts were made ischemic by reducing the buffer flow to 1 ml/min for 30 minutes. During this ischemic period the control and heat shocked hearts stopped contracting. Upon reperfusion at 10 ml/min the heat shocked hearts recovered their contractile force to a significantly higher level than the control hearts (Currie et al., 1988). In addition, release of creatine kinase was significantly lower in the heat shocked hearts than in the controls, suggesting less cellular injury in the heat shocked

72

hearts. While maximal contractile recovery from 30 min of ischemia was seen in 24 and 48 hr post-heat shocked hearts, by 96 hours the improved contractile recovery was decaying (Karmazyn et al., 1990).

More recently, there has been considerable interest in induction of the heat shock response and the ability of cells in organs to protect themselves from metabolic injury (Donnelly et al., 1992; Yellon et al., 1992; Currie et al., 1993; Yellon and Latchman, 1992; Das et al., 1995; Knowlton, 1995; Mestril and Dillmann, 1995). In *in vivo* experiments, myocardial infarct size was significantly reduced in heat shock treated animals (Donnelly et al., 1992; Currie et al., 1993; Marber et al., 1993). In collaboration with Dr. John Kingma, Université Laval, it was shown that induction of the heat shock response (and 24 hr of recovery) in rabbits significantly reduced infarct size following 30 min of occlusion of the left anterior descending artery (Currie et al., 1993). No reduction in infarct size was seen with 40 hr of recovery from the heat shock treatment or if the occlusion was extended to 45 minutes. This result suggested that the heat shock induced myocardial protection was transient and decayed by 40 hr post-heat shock and that the induced myocardial protection delayed (but did not prevent) the onset of irreversible injury.

Hsp70 has been implicated in myocardial protection (Currie et al., 1988; Karmazyn et al., 1990; Yellon and Latchman, 1992). Cells transfected with the *hsp70* gene under the control of constitutive promoters were protected in culture against thermal stress (Angelidis et al., 1991; Li et al., 1991; Heads et al., 1994). Murine cells expressing high levels of the human Hsp70 were protected from severe metabolic stress (Williams et al., 1993). Similarly, cultured myogenic cells overexpressing an exogenous *hsp70* gene have improved survival to simulated ischemia (Mestril et al., 1994). From these studies it seems reasonable to suggest that overexpression of Hsp70 conditions the cells and extends the period during metabolic stress before cells are irreversibly injured. The protective role of Hsp70 in cell culture studies seems well established.

In animal studies, there is circumstantial evidence for a role for Hsp70 in cell protection. Several studies have shown that induction of the heat shock response indicated by expression of Hsp70, significantly reduced infarct size in the hearts of live animals (Donnelly et al., 1992; Currie et al., 1993; Marber et al., 1993). Similarly, heat shock pretreatment, with expression of Hsp70, has been shown to reduce arrhythmias in hearts due to reperfusion injury (Steare and Yellon, 1993). These effects have been suggested to be related to the synthesis of heat shock proteins, and especially Hsp70. For example, Marber et al., (1994) demonstrated that heat shock-induced protection was related to the amount of Hsp70 but not Hsp60. Hutter et al., (1994) examined the infarct size induced by 35 minutes of left coronary artery occlusion in rats pretreated with 40°C, 41°C, and 42°C hyperthermia. Measurement of Hsp70 by Western blot revealed a progressive increase in Hsp70 with increasing temperature. While no difference was detected between control and 40° C pretreated rats, infarct size was significantly reduced in 41°C pretreated rats and the greatest reduction in infarct size was observed in 42° C pretreated rats. This result was the first direct correlation of the amount of myocardial Hsp70 and the degree of myocardial protection (Hutter et al., 1994). Recently, in transgenic mice overexpressing Hsp70, the protective role of Hsp70 has been examined.

HSP70 TRANSGENIC MICE AND MYOCARDIAL PROTECTION

Recently, the role of high levels of the human inducible Hsp70 in transgenic mouse hearts has been examined (Plumier et al., 1995). Overexpression of the human Hsp70 did not appear to affect normal protein synthesis or the stress response in transgenic mice compared with the non-transgenic mice. After 30 min of ischemia, upon reperfusion, transgenic hearts versus non-transgenic hearts showed significantly improved recovery of contractile force, rate of contraction and rate of relaxation. Creatine kinase, an indicator of cellular injury, was released at a high level upon reperfusion from the non-transgenic hearts, but not the transgenic hearts. It was concluded that high level constitutive expression of the human inducible Hsp70 played a direct role in the protection of the myocardium from ischemia and reperfusion injury. Simulaneously, Wolfgang Dillmann and his group (Marber et al., 1995) developed transgenic mice overexpressing the rat highly inducible Hsp70 under the control of a cytomegalovirus enhancer and β-actin promoter. These transgenic mouse hearts had significantly reduced infarct size after 20 minutes of global ischemia and creatine kinase release was significantly reduced during the reperfusion period. These two studies using Hsp70 transgenic mice suggest to us that overabundance of a physiological (transgene) protein was not necessarily stressful to cells and that Hsp70 did not interfere with developmental processes. Yet the overabundance of either the human or rat Hsp70 seems to be functional, as demonstrated by cellular protection from ischemia-reperfusion injury.

HEAT SHOCK, ANTIOXIDATIVE ENZYMES AND ENDOGENOUS CELLULAR PROTECTION IN THE HEART

Hypoxia followed by reoxygenation was first reported to induce a heat shock response in Drosophila cells (Ropp et al., 1983). Oxidative stress (hydrogen peroxide) was shown to induce some of the heat shock proteins and to convey a measure of protection against thermal and oxidative injury in bacteria (Christman et al., 1985; Morgan et al., 1986) and mammalian fibroblasts (Spitz et al., 1987). As mentioned above, we showed that induction of the heat shock response could significantly improve functional recovery of hearts from ischemia-reperfusion injury (Currie et al., 1988). At this time, others were showing that addition of antioxidative enzymes to the perfusion buffer of isolated hearts could improve recovery from ischemic injury during reperfusion (Das et al., 1986; Otani et al., 1986). We considered whether our heat shocked rat hearts had increased capacity to metabolize reactive oxygen species that would be generated during reperfusion with the re-introduction of molecular oxygen. Measurement of antioxidative enzymes in these heat shocked hearts revealed that catalase activity was approximately 2 times elevated, while there was no clear change in the activity of either glutathione peroxidase or superoxide dismutase. While this was a rather modest increase in catalase activity, we argued that it was important since it was inside the cells where oxygen free radicals were generated upon reperfusion. Therefore relatively modest increases in endogenous antioxdative enzyme activity could be as effective as relatively larger amounts of antioxidants in the perfusion buffer that would be resticted to the inside of the microvessels (Currie et al., 1988).

Heat shock treatment modulates the activity of cellular antioxidative enzymes and appears to play a role in myocardial protection (Karmazyn et al., 1990). In isolated rat hearts subjected to 30 min of low flow ischemia, recovery of ventricular function was strongest at 24 and 48 hours after heart shock treatment when Hsp70 and catalase activity were highest. As Hsp70 and catalase activity returned to control levels, so did the improved contractile recovery of the heat shocked hearts. In these experiments the compound 3-amino-1,2,4- triazole was used to suppress catalase activity. This compound had been reported to irreversibly inactive catalase (Darr and Fridovich, 1986). Injection of this compound, 3-amino triazole, into 24 hr post heat shocked rats, 30 minutes before isolation of the hearts effectively decreased catalase activity to the control level. Co-incidently, the improved contractile recovery of the hearts from ischemic injury was abolished. This suggested that the elevated catalase activity in heat shocked hearts played a role in the improved myocardial recovery. In rabbit hearts heat shock treatment also improves contractile function after ischemic injury (Yellon et al., 1992). In fact in these rabbit hearts, evidence has been presented that the heat shocked hearts have less oxidative injury during reperfusion that the control hearts. Oxidized glutathione accumulation and release was at a significantly lower level in the heat shocked hearts as compared to the control hearts.

In a recent study, heat shock treatment elevated catalase activity and lead to a significant reduction in infarct size in rat hearts after 35 min of coronary artery occlusion (Auyeung et al., 1995). Treatment of these rats with 3-amino-1,2,4-triazole significantly reduced catalase activity in both the heat shocked hearts and in the non-heat shocked hearts. Interestingly, the inhibition of catalase activity with 3-amino-1,2,4-triazole did not abolish the reduction of infarct size seen after heat shock treatment. In this study the data suggests that the elevation of catalase activity did not contribute to the reduction of infarct size and hence myocardial protection seen after heat shock treatment of rats. In a similar set of experiments, the role of elevated catalase activity has been examined in 24 hr post-heat shock rabbits (Kingma et al., 1996). Twenty-four hr after heat shock treatment rabbits underwent 30 min of regional myocardial ischemia and 3 hr of reperfusion. Catalase activity was irreversibly inactivated using 3-amino-1,2,4-triazole 30 min before the onset of ischemia. Inhibition of catalase activity in 24 hr post-heat shocked rabbits with 3-amino-1,2,4-triazole disrupted the hyperthermia-induced cardioprotection. In this latter study, catalase appears to contribute to hyperthermia-induced cardioprotection. While these studies (Auyeung et al., 1995; Kingma et al., 1996) agree that catalase activity is elevated in the heart after heat shock treatment, it seems that the role of catalase in myocardial protection is unresolved and more studies are required. However, whether catalase is involved in myocardial protection, it seems likely that more that one mechanism may contribute to cardioprotection.

Other evidence also suggests that there is increased antioxidative enzyme activity after heat shock treatment. But whether the increased antioxidative capacity is of benefit depends on the circumstances. The heat shock elevation of catalase activity did not appear to play a role in the functional recovery of hearts after 4 hours of cardioplegic arrest at 4°C. Treatment with 3-amino-triazole, which inhibited catalase activity had no effect on the functional recovery of the hearts (Amrani et al., 1993). However, endothelial function in these hearts was correlated with catalase activity. In other experiments, heat shock treatment significantly increased catalase activity and improved post-ischemic function in non-hypertrophied isolated ejecting rat hearts (Cornelussen et al., 1994). While the heat shock treatment improved post-ischemic function in hypertrophied hearts, catalase activity was not increased. This suggests that mechanisms other than catalase were involved in the improved post-ischemic recovery. In other experiments (with no heat shock treatment), 3-amino-triazole has also been used to suppress the normal endogenous catalase activity. While catalase levels were reduced significantly in 3-amino-triazole treated hearts, these hearts were not rendered sensitive to either 35 min of 37°C cardioplegia with reperfusion (ischemia-reperfusion injury) or to hydrogen peroxide induced injury (Konorev et al., 1993). Again this suggests that mechanisms other than catalase were involved in myocardial protection. Heat shock treatment and the subsequent elevation of heat shock proteins and catalase activity appeared to play a role in the reduction of ventricular arrhythmias during reperfusion (Steare and Yellon, 1993). Since 3-amino-triazole did not block the protection, catalase was thought not to be directly involved in reducing the number of arrhythmias. In other experiments where heat shock treatment elevated catalase activity, hearts were not protected from exogenously applied hydrogen peroxide (Steare and Yellon, 1994). It has been suggested that elevation of endogenous antioxidants was very important in protecting cells from endogenous free radical generation during reperfusion (Currie et al., 1988). Endogenous catalase not protecting heart from exogenous hydrogen peroxide re-enforces the notion that location of protective mechanisms is very important (Steare and Yellon, 1994; 1995). Finally, it has been suggested that heat shock treatment of rats does not increase catalase activity nor significantly improve post-ischemic myocardial recovery (Wall et al., 1993).

Other antioxidants have also been reported to be elevated after hyperthermia. Elevation of body temperature of pigs treated with amphetamine caused a marked increase in activity of copper/zinc-superoxide dismutase and catalase 48 hours later (Maulik et al., 1994). Treatment of rats with interleukin-1α similarly stimulated a elevation of the antioxidative enzymes superoxide dismutase, catalase, glutathione peroxidase that seemed to play a role in protectioning the heart from ischemic injury (Maulik et al., 1993).

Interestingly, in transgenic mice overexpressing glutathione peroxidase expressed less Hsp70 after heat shock treatment as compared to nontransgenic mice (Mirochnitchenko et al., 1995). On the other hand, over-production of copper zinc superoxide dismutase had no effect on the level of Hsp70 after heat shock treatment (Mirochnitchenko et al., 1995). The glutathione peroxidase transgenic mice also had lower levels of tissue peroxides after heat shock that the non transgenic mice. Since the level of expression of Hsp70 was correlated with the level of metabolic stress, these glutathione peroxidase transgenic mice appear to have experience less metabolic stress that the nontransgenic mice.

It has also been shown that controlled amounts of oxidative stress increase antioxidative enzymes such as catalase, superoxide dismutase, glutathione reductase and glutathione peroxidase and that these antioxidants enhanced myocardial tolerance to ischemia (Maulik et al., 1995). In these experiments, rats were treated with endotoxin or its non-toxic derivative, lipid A. Similarly, antioxidants have been reported to be elevated after ischemic preconditioning. The activity of manganese-superoxide dismutase, peroxisomal catalase, and glutathione peroxidase were elevated at 1 hour after 4 cycles of 5 min of ischemia and 10 min of reperfusion in rat hearts (Das et al., 1993).

CONCLUSIONS AND FUTURE DIRECTIONS

The transgenic mouse experiments (Marber et al., 1995; Plumier et al., 1995) strongly suggest that Hsp70 plays a role in recovery of the heart from ischemic injury. It is also clear that antioxidative enzymes help to reduce injury caused by oxygen free radicals during reperfusion of ischemic tissue. Ultimately, other mechanisms that protect post-mitotic cells from injury will be identified. Since post-mitotic cells can not replace themselves it seems reasonable that they should have multiple mechanisms to protect themselves from changes in their local environment. Also, it seems that cells have protective mechanisms that are effective within minutes (such as after ischemic preconditioning) and others that require time for gene expression (such as after heat shock treatment or ishemic injury). Finally, inducible endogenous protective mechanisms can not protect cells from severe injury and death. However it is reasonable to suggest that cells can adapt their metabolism to extend the period of time during metabolic distress such as ischemia before there is irreversible cell injury.

Now the goal should be to identify clearly all the mechanisms that cells use to adapt and facilitate recovery of metabolic processes after being challenged by changes in their environment. While we know that heat shock, or brief ischemia can lead to metabolic changes that are advantagous to the recovery and survival of cells, now we must find less noxious ways of turning on these protective mechanisms. In fact, there are several recent papers that demonstrate that the expression of Hsp70 can be increased by administration of pharmaceutical compounds. Indomethacin has been shown to activate the DNA-binding activity of heat shock factor 1. This has the effect of lowering the temperature threshold for heat shock factor 1 activation and synthesis of Hsp70 (Lee et al., 1995). In addition, herbimycin-A has been shown to increase expression of Hsp70 in cultured primary cardiomyoctes (Morris et al., 1996). In these studies, the increased expression of Hsp70 was associated with resistance to metabolic injury. In animal studies, other compounds such as amphetamine (Maulik et al., 1994) and d-lysergic acid diethylamide (LSD) which clearly elevated body temperature (Cosgove and Brown, 1983) have been used to induce a heat shock response. Of course, the goal is for clinical manipulation of the stress response and/or other protective mechanisms to improve cell survival (Minowada and Welch, 1995). Improvement in cell survival and function are likely in at least two situations. Presently, we are learning how to manipulate protective mechanisms prior to planned insults (such ischemia during coronary artery by-pass surgery or transplantation). Secondly, and more challenging, we must explore ways of enhancing these protective mechanisms after an unplanned insult (such as sudden ischemic attacks in the heart) to recover cells that are entering into programmed cell death.

REFERENCES

Amrani M, Allen NJ, O'Shea J, Corbett J, Dunn MJ, Tadjkarimi S, Theodoropoulos S, Pepper J, Yacoub MH. Role of catalase and heat shock protein on recovery of cardiac endothelial and mechanical function after ischemia. Cardioscience 1993;4:193-198

Angelidis CE, Lazaridis I, Pagoulatos GN. Constitutive expression of heat-shock protein 70 in mammalian cells confers thermotolerance. Eur J Biochem 1991;199:35-39

Auyeung Y, Sievers RE, Weng D, Barbosa V, Wolfe CL. Catalase inhibition with 3-amino-1,2,4-triazole does not abolish infarct size reduction in heat-shocked rats. Circulation 1995;92:3318-3322

Christman MF, Morgan RW, Jacobson FS, Ames BN. Positive control of a regulon for defenses against oxidative stress and some heat shock proteins in Salmonella typhimurium. Cell 1985;41:753-762

Cornelussen R, Spiering W, Webers JHG, de Bruin WG, Reneman RS, Van der Vusse GJ, Snoeckx LHEH. Heat shock improves ischemic tolerance in hypertropied rat hearts. Am J Physiol 1994;267:H1941-H1947

Cosgrove JW, Brown IR. Heat shock in the mammalian brain and other organs following a physiologically relevant increase in body temperature induced by LSD. Proc Natl Acad Sci USA 1983;80:569-573

Currie RW. Effects of cold ischemia and perfusion temperature on protein synthesis in isolated and perfused rat hearts. J Mol Cell Cardiol 1987;19:795-808

Currie RW. Protein synthesis in perfused rat hearts after in vivo hyperthermia and in vitro cold ischemia. Biochem Cell Biol 1988;66:13-19

Currie RW, Karmazyn M. Improved post-ischemic ventricular recovery in the absence of changes in energy metabolism in working rat hearts following heat shock. J Mol Cell Cardiol 1990;22:631-636

Currie RW, White FP. (1981) Trauma-induced protein in rat tissues: A physiological role for a "heat shock" protein? Science 1981;214:72-73

Currie RW, Karmazyn M, Kloc M, Mailer K. Heat-shock response is associated with enhanced post-ischemic ventricular recovery. Circulation Res 1988;63:543-549

Currie RW, Tanguay RM. Kingma JG. Heat-shock response and limitation of tissue necrosis during occlusion/reperfusion in rabbit hearts. Circulation 1993;87:963-971

Darr D, Fridovich I. Irreversible inactivation of catalase by 3-amino-1,2,4-triazole. Biochem Pharmacol 1986;35:3642

Das DK, Engelman RM, Otani H, Rousou JA, Breyer RH, Lemeshow S. Effect of superoxide dismutase and catalase on myocardial energy metabolism during ischemia and reperfusion. Clin Physiol Biochem 1986;4:187-198

Das DK, Englelman RM, Kimura Y. Molecular adaptation of cellular defences following preconditioning of the heart by repeated ischemia. Cardiovascular Res 1993;27:578-584

Das DK, Maulik N, Moraru II. Gene expression in acute myocardial stress. Induction by hypoxia, ischemia, reperfusion, hyperthermia and oxidative stress. J Mol Cell Cardiol 1995;27:181-193

Dillmann WH, Mehta HB, Barrieux A, Guth BD, Neeley WE, Ross J. Ischemia of the dog heart induces the appearance of a cardiac mRNA coding for a protein with migration characteristics similar to heat-shock/stress protein 71. Circ Res 1986;59:110-114

Donnelly TJ, Sievers RE, Vissern FLJ, Welch WJ, Wolfe CL. Heat shock protein induction in rat hearts. A role for improved myocardial salvage after ischemia and reperfusion? Circulation 1992;85:769-778

Heads RJ, Latchman DS, Yellon DM. Stable high level expression of a transfected human Hsp70 gene protects a heart-derived muscle cell line against thermal stress. J Mol Cell Cardiol 1994;26:695-699

Hightower LE. Cultured animal cells exposed to amino acid analogues or puromycin rapidly synthesize several polypeptides. J Cell Physiol 1980;102:407-427

Hutter MM, Sievers RE, Barbosa V, Wolfe CL. Heat-shock protein induction in rat hearts: a direct correlation between the amount of heat-shock protein induced and the degree of myocardial protection. Circulation 1994;89:355-360

Karmazyn M, Mailer K, Currie RW. Acquisition and decay of enhanced post-ischemic ventricular recovery is associated with the heat-shock response. Am J Physiol 1990;259:H424-H431

Kingma JG, Simard D, Rouleau JR, Tanguay RM, Currie RW. Contribution of catalase to hyperthermia-mediated cardioprotection after ischemia-reperfusion in rabbits. Am J Physiol 1996;(Accepted)

Kinouchi H, Sharp FR, Koistinaho J, Hicks K, Kamii H, Cha PH. Induction of heat shock hsp70 mRNA and Hsp70 kDa protein in neurons in the 'penumbra' following focal cerebral ischemia in the rat. Brain Res 1993;619:334-338

Knowlton AA. The role of heat shock proteins in the heart. J Mol Cell Cardiol 1995;27:121-131

Knowlton AA, Brecher P, Apstein CS. Rapid expression of heat shock protein in the rabbit after brief cardiac ischemia. J Clin Invest 1991;87:139-147

Konorev EA, Struck AT, Baker JE, Ramanujam S, Thomas JP, Radi R, Kalyanaraman B. Intracellular catalase inhibition does not predispose rat heart to ischemia-reperfusioon and hydrogen peroxide-induced injuries. Free Radic Res Comm 1993;19:397-407

Lee BS, Chen J, Angelidis C, Jurivich DA, Morimoto RI. Pharmacological modulation of heat shock factor 1 by antiinflammatory durgs results in protection against stress-induced cellular damage. Proc Natl Acad Sci USA 1995;92:7207-7211

Li GC, Li L, Liu YK, Mak JY, Chen LL, Lee WM. Thermal response of rat fibroblasts stably transfected with the human 70-kDa heat shock protein-encoding gene. Proc Natl Acad Sci USA 1991;88:1681-1685

Locke M, Noble EG, Atkinson BG. Exercising mammals synthesize stress proteins. Am J Physiol 1990;258(Cell Physiol 27):C723-C729

Locke M, Noble EG, Tanguay RM, Field MR, Ianuzzo SE, Ianuzzo CD. Activation of heat-shock transcription factor in rat heart after heat shock and exercise. Am J Physiol 1995;268(Cell Physiol 37):C1387-C1394

Marber MS, Latchman DS, Walker JM, Yellon DM. Cardiac stress protein elevation 24 hours after brief ischemia or heat stress is associated with resistance to myocardial infarction. Circulation 1993;88:1264-1272

Marber MS, Mestril R, Chi SH, Sayen MR, Yellon DM, Dillmann WH. Overexpression of the rat inducible 70-kD heat stress protein in a transgenic mouse increases the resistance of the heart to ischemic injury. J Clin Invest 1995;95:1446-1456

Marber MS, Walker JM, Latchman DS, Yellon DM. Myocardial protection after whole body stress in the rabbit is dependent on metabolic substrate and is related to the amount of the inducible 70-kD heat stress protein. J Clin Invest 1994;93:1087-1094

Maulik N, Engelman RM, Wei Z, Lu D, Rousou JA, Das DK. Interleukin-1a preconditioning reduces myocardial ischemia reperfusion injury. Circulation 1993;88:387-394

Maulik N, Watanabe M, Engelman DT, Engelman RM, Das DK. Oxidative stress adaptation improves postischemic ventricular recovery. Mol Cell Biochem 1995;144:67-74

Maulik N, Wei Z, Liu X, Engelman RM, Rousou JA, Das DK. Improved postischemic ventricular functional recovery by amphetamine is linked with its ability to induce heat shock. Mol Cell Biochem 1994;137:17-24

Mehta HB, Popovitch BK Dillmann WH. Ischemia induces changes in the level of mRNAs coding for stress protein 71 and creatine kinase M. Circ Res 1988;63:512-517

Mestril R, Dillmann WH. Heat shock proteins and protection against myocardial ischemia. J Mol Cell Cardiol 1995;27:45-52

Mestril R, Chi S-H, Sayen MR, O'Reilly K, Dillmann WH. Expression of inducible stress protein 70 in rat heart myogenic cells confers protection against simulated ischemia-induced injury. J Clin Invest 1994;93:759-767

Minowada G, Welch WJ. Clinical implications of the stress response. J Clin Invest 1995;95:3-12

Mirault M-E, Goldschmidt-Clermont M, Moran L, Arrigo A-P, Tissiere A. The effect of heat shock on gene expression in *Drosophila melanogaster*. Cold Spring Harbor Symp Quant Biol 1978;42:819-827

Mirochnitchenko O, Palnitkar U, Philbert M, Inouye M. Thermosensitive phenotype of transgenic mice overproducing human glutathione peroxidase. Proc Natl Acad Sci USA 1995;92:8120-8124

Mitchell HK, Moller G, Petersen NS , Lipps-Sarmento L. Specific protection from phenocopy induction by heat shock. Dev Genet 1979;1:181-192

Morgan RW, Christman MF, Jacobson FS, Storz G, Ames BN. Hydrogen peroxide inducible proteins in Salmonella typhimurium overlap with heat shock and other stress proteins. Proc Natl Acad Sci USA 1986;83:8059-8063

Morris SD, Cumming DVE, Latchman DS, Yellon DM. Specific induction of the 70-kD heat stress proteins by the tyrosine kinase inhibitor herbimycine-A protects rat neonatal cardiomyocytes. A new pharmacological route to stress protein expression? J Clin Invest 1995;97:706-712

Otani H, Umemoto M, Kagawa K, Nakamura Y, Omoto K, Tanaka K, Sato T, Nonoyama A, Kagawa T. Protection against oxygen-induced reperfusion injury of the isolated canine heart by superoxide dismutase and catalase. J Surgical Res 1986;41:126-133

Plumier J-CL, Robertson HA, Currie RW. Differential accumulation of mRNA for immediate early genes and heat shock genes in heart after ischemic injury. J Mol Cell Cardiol 1996;(accepted)

Plumier J-CL, Ross BM, Currie RW, Angelidis CE, Kazlaris H, Kollias G, Pagoulatos GN. Transgenic mice expressing the human HSP70 have improved post-ischemic myocardial recovery. J Clin Invest 1995;95:1854-1860

Ropp M, Courgeon AM, Calvayrac R, Best-Pomme M. The possible role of superoxide ion in the induction of the heat-shock and specific proteins in aerobic Drosophila cells during return to normoxia after a period of anaerobiosis. Can J Biochem Cell Biol 1983;61:456-461

Spitz DR, Dewey WC, Li GC. Hydrogen peroxide or heat shock induces resistance to hydrogen peroxided in Chinese hamster fibroblasts. J Cell Physiol 1987;131:364-373

Steare SE, Yellon DM. The protective effect of heat stress against reperfusion arrhythmias in the rat. J

Mol Cell Cardiol 1993;27:65-74

Steare SE, Yellon DM. Increased endogenous catalase activity caused by heat stress does not protect the isolated heart against hydrogen peroxide. Cardiovasc Res 1994;28:1096-1101

Steare SE, Yellon DM. The potential for endogenous myocardial antioxidants to protect the myocardium against ischaemia-reperfusion injury: refreshing the parts exogenous antioxideants cannot reach? J Mol Cell Cardiol 1995;27:65-74

Wall SR, Fliss H, Korecky B. Role of catalase in myocardial protection against ischemia in heat shocked rats. Mol Cell Biochem 1993;129:187-194

White FP. Differences in protein synthesized in vivo and in vitro y cells associated with the cerebral mirovasculature. A protein synthesized in response to trauma? Neuroscience 1980;5:1793-1799

Williams RS, Thomas JA, Fina M, German Z, Benjamin IJ. Human heat shock protein 70 (hsp70) protects murine cells from injury during metabolic stress. J Clin Invest 1993;92:503-508

Yellon DM, Latchman DS. Stress proteins and myocardial protection. J Mol Cell Cardiol 1992;24:113-124

Yellon DM, Pasini E, Cargnoni A, Marber MS, Latchman DS, Ferrari R. The protective role of heat stress in the ischaemic and reperfused rabbit myocardium. J Mol Cell Cardiol 1992;24:895-907

5

CHANGES IN HEAT SHOCK PROTEINS IN CARDIAC HYPERTROPHY

Shogen Isoyama, M.D.
First Department of Internal Medicine, Tohoku University School of Medicine, Sendai 980-77, Japan

Address for Correspondence: Shogen Isoyama, M.D.
First Department of Internal Medicine, Tohoku University School of Medicine
1-1 Seiryo-machi, Aoba-ku, Sendai 980-77, Japan
Tel 81-22-717-7153
Fax 81-22-717-7156

INTRODUCTION

Hearts or myocytes respond immediately to various types of stimuli, which are either nontrophic or trophic to myocytes, with the induction of heat shock proteins (HSPs) and many other genes. For example, the induction of HSPs is observed after an episode of ischemia or hypoxia to which the heart does not usually respond with myocyte hypertrophy, and after pressure- or volume-overload to which the heart responds with hypertrophy, later. In addition, not only HSPs but also many other genes such as proto-oncogenes are usually induced. It is unclear whether the induction of HSPs is essential for the development of myocardial hypertrophy, or whether HSPs have a role in the development of myocardial hypertrophy in combination with other genes.

After the establishment of myocardial hypertrophy, many alterations in myocardial function and structure and in the regulation of gene induction occur. How the myocardium is altered depends on what types of stimuli have caused the hypertrophy, i. e., pressure- or volume-overload, exercise or hormonal stimulation. It also depends on whether the model of myocardial hypertrophy is genetic or nongenetic. Therefore, HSP induction may be modulated by the presence of myocardial hypertrophy in a type-specific manner.   If HSPs have a protective role against cell injury by various kinds of stress, the high vulnerability to ischemia of the heart hypertrophied by pressure-overload may be correlated with alterations in HSP induction.

The purpose of this chapter is to discuss the induction of HSPs by trophic stimuli, its role in the development of myocardial hypertrophy, and alterations of HSP induction in established myocardial hypertrophy.

HSP INDUCTION DURING THE DEVELOPMENT OF MYOCARDIAL HYPERTROPHY

Mechanical Stimulus for the Induction of HSPs or Myocardial Hypertrophy

In vivo Hearts

As summarized in Table 1, the induction of HSPs by mechanical overload has been studied in three types of experimental models: in vivo hearts, isolated perfused hearts and cultured myocytes.   In an in vivo experimental model of rodents, HSPs and proto-oncogenes were induced in the heart immediately after imposition of pressure-overload by aortic constriction, and, later, myocardial hypertrophy was induced with isoform shifts in myosin and alpha-actin (Delcayre et al., 1988; Izumo et al.,1988; Komuro et al., 1988; Nadal-Ginard and Mahdavi, 1989; Snoeckx et al., 1991; Takahashi et al., 1992).

The onset and rate of a pressure increase depend on the type of experimental model: an abrupt increase in the ascending aortic banding model and a gradual increase in the banding model of the abdominal aorta or the renal artery, or the model of renal wrapping. The time-course of changes in HSP induction will depend upon the way the arterial pressure is increased.   In the rat model of ascending aortic banding, HSP70 mRNA was detected within 30 minutes, and reached to very high levels in 2 to 3 hours (Izumo et al., 1988).   This rapid induction of HSP70 mRNA is similar to that by coronary occlusion (Knowlton et al., 1991a; Nitta et al., 1994).   As for the HSP induction at the protein level, immunohistological examination revealed that HSP70 as well as other HSPs of 68 and 58 kD were detected in myocytes 3 hours after ascending aortic banding in association with the induction of c-fos, and that the protein disappeared 12 hours later (Snoeckx et al., 1991).   In the study of Delcayre et al. (1988), HSP70 was detected in myocytes isolated from hearts with ascending aortic banding or aortic regurgitation for 2 to 4 days.   The HSP synthesis was no longer observed 7 days after aortic banding (Delcayre et al., 1988). In in vivo hearts, HSP70 was induced not only in the myocytes but also in the nonmuscle cells after hemodynamic or surgical stress (Snoeckx et al., 1991).

Table I

Model	Mechanical Load	Reponses	References
In Vivo Hearts	Coarctation	HSPs	Delcayre et al. 1988
		c-fos, c-myc	Snoeckx et al. 1991
		c-jun, c-Ha-ras	Takahashi et al. 1992
			Komuro et al. 1988
			Izumo et al. 1988
	Aortic Regurgitation	HSPs	Delcayre et al. 1988
	Coronary Occlusion	HSPs, Proto-oncogenes	Nitta et al. 1994
Isolated Hearts	Increased Perfusion	c-fos, c-myc, HSP68(70)	Bauters et al. 1988
		MHC isoform	Delcayre et al. 1992
		Amino Acid Incorporation	Kira et al. 1984
	Increased Systolic/ Diastolic Pressure	c-fos, c-myc, c-jun	Shida et al. 1993
			Schunkert et al. 1991
	Decreased Fiber Shortening	Induction of HSP 70	Knowlton et al. 1991b
	Stretch of Ventricular Wall	HSP 70	Knowlton et al. 1991b
Cultured Myocytes	Stretch	No Induction of HSP 70	Izumo et al. 1988
		c-fos, c-jun	Komuro et al. 1990,91
	Deformation	Growth	Mann et al. 1989
	Contraction		McDermott et al. 1989
	Hypoxia	HSP 70	Iwaki et al. 1993

What component of mechanical overload in vivo is responsible for the induction of HSPs or myocardial hypertrophy?   Aortic constriction in vivo includes the elevation of coronary perfusion pressure and systolic left ventricular pressure, possibly myocardial ischemia, especially in the endomyocardium,   and neurohormonal changes such as the elevation of circulating catecholamine levels and activation of circulating and   local renin-angiotensin system.   Aortic regurgitation increases diastolic and systolic wall stress, and possibly causes myocardial ischemia due to reduced aortic diastolic pressure and increased myocardial oxygen demand (Isoyama et al., 1988). Neurohormonal activation by hemodynamic overload would have additive or synergistic effects on the induction of HSPs as in the case of proto-oncogene induction by combined stimulation of hemodynamic overload and norepinephrine (Kolbeck-Ruhmkorff et al.,1995).   How each of those components activates HSP induction is discussed below.

Isolated, perfused hearts

How systolic or diastolic pressure/wall stress, fiber shortening by contraction, stretch of the ventricular wall and the perfusion condition affect the induction of HSPs or proto-oncogenes has been studied using an isolated, perfused heart preparation. There are several advantages in the isolated perfused heart preparation.   First, the hearts are free from the circulating hormonal and central neural control, and therefore, it is easy to minimize or negate the neurohormonal effects on the gene induction. Second, the coronary perfusion condition can be independent of the pressure generation by ventricles.

In isolated, isovolumically contracting hearts, the proto-oncogene (c-jun, c-fos and c-myc) mRNA levels could be correlated with the increase in developed pressure or systolic and diastolic wall stress (Schunkert et al., 1991; Shida and Isoyama, 1993). A greater increase in systolic wall stress produced by inflating a balloon in the left ventricle elevated mRNAs to higher levels.   Furthermore, Kolbeck-Ruhmkorff and Zimmer (1995) reported that simultaneous increases in preload and afterload resulted in an earlier, more pronounced and longer-lasting induction of c-fos and c-myc mRNAs in working rat hearts perfused with crystalloid solution.   However, the absence of increased induction of proto-oncogene mRNAs by the inflation of a balloon in the left ventricle under a noncontractile state resulted from the prevention of systolic cross-bridge cycling and force generation (Schunkert et al.,1991).   Thus, an increase in systolic pressure or wall stress is an important factor which determines the mRNA levels of immediate-early response genes, but an increase in diastolic pressure or wall stress alone does not seem to be an inducer of those genes.   However, there are no reports showing a correlation between the changes in systolic or diastolic pressure/wall stress and the level of HSP induction.

Using an isolated, perfused heart preparation, several investigators have reported a relationship between the perfusion condition and the induction of HSPs and/or proto-oncogenes. Changes in the perfusion condition implicate the two important stimuli for the gene induction: ischemia by reduction of the perfusate flow and mechanical (erectile) effects on myocytes by increased perfusion pressure. Many studies have shown that brief zero-flow ischemia induces HSPs in in vivo hearts (Iwabuchi et al., 1996; Knowlton et al., 1991a; Mestril and Dillman, 1995; Nitta et al., 1994; Tajima and Isoyama, 1995). In isolated, erythrocyte-perfused hearts, Knowlton et al. (1991b) failed to observe an effect of long-lasting low-flow ischemia (85-90% decrease in flow) by reduction of the perfusion pressure on the HSP70 mRNA induction, probably because the mRNA had been already maximally induced by factors other than ischemia. Thus, the induction of HSPs by ischemia has not been demonstrated in isolated hearts.

Considering the HSP induction by ischemia in in vivo hearts and by hypoxia in cultured myocytes (Iwaki et al., 1993), it is easy to suppose that both types of ischemia, low- and zero-flow ischemia, are potent inducers, even in isolated hearts.

In hearts perfused with crystalloid solution, an elevation of the perfusion pressure from 60 to 120 mm Hg increased the induction of mRNAs coding for c-fos and c-myc genes (Bauters et al., 1988; Delcayre et al., 1992) and HSP68 (Delcayre et al., 1992; Swynghedauw et al., 1990) in either beating or arrested hearts. The elevation of perfusion pressure also increased beta-myosin heavy chain mRNA induction and the synthesis rate of total proteins or myosin heavy chain measured by amino acid incorporation (Delcayre et al., 1992; Kira et al., 1984). The flow rates of the perfusate are much higher in hearts perfused with crystalloid solution than in in vivo hearts. Therefore, the effects of elevated perfusion pressure in hearts perfused with crystalloid solution might be overestimated if a high flow rate affects the gene induction through the garden hose effect.

Knowlton et al. (1991b) reported that single stretch by placement of a drainage cannula through the apex of the left ventricle resulted in a three fold increase in HSP70 mRNA. A decrease in systolic fiber shortening by inflating a balloon in the left ventricle elevated the level further. In this study, however, the effect of myocardial fiber shortening on the gene induction was not examined between hearts with and without fiber shortening at the same diastolic pressure.

Cultured Myocytes

The myocardial tissue consists of various types of cells in addition to myocytes: endocardial and vascular endothelial cells, vascular smooth muscle cells, fibroblasts, and so on. These cells would respond to mechanical stimuli and may then modify the response of myocytes. The effect of mechanical stimuli on the induction of HSPs or other genes has been studied in cultured neonatal myocytes grown on a stretchable substrate in a serum-free medium, thereby minimizing the effect of other cells (Komuro et al.,1990;1991; 1993; Sadoshima et al., 1992). Deformation or stretching of myocytes (20% in length), the contractile action induced by electrical pacing and a hypoxic environment are suggested to be primary stimuli responsible for the induction of myocardial hypertrophy (Mann et al., 1989; McDermott and Morgan, 1989). In contrast to observations at the organ level, the stretching of myocytes induced mRNAs of proto-oncogenes such as c-fos, c-jun and c-myc, but did not induce HSP70 mRNA in the study of Izumo et al. (1988). They suggested that these differing results between the organ and the cell level might be derived from the differences in the oxygenation conditions of the myocytes in the two experimental models. Myocytes, especially in the endomyocardium of pressure-overloaded hearts in vivo, might be hypoxic because of increased oxygen demand and/or perfusion abnormalities by compression of the coronary vasculature, while cultured myocytes might not be so hypoxic during stretch. Sadoshima et al. (1993) and Kojima et al. (1994) reported that angiotensin II released by stretching cultured neonatal myocytes affects their growth through an autocrine mechanism. This autocrine mechanism may also modulate the HSP induction after imposition of mechanical overload. It is unclear whether observations in neonatal or fetal myocytes can be extrapolated to those in adult myocytes or hearts.

Nonmechanical Stimulus for the Induction of HSPs

Stimulation by hormones which have trophic effects on myocytes induces HSPs. Knowlton et al. (1995) observed that T_3 treatment increased the induction of HSP70 24-48 hours after the initiation of treatment, and that this preceded the development of hypertrophy. This increase in HSP70 mRNA was much later than that reported with aortic banding. In the study of Moalic et al. (1989), alpha-adrenergic stimulation by phenylephrine infusion, or vasopressin infusion has been observed to induce mRNAs of HSP70 and 68 as well as c-myc and c-fos genes. In this study, however, it is unclear how the elevation of arterial blood pressure modified the gene induction. In hearts with pressure- or volume-overload by aortic consriction or regurgitation, it is very likely that catecholamines elevated by hemodynamic changes or surgical stress play a role in the induction of HSPs, since the combination of hormonal stimulation by norepinephrine in the perfusate and mechanical load has been shown to have an additive effect on proto-oncogene induction (Kolbeck-Ruhmkorff and Zimmer, 1995).

Exercise in the Induction of HSPs

Chronic exercise is one of the inducers of myocardial hypertrophy. Single bouts of running exercise induced HSP70 mRNA in rat hearts (Locke et al., 1990; 1995). Exercise causes alterations in many aspects: an increase in the hemodynamic load for the heart, activation of hormonal (adrenergic) conditions, elevation of body temperature, an increase in intracellular calcium, changes in blood and tissue pH and so on. It is unclear what component(s) of exercise is responsible for the HSP induction.

The Role of HSPs in the Induction of Myocardial Hypertrophy

In a study of cultured myocytes, stretching induced mRNAs of proto-oncogenes such as c-fos, c-jun, c-myc, Egr-1 and JE, but did not induce HSP70 mRNA (Sadoshima et al., 1992). At the organ level, however, the induction of HSP70 is temporally associated with that of immediate-early response genes following the application of stimuli independently of whether these result in the hypertrophic growth of myocytes. Also, it has been immunohistologically observed that HSP70 and c-fos were often colocalized in the same nuclei of myocytes (Snoeckx et al., 1991). The induction of HSPs and proto-oncogenes is not an obligatory process for the development of myocyte hypertrophy, as has been reported in the case of proto-oncogene induction by the addition of extracellular ATP into the medium for the culture of neonatal myocytes (Zheng et al., 1994). In addition, transient stimuli are sufficient for the gene induction as discussed above, but not for the development of myocardial hypertrophy. The functional significance of HSP70 in pathways that modulate the growth of the heart remains to be determined. The concomitant induction of HSPs with proto-oncogenes such as c-fos and c-myc may be coincidental, or, as suggested in other biological systems, it may reflect synergistic actions (Kingston et al., 1984; Milarski et al., 1989; Nadal-Ginard and Mahdavi, 1989; Sanders and Benjamin 1991).

HSP INDUCTION IN ESTABLISHED CARDIAC HYPERTROPHY

Cardiac Hypertrophy in a Genetically Hypertensive Model

It is known that genetically hypertensive animals have greater sensitivity to changes in the environmental temperature. In spontaneously hypertensive rats, the body temperature was more easily elevated compared with Wistar-Kyoto rats, probably because of a thermoregulation abnormality (Malo et al., 1989). In genetically hypertensive animals, the overinduction of HSP70 mRNA was observed in hearts as well as in other organs such as the brain and kidney (Hamet et al., 1990; Iwabuchi et al., 1996) when the whole body was subjected to high environmental temperature. This greater thermosensitivity resulted not only from changes in the thermoregulation of the whole body, but also from properties at the cell level. In a culture system, the overinduction was also observed in fibroblasts (Lukashev et al., 1991) and aortic smooth muscle cells (Hashimoto et al., 1991) obtained from spontaneously hypertensive rats, and in lymphocytes obtained from hypertensive human, especially in women (Kunes et al., 1992). The increased thermosensitivity is genetically linked to hypertension and is characterized by an overinduction of heat shock proteins at the molecular level. The induction was decreased with age from the developmental (2 months), matured (6 months) and to the old phase (18 months). The overinduction of HSP70 by thermal stimulation was observed in all age groups (Bongrazio et al., 1994).

Recently, the present author and co-workers have examined whether the hearts of spontaneously hypertensive rats respond with the overinduction of HSP70 to stimuli other than heat (Iwabuchi et al., 1996). The chest was opened under general anesthesia and artificial ventilation, and a snare was placed around the coronary arterial branches. Seven days later, brief coronary occlusion (5 minutes) was applied without chest opening. The overinduction of HSP70 and HSC70 (heat shock cognate protein 70, or constitutive HSP70) mRNAs was also observed after the application of coronary occlusion in spontaneously hypertensive rats vs. Wistar-Kyoto Rats. The overinduction of HSPs may be a general response to other types of stimuli in spontaneously hypertensive rats. Given the overinduction of HSPs at the protein level after thermal stimulation (Bongrazio et al., 1994) and at the mRNA level after coronary occlusion (Iwabuchi et al., 1996), the main cause of the overinduction of HSPs seems to be activation of the transcriptional process.

HSPS IN A NONGENETIC MODEL OF CARDIAC HYPERTROPHY

The induction of HSP70 and HSC70 in established, pressure overload-type cardiac hypertrophy was examined after application of brief ischemia (Tajima and Isoyama, 1995). In Wistar rats, the chest was opened under general anesthesia and artificial ventilation, and the ascending aorta was banded so that the internal diameter of the ascending aorta was 1.4 mm. The peak systolic left ventricular pressure measured 4 weeks later was increased to nearly 200 mm Hg (Isoyama et al., 1989; Sato et al., 1990). Four-week banding produced left ventricular hypertrophy at the cellular (23% increases in myocyte width above controls) and organ level (25% increases in left ventricular muscle weight/body weight ratio above controls). During the procedures for aortic banding a snare was created around the left coronary arterial branches with a nylon thread and a small polyethylene tube (Nitta et al., 1994). The end of the thread and one side of the tube was placed just under the skin and the chest was closed. Five-minute ischemia was applied without opening the chest under diethyl-ether anesthesia. Although both ascending aortic banding and surgical stress could have induced HSPs in the early phase of pressure-overload as discussed above, the induction of HSP70 mRNA or protein was not detected 4 weeks after the surgery.

In hearts without myocardial hypertrophy the induction of HSP70 mRNA was detected 0.5 hours after the application of 5-minute ischemia, peaked at 1 hour, and declined thereafter. Compared with normal hearts, the induction peaked more rapidly (0.5 hours after ischemia) in hypertrophied hearts, and declined thereafter. More interestingly, HSP70 mRNA induction was substantially attenuated in hypertrophied hearts. The HSP induction at the protein level was also attenuated in parallel with the attenuation of mRNA induction. However, this attenuation in cardiac hypertrophy was dependent on the severity of ischemia. When a longer duration of ischemia (10-minute ischemia) was applied, HSP70 and HSC70 mRNAs in hypertrophied hearts was induced to a level similar to that in non-hypertrophied hearts. As for the induction of HSC70 by brief ischemia, the severity-dependent attenuation was also observed in hypertrophied hearts at the mRNA level. As in the case of HSP70, the induction in hypertrophied hearts peaked more rapidly compared with that in nonhypertrophied hearts, and declined thereafter.

At present, there are no data available concerning how the induction of HSPs is altered in hearts hypertrophied by volume-overload, exercise or hormonal stimulation,.

HSPS IN CARDIAC HYPERTROPHY OF AGED MAMMALS

In the aged heart, myocyte loss occurs and the remaining cells are hypertrophic. This loss and hypertrophy is remarkable in the left ventricle (Isoyama, 1996; Lakatta, 1993). The HSP induction in cardiac hypertrophy of aged mammals has been studied after thermal stimulation and application of brief ischemia (Isoyama, 1996; Nitta et al., 1994). The studies revealed that HSP induction at the mRNA and protein level was attenuated in hearts as well as in other cells or organs such as fibroblasts, neutrophils, smooth muscle cells, hepatocytes, brain, skin, liver, adrenal gland, lung, aorta and kidney (Isoyama, 1996).

In the rat heart, 10-minute ischemia, which was applied without chest opening, induced the HSP70 and HSC70 mRNAs. The level of HSP70 mRNA peaked 2 hours after the application and declined thereafter. On the other hand, HSC70 mRNA peaked at 4 hours and gradually declined thereafter. The induction of both HSP70 and HSC70 mRNAs was attenuated in aged hearts (18 months of age), compared with that in young hearts (2 months of age). The time course of changes was similar to that in young hearts. When 20-minute ischemia was applied, HSP70 and HSC70 mRNAs were induced to a similar level in young hearts. Thus, the age-related attenuation was observed after brief ischemia, but was not observed after more severe ischemia. In addition, the mRNA induced after more severe ischemia was linked to the translational process in aged hearts. Twenty-four hours after the application of ischemia, Western blotting revealed that HSP70 was induced to a level comparable to that in young hearts. Immunohistological study showed that each myocyte responded to ischemia with the induction of HSP70. Therefore, the age-related attenuation seems to result from the characteristics of each myocyte, but not from a decrease in the number of responding myocytes. It is not clear how adult-aging modifies the HSP induction in the heart by extracardiac factors in vivo.

It is not clear whether the age-related attenuation in the induction of HSPs by thermal stimulation or ischemia resulted from the adult-aging of the heart per se or from the presence of myocardial hypertrophy produced as a result of adult-aging. Probably, both of them would be rsponsible for the attenuation in the induction of HSPs in aged hearts, considering the fact that, in the right ventricle in which age-related myocardial hypertrophy is relatively moderate, attenuated hypertrophic responses to pressure overload are also observed (Kuroha et al., 1991).

Of interest, the attenuation in the aged organs disappeared after stimulation by much higher temperatures (Blake et al., 1991). This severity-dependent attenuation in the aged organs is consistent with the HSP induction by ischemia in hearts (Nitta et al., 1994), and with the proto-oncogene induction by hemodynamic stress in hearts hypertrophied by pressure-overload (Tajima et al., 1995).

BIOLOGICAL ROLE OF HSPS IN ESTABLISHED CARDIAC HYPERTROPHY

From the Framingham study it has been shown that myocardial hypertrophy is one of the major risk factors for such cardiac events as sudden death, myocardial infarction and heart failure (Levy et al., 1990). In animal hearts with myocardial hypertrophy, coronary occlusion induced a greater necrotic area relative to risk area, compared with that in hearts without hypertrophy (Marcus et al., 1987). Several mechanisms responsible for the higher vulnerability to ischemia in hypertrophied hearts have been suggested: abnormalities in the coronary circulation such as decreased dilator reserve and impaired autoregulation of coronary blood flow (Isoyama et al., 1989; 1992; Marcus et al., 1987; Sato et al., 1990), alterations in energy metabolism (Snoeckx et al., 1990) and a diminution of oxygen-radical scavengers (Batist et al., 1989).

A number of studies support the claim that HSP70 provides protection against the effects of oxygen deprivation such as ischemia and hypoxia in the hearts of several animal species, including humans. Although the exact mechanism of HSP70-mediated cardiac protection is not entirely clear, the most popular hypotheses are (i) the specific reduction of oxygen-free radical damage and (ii) the maintenance of intracellular homeostasis and protein folding. The attenuation in HSP70 induction therefore could contribute to higher vulnerability to hemodynamic stress such as ischemia in hearts hypertrophied by pressure-overload (Levy et al., 1990) and in aged hearts (Weisfeldt et al., 1992). It is also known that the hearts of genetically hypertensive animals are vulnerable to ischemia. It is difficult to consider the overinduction of HSP70 in hearts of genetically hypertensive animals as a detrimental phenomenon. Further studies are needed to clarify the pathophysiological significance of the overinduction of HSP70 in such hearts.

CONCLUSION

In this chapter, the induction of HSPs by trophic stimuli and the role of HSPs in the development of myocardial hypertrophy were discussed. Immediately (at least within 30 minutes) after the imposition of pressure- or volume-overload, or exercise, HSP mRNAs are induced with mRNAs of other types of genes such as proto-oncogenes in the rodent heart. Several hours later, the synthesis of HSPs at the protein level are detected, but are not detected several days after the imposition of stimuli. Although this process at the molecular level mimics the proliferation process of other cells, the induction of HSPs may not be essential for the development of myocardial hypertrophy.

In established myocardial hypertrophy, the HSP induction by heat or ischemia is altered: it was upregulated in a genetic model of hypertension and downregulated in a nongenetic (coarctation) model, and in aged subjects. Further studies are needed to clarify the biological significance of this difference of induction in the two models of hypertrophy.

ACKNOWLEDGEMENT

This study was partly supported by Grant-in-Aid for Scientific Research (No. 06670688) from the Ministry of Education, Science and Culture of Japan.

REFERENCES

Batist G, Mersereau W, Malashenko B-A, Chiu RC-J. Response to ischemia-reperfusion injury in hypertrophic heart. Role of free-radical metabolic pathways. Circulation 1989;80 (suppl III):III-10-III-13

Bauters C, Moalic JM, Bercovici J, Mouas C, Emanoil-Ravier R, Schiaffino S, Swyghedauw B: Coronary flow as a determinant of c-myc and c-fos proto-oncogene expression in an isolated adult heart. J Mol Cell Cardiol 1988;20:97-101

Blake MJ, Fargnoli J, Gershon D, Holbrook NJ. Concomitant decline in heat-induced hyperthermia and HSP70 mRNA expression in aged rats. Am J Physiol 1991;260 (Regulatory Integrative Comp Physiol 29):R663-667

Bongrazio M, Comini L, Gaia G, Bachetti T, Ferrari R . Hypertension, aging, and myocardial synthesis of heat-shock protein 72. Hypertension 1994;24: 620-624

Delcayre C, Samuel J-L, Marrotte F, Best-Belpomme M, Mercadier J J, Rappaport L. Synthesis of stress proteins in rat cardiac myocytes 2-4 days after imposition of hemodynamic overload. J Clin Invest 1988; 82:460-468

Delcayre C, Klug D, Thien NV, Mouas C, Swynghedauw B. Aortic perfusion as early determinant of beta-isomyosin expression in perfused hearts. Am J Physiol 1992;263 (Heart Circ Physiol 32):H1537-H1545

Hamet P, Malo D, Tremblay J. Increased transcription of a major stress gene in spontaneously hypertensive mice. Hypertension 1990;15:904-908

Hashimoto T, Mosser RD, Tremblay J, Hamet P. Increased accumulation of hsp70 messenger RNA due to enhanced activation of heat-shock transcription factor in spontaneously hypertensive rats. J Hypertens 1991;9 (suppl 6):S170-S171

Isoyama S, Grossman W, Wei JY: Effects of age on myocardial adaptation to volume-overload in the rat. J Clin Invest 1988;81:1850-1857

Isoyama S, Ito N, Kuroha M, Takishima T. Complete reversibility of physiological coronary vacular abnormalities in hypertrophied hearts produced by pressure-overload in the rat. J Clin Invest 1989;84:288-294

Isoyama S, Ito N, Satoh K, Takishima T. Collagen deposition and the reversal of coronary reserve in cardiac hypertrophy. Hypertension 1992;20:491-500

Isoyama S. Age-related changes before and after imposition of hemodynamic stress in the mammalian heart. Life Sci 1996; 58:1601-1614

Iwabuchi K, Isoyama S, Tajima M. unpublished data.

Iwaki K, Chi S-H, Dillmann WH, Mestril R. Induction of HSP70 in cultured rat neonatal cardiocytes by hypoxia and metabolic stress. Circulation 1993;87:2023-2032

Izumo S, Nadal-Ginard B, Mahdavi V (1988) Protooncogene induction and reprogramming of cardiac gene expression produced by pressure overload. Proc Natl Acad Sci USA 1988;85:339-343

Kingston RE, Baldwin AS Jr, Sharp PA: Regulation of heat shock protein 70 gene expression by c-myc. Nature 1984;312:280-282

Kira Y, Kochel PJ, Gordon EE, Morgan HE. Aortic pressure as a determinant of cardiac protein synthesis. Am J Physiol 1984;246 (Cell Physiol 15):C247-C258

Knowlton AA, Brecher P, Apstein CS. Rapid expression of heat shock protein in the rabbit after brief cardiac ischemia. J Clin Invest 1991a;87:139-147

Knowlton AA, Eberli FR, Brecher P, Romo GM, Owen A, Apstein CS. A single myocardial stretch or decreased systolic fiber shortening stimulates the expression of heat shock protein 70 in the isolated, erythrocyte-perfused rabbit heart. J Clin Invest 1991b;88:2018-2025

Knowlton AA. The role of heat shock proteins in the heart. J Mol Cell Cardiol 1995; 27:121-131

Kojima M, Shiojima I, Yamazaki T, Komuro I, Yunzeng Z, Ying W, Mizuno T, Ueki K, Tobe K, Kadowaki T, Nagai R, Yazaki Y. Angiotensin II receptor agonist TCV-116 induces regression of hypertensive left ventricular hypertrophy in vivo and inhibits intracellular signaling pathway of stretch-mediated cardio-myocyte hypertrophy in vitro. Circulation 1994;89:2204-2211

Kolbeck-Ruhmkorff C, Zimmer H-G. Proto-oncogene expression in the isolated working rat heart: combination of pressure and volume overload with norepinephrine. J Mol Cell Cardiol 1995,27:501-511

Komuro I, Kurabayashi M, Takaku F, Yazaki Y. Expression of cellular oncogenes in the myocardium during the developmental stage and pressure-overloaded hypertrophy of the rat heart. Circ Res 1988;62:1075-1079

Komuro I, Kaida T, Shibasaki Y, Kurabayashi M, Katoh Y, Hoh E, Takaku F, Yazaki Y: Stretching cardiac myocytes stimulates protooncogene expression. J Biol Chem 1990;265:3591-3598

Komuro I, Katoh Y, Kaida T, Shibazaki Y, Kurabayashi M, Hoh E, Takaku F, Yazaki Y. Mechanical loading stimulates cell hypertrophy and specific gene expression in cultured rat cardiac myocytes. J Biol Chem 1991;266:1265-1268

Komuro I, Yazaki I. Control of cardiac gene expression by mechanical stress. Annu Rev Physiol 1993;55:55-75

Kunes J, Poirier M, Tremblay J, Hamet P. Expression of hsp70 gene in lymphocytes from normotensive and hypertensive humans. Acta Physiol Scand 1992;146:307-311

Kuroha M, Isoyama S, Ito N, Takishima T. Effects of age on right ventricular hypertrophic response to pressure-overload in rats. J Mol Cell Cardiol 1991;23:1177-1190

Lakatta EG. Cardiovascular regulatory mechanisms in advanced age. Physiol Rev 1993;73:413-467

Levy D, Garrison RJ, Savage DD, Kannel WB, Castelli WP. Prognostic implications of echocardiographically determined left ventricular mass in the Framingham Heart Study. N Engl J Med 1990;322:1561-1566

Locke M, Noble EG, Atkinson BG. Exercising mammals synthesize stress proteins. Am J Physiol 1990;258(Cell Physiol 27):C723-C729

Locke M, Noble EG, Tanguay RM, Feild MR, Ianuzzo SE, Ianuzzo CD. Activation of heat-shock transcription factor in rat heart after heat shock and exercise. Am J Physiuol 1995;268 (Cell Physiol 37):C1387-C1394

Lukashev ME, Klimanskaya IV, Postnov YV. Synthesis of heat-shock proteins in cultured fibroblasts from normotensive and spontaneously hypertensive rat embryos. J Hypertens 1991;9(suppl 6):S182-S183

Malo D, Schlager G, Tremblay J, Hamet P. Thermosensitivity, a possible new locus involved in genetic hypertension. Hypertension 1989;14:121-128

Mann DL, Kent RL, Cooper G IV: Load regulation of the properties of adult feline cardiocytes: growth induction by cellular deformation. Circ Res 1989;64:1079-1090

Marcus ML, Harrison DG, Chilian WM, Koyanagi S, Inou T, Tomanek RJ, Martins JB, Eastham CL, Hiratzka LF. Alterations in the coronary circulation in hypertrophied ventricles. Circulation 1987;75 (suppl I):I-19-I-25

McDermott PJ, Morgan HE. Contraction modulates the capacity for protein synthesis during growth of neonatal heart cells in culture. Circ Res 1989;64:542-553

Mestril R, Dillmann WH. Heat shock proteins and protection against myocardial ischemia. J Mol Cell Cardiol 1995;27:45-52

Milarski KL, Welch WJ, Morimoto RI: Cell cycle-dependent association of HSP70 with specific cellular proteins. J Cell Biol 1989;108:413-423

Moalic JM, Bauters C, Himbert D, Bercovici J, Mouas C, Guicheney P, Baudoin-Legros M, Rappaport L, Emanoil-Ravier R, Mezger V, Swynghedauw B: Phenylephrine, vasopressin and angiotensin II as determinants of proto-oncogene and heat shock protein gene expression in adult rat heart and aorta. J Hypertens 1989; 7:195-201

Nadal-Ginard B, Mahdavi V: Molecular basis of cardiac performance. Plasticity of the myocardium generated through protein isoform switches. J Clin Invest 1989;84:1693-1700

Nitta Y, Abe K, Aoki M, Ohno I, Isoyama S. Diminished heat shock protein 70 mRNA induction in aged rat hearts after ischemia. Am J Physiol 1994;267 (Heart Circ Physiol 36):H1795-H1803

Rothman JE. GTP and methionine bristles. Nature 1989;340:433-434

Sadoshima J, Jahn L, Takahashi T, Kulik TJ, Izumo S. Molecular characterization of the stretch-induced adaptation of cultured cardiac cells. An in vitro model of load-induced cardiac hypertrophy. J Biol Chem 1992; 267:10551-10560

Sadoshima J, Xu Y, Slayter H, Izumo S. Autocrine release of angiotensin II mediates stretch-induced hypertrophy of cardiac myocytes in vitro. Cell 1993;75:977-984

Sanders W, Benjamin IJ: Stress proteins and cardiovascular disease. Mol Biol Med 1991;8:197-206

Sato F, Isoyama S, Takishima T. Normalization of impaired coronary circulation in hypertrophied rat hears. Hypertension 1990;16:26-34

Schunkert H, Jahn L, Izumo S, Apstein CS, Lorell BH. Localization and regulation of c-fos anf c-jun protooncogene induction by systolic wall stress in normal and hypertrophied rat hearts. Proc Natl Acad Sci USA 1991;88:11480-11484

Shida M, Isoyama S. Effects of age on c-fos and c-myc gene expression in response to hemodynamic stress in isolated perfused rat hearts. J Mol Cell Cardiol 1993;25:1025-1035

Snoeckx LHEH, van der Vusse GJ, Counans WA, Reneman RS. The effects of global ischemia and reperfusion on compensated hypertrophied rat hearts. J Mol Cell Cardiol 1990;22:1439-1452

Snoeckx LHEH, Contard F, Samuel JL, Marotte F, Rappaport L. Expression and cellular distribution of heat-shock and nuclear oncogene proteins in rat hearts. Am J Physiol 1991;261 (Heart Circ Physiol 30):H1443-H1451

Swynghedauw B, Moalic JM, Delcayre C. "The origin of cardiac hypertrophy." In *Cardiac Hypertrophy and Failure*, Swynghedauw B ed. INSERM/John Libbey Eurotext, Montrouge, France: 1990.

Tajima M, Isoyama S. The effect of ACE inhibitor or AT1 blocker treatment on HSP expression after ischemia in hypertrophied hearts. J Mol Cell Cardiol 1995;27:A514

Takahashi T, Schunkert H, Isoyama S, Wei JY, Nadal-Ginard B, Grossma W, Izumo S: Age-related differences in the expression of proto-oncogene and contractile protein genes in response to pressure overload in the rat myocarium. J Clin Invest 1992;89:939-946

Weisfeldt ML, Lakatta EG, Gerstenblith G. "Aging and the heart." *In Heart Disease: A textbook of Cardiovascular Medicine*, Braunwald E ed. Saunders, Philadelphia, PA U.S.A.: 1992

Williams RS, Benjamin IJ. Stress proteins and cardiovascular disease. Mol Biol Med 1991;8:197-206

Zheng J-S, Boluyt MO, O'Neill L, Crow MT, Lakatta EG. Extracellular ATP induces immediate-early gene expression but not cellular hypertrophy in neonatal cardiac myocytes. Circ Res 1994;74:1034-1041

6

HEAT SHOCK PROTEIN EXPRESSION IN THE AGING CARDIOVASCULAR SYSTEM

Nikki J. Holbrook, Timothy W. Fawcett, and Robert Udelsman*. Gene Expression and Aging Section, National Institute on Aging, Baltimore, MD 21224 and *Department of Surgery, Johns Hopkins University, Baltimore, MD 21225

Mammalian aging is accompanied by a progressive decline in most physiologic functions and in particular by a decreased ability to maintain homeostasis when faced with conditions of stress (Shock et al., 1984; Martin et al., 1993). The cardiovascular system is no exception as aging constitutes a major risk factor for the development of cardiovascular disease, with the incidence of hypertension, atherosclerosis, stroke and myocardial infarction all increasing markedly with advancing age (Wei and Gersh, 1987; Stout, 1987; Wei, 1992). The mechanisms responsible for these age-related changes are not clear, but significant histological, biochemical and functional alterations occur in both the myocardium (e.g. left ventricular hypertrophy, diminished sensitivity to β-adrenergic hormones, and interstitial fibrosis) and vasculature (e.g. thickening of vessel walls, smooth muscle cell relocation and reduced compliance) with aging (reviewed in Lakatta, 1993; Isoyama et al., 1994; Crow et al., 1996). In addition, and perhaps of greatest significance, elderly patients are much more vulnerable to acute cardiovascular stress. Aged hearts are more susceptible to post ischemic injury than are young hearts, and older individuals display an increased tendency to develop cardiac failure following hemodynamic stress (Isoyama et al., 1994).

Heat shock proteins (HSPs) play a critical role in maintaining cellular homeostasis during episodes of acute stress and serve an adaptive function conferring a survival advantage to cells in situations of continued, repetitive or chronic stress (Craig et al., 1994; Welch, 1993; Morimoto et al., 1994). We hypothesized that the ability to express these stress proteins is a major factor in resistance to disease and aging, and that a diminution of their expression leads to an increased vulnerability to stress. Using a variety of model systems and cell types, we and others have demonstrated that the ability to mount the so-called heat shock response is indeed diminished with aging (for review see Richardson and Holbrook, 1996).   Given the role of HSPs in myocardial protection (addressed throughout this book), it seems likely that an attenuation of HSP expression could contribute to the age-related decline in cardiovascular function. Only recently have studies begun to address the relationship between HSP expression and age-associated cardiovascular dysfunction, and most of these have restricted their examination to members of the HSP70 family.

This chapter will be divided into two parts. In the first we review recent studies demonstrating age-related alterations in HSP70 expression in the heart and relate these changes to alterations in other tissues. In addition, we summarize evidence pointing to a common mechanism accounting for the decline in mammalian age-associated HSP expression. This mechanism is likely to account for changes seen in the heart. In the second part we review our studies examining HSP70 expression in vessels in response to restraint or immobilization stress, focusing on the physiological and molecular mechanisms serving to control the response as well as additional unique factors contributing to its decline during aging.

STRESS-INDUCED HSP EXPRESSION DECLINES IN THE AGED HEART

Several recent studies, using different strains of rats have provided evidence for an age-related decline in heat-induced HSP70 expression in heart tissue. Kregel et al. (1995) compared HSP70 protein levels in left ventricles of mature (12 month old) and aged (24 month old) Fischer 344 rats. In the absence of heat exposure, HSP70 protein levels did not differ significantly between the two age groups although they were somewhat higher in the aged rats. In response to mild heat stress ($41°C$ for 30 min), hearts of mature animals showed a 187% increase in protein levels while those of aged animals increased by only 67%. In another study, Gaia et al. (1995) compared basal and heat-induced HSP70 protein levels in young (2 month) and old (18 month) Wistar Kyoto rats. While they also found no significant differences in basal HSP70 expression (the protein being virtually undetectable in either age group in the absence of stress), in response to hyperthermia ($42°$ C for 15 min), left ventricles of young animals showed approximately 2-fold higher levels of HSP70 protein induction compared to old rats.

The age-related difference in HSP70 expression in the heart is not limited to heat stress, but also occurs with transient ischemic injury. Nitta et al. (1994) examined the kinetics of HSP70 mRNA induction in left ventricles of hearts of young (2 month old) and aged (18 month old) rats following either a 10 or 20 min period of ischemia achieved through occlusion of a coronary artery. Although little HSP70 mRNA was present in hearts of unstressed animals, HSP70 mRNA was markedly induced in young hearts subjected to either 10 or 20 min of ischemia. Aged hearts showed only a slight induction of HSP70 with 10 min of ischemia (peak expression levels were approximately one-sixth those seen in young animals), although a 20 min ischemic insult resulted in a similar level of HSP70 expression in the two age groups. Age-related differences were also observed for HSC70, another member of the HSP70 family, which is expressed constitutively in most tissues but whose expression is also inducible in response to stress. The induction of HSP70 mRNA expression was likewise accompanied by increased expression of HSP70 protein. The fact that aged animals could achieve high levels of HSP70 induction given a longer period of stress led these authors to suggest that aging was associated with a defect in the mechanism responsible for sensing ischemic injury rather than the ability to express HSPs.

Hypertension is associated with many features characteristic of the aged heart. It is well documented that genetically hypertensive animals, such as spontaneously hypertensive rats (SHR) show greater sensitivity to environmental temperatures compared to their normotensive counterparts (McMurty et al., 1981; Hamet et al., 1985). Based on this information one might have expected that SHR rats (even in the absence of aging) would show reduced levels of HSP expression compared to normotensive animals. This, however, is not the case, as several different groups have shown elevated expression of HSP70 in cells and tissues of SHR rats (Hamet et al., 1990; Bongrazio et al., 1994). In comparative studies examining HSP70 induction in response to thermal stress in young versus aged SHR and control rats, Bongrazio et al. (1994) found that young (2 months) SHR responded to hyperthermic stress with 3-4 fold higher levels of HSP70 expression compared to age-matched controls. However, the differences between normo- and hypertensive rats were diminished to about 2-fold in adult rats (6 months) and were totally absent in aged rats (18 months). Thus, an age-related decline in HSP70 expression occurs in both SHR and normotensive controls, but the magnitude of the change is greater in the SHR rats. The basis for the elevated HSP70 expression seen in response to thermal stress in young SHR is unclear, but apparently is not related directly to hypertension since the differences are seen before significant hypertension and myocardial hypertrophy appears in these animals, and is maintained in other SHR tissues that are not directly associated with the hypertensive state (Kunes et al., 1992; Lukashey et al., 1991).

Mechanisms Contributing to the Age-Related Decline in HSP Expression

The finding of an age-related decline in HSP70 expression in the heart is consistent with observations made in a variety of other mammalian tissues as summarized in Table1 for heat stress and reviewed in detail by Richardson and Holbrook (1996).

Table 1. Mammalian Cells and Tissues which Display an Age-Related Reduction in Heat-Induced HSP70 Expression. Studies measured either mRNA or protein expression. See individual references for details.

Strain/Tissue Type	% Decline	References
Human- mononuclear cells	30	Deguchi et al., 1988
Rhesus monkey - splenocytes	75	Pahlavani et al., 1995
Wistar rat - lung and skin	decrease	Fargnoli et al., 1990
Fischer 344 - hippocampus	50-75	Pardue et al., 1992
Fischer 344 - hepatocytes	40-45	Heydari et al., 1993
Fischer 344 - splenocytes	37-52	Pahlavani et al., 1995
Fischer 344 - liver	>40	Kregel et al., 1995
Fischer 344 - heart	25	Kregel et al., 1995
Wistar Kyoto - heart	25	Gaia et al., 1995

An age-related decline in HSP70 expression occurs in response to heat in a variety of mammalian cell types and tissues. As noted above for the heart, the age-related attenuation in HSP expression in other tissues is not limited to heat stress but occurs following exposure to a variety of stressors capable of eliciting the response, e.g. arsenite-induced HSP70 expression in *in vitro* aged fibroblasts (Luce and Cristofalo, 1992), mitogen-induced HSP70 expression in lymphocytes (Faassen et al., 1989; Effros et al., 1994), and restraint-induced HSP expression in the adrenal gland and aorta of rats (Blake et al., 1991, and Udelsman et al., 1993). Although the magnitude of the age-related decline varies between individual tissues and studies, in general the response is reduced by about half in 23-24 month old rats compared to 4-6 month old rats.

The fact that so many tissues display an age-related diminution in HSP expression suggests that the decline reflects an intrinsic component common to all tissues. Stress-induced HSP70 expression is regulated primarily at the level of transcription and is mediated by the heat shock transcription factor 1 (HSF1) which interacts with a specific regulatory element, the heat shock element (HSE), present in the promoters of HSP genes (Baler et al., 1993; Morimoto, 1993). HSF1 is present constitutively , but in an inactive state (i.e non-DNA binding) in the absence of stress. Stress results in the activation of HSF1 to a form that binds the HSE. Although the activation process is still poorly understood, it requires the oligomerization of HSF1 monomers to a trimeric state and is generally associated with hyperphosphorylation of the transcription factor (Baler et al., 1993; Sistonen et al., 1994).

Using nuclear run-on assays, a number of studies have provided evidence that the age-related attenuation in HSP70 expression following heat or other stresses, is associated with reduced transcription of the gene (Heydari et al., 1994; Deguchi et al., 1988; Liu et al., 1989). Furthermore, using gel mobility shift assays, four different model systems have provided evidence that the age-related decline involves reduced binding of HSF1 to DNA. Heydari et al. (1993) showed 40% lower heat stress-induced HSE-binding activity in hepatocytes of old (24 month) rats compared to those of young (4-6 month) rats, while Pahlavani et al. (1995) reported a 55% decline in heat-induced HSE binding activity in old splenocytes compared to their young counterparts. We have observed a significant age-related decline in restraint (immobilization) stress-induced HSF1 DNA-binding in adrenal extracts from two different rat strains; 60% and 40% declines for Fischer 344 and Wistar rats, respectively (Fawcett et al., 1994). Finally, Choi et al. (1990) demonstrated a reduction in HSE binding activity associated with *in vitro* aging of cultured human diploid fibroblasts. Importantly, in all cases the magnitude of change in DNA binding activity is consistent with the reduction seen in HSP expression. Thus, the current data suggest that the reduced ability of cells from old animals to express HSP70 in response to stress occurs because less HSF1 is binding to the HSP70 (or other HSP genes) promoter. Therefore, one must ask why there is less HSF1 binding activity in aged cells? One possibility is simply that HSF1 protein levels decline with age. However, studies comparing HSF1 protein levels in adrenal tissue and hepatocytes of old and young rats, showed no significant differences between the two age-groups. In fact, if anything, the HSF1 levels appear to somewhat higher in aged tissues (Fawcett et al., 1994; Richardson and Holbrook, 1996). An alternative explanation for the reduced DNA binding activity is that, although actual HSF1 protein amounts do not decline with aging, there is a decrease in stress-induced posttranslational activation of HSF1 to a DNA binding form. This decrease in activation could come about either through modification of the HSF1 protein itself which impedes its activation capacity, or alterations in the signaling processes that lead to activation.

Thus, while there are to date no reports in which stress-induced levels of HSF activity have been measured in the hearts of old and young animals, it is likely that the decreased HSP70 expression seen with aging reflects a general decline in DNA binding activity as seen for other tissues.

RESTRAINT-INDUCED HSP EXPRESSION IN VASCULATURE

Several years ago, we demonstrated that restraint or immobilization stress resulted in a marked induction of HSP70 and HSP27 expression in rat aorta (Udelsman et al., 1993). The response was rapid, with maximum mRNA levels achieved within 30 min of placing animals in the restraint devices, and was followed by an increase in HSP70 protein expression which peaked between 3 and 6 h following one hour of restraint (Figure 1). A similar response was found to occur in response to surgical stress (Udelsman et al., 1991). Further characterization of the response revealed that induction was not confined to the aorta, but also occurred in other vessels including the vena cava, although to a lesser extent. Importantly, however, the induction was absent in heart tissue. Interestingly, *in situ* hybridization analysis showed that the vascular expression occurred in the smooth muscle cells of the media with little expression evident in either the luminal endothelial cell layer or external adventitia.

Restraint differs from most stress paradigms used to elicit HSP expression in that it is not associated with overt damage to tissues. Viewed more as a behavioral stress, it has been utilized extensively to induce physiologic stress response syndromes in animals and to examine the central and peripheral mechanisms associated with stress-related

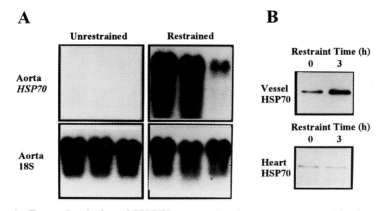

Figure 1. Restraint-induced HSP70 expression in rat aorta. (A) Northern analysis of HSP70 mRNA expression in control rats and rats subjected to 30 min of restraint. (B) Western analysis of HSP70 protein expression in control rats and rats subjected to 30 min of restraint.

disorders such as gastric ulcers (Pare and Glavin, 1986). In our early studies we demonstrated that vascular HSP70 induction following restraint was associated with activation of the sympathetic nervous system. It could be blocked by pretreatment of rats with prasozin (an alpha$_1$ adrenergic blocking agent), and elicited by treatment with phenylephrine, leading us to suggest that the response to restraint was mediated through alpha$_1$ adrenergic receptors. Subsequent studies by others revealed that the response could be mimicked by treatment with other agents such as dopamine and cocaine (Blake et al., 1993; Blake et al., 1994). Since these agents exert their effects through interaction with receptors distinct from the alpha$_1$ adrenoreceptor we began to question whether the induction in the aorta was occurring as a direct response to the treatment, or was in fact occurring secondary to an effect common to all of these agents. Realizing that a universal effect of each of these agents, as well as restraint, is an increase in blood pressure we investigated this relationship more directly.

Evidence that HSP70 is in fact induced in the aorta in response to acute hypertension is supported by a number of observations (Xu et al.,1995). First, as shown in Figure 2, a variety of vasoactive agents (phenylephrine, dopamine, angiotensin II, vasopressin and endothelin), all of which cause acute hypertension, likewise result in HSP70 expression in the aorta. Second, the dose-response relationships and potencies of the agents tested for inducing HSP70 are directly correlated with their relative effects on blood pressure. Third, the vasodilator, sodium nitroprusside, which acts nonspecifically to prevent an increase in blood pressure in response to hypertensive agents, blocked the induction of HSP70 expression. Finally, this *in vivo* response could not be mimicked by treatment of primary smooth muscle cultures with the vasoactive agents.

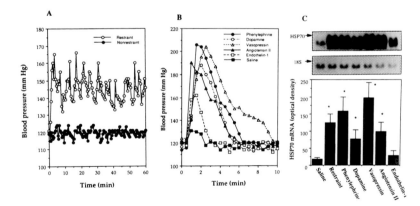

Figure 2. Effects of restraint and hypertensive agents on blood pressure and aortic HSP70 mRNA expression. (A) and (B); systolic blood pressure of Fischer 344 rats during 60 min restraint or following treatment with hypertensive agents. (C) Northern blot analysis of HSP70 mRNA expression. Doses were as follows: phenylephrine, 140 µg/kg; dopamine, 250 µg/kg; vasopressin, 2 µg/kg; angiotensin II, 2 µg/kg; and endothelin-1, 1 µg/kg. N=3 for each treatment group. * indicates values significantly different from control, P<0.05. (Reproduced with permission from Xu et al., 1995).

Additional evidence supporting this view was obtained by Blake et al. (1995) who demonstrated that chronic exposure of rats to restraint, results in an attenuation in both restraint-induced changes in blood pressure and loss in HSP70 induction. Also consistent with our findings are earlier studies by Moalic et al. (1989), who showed that HSP70 mRNA expression was induced in rat aorta following i.v. injection of either phenylephrine, vasopressin, or angiotensin II. However, these investigators proposed that HSP induction occurred as a primary response to ligand-receptor interactions rather than to changes in arterial blood pressure. While we cannot exclude the possibility that direct effects of these vasoactive agents on the aorta contribute to the response, for the reasons summarized above, they are unlikely to be the main determinant of aortic HSP70 expression in response to the hypertensive agents.

In view of the effect of acute elevations in blood pressure on HSP70 expression, and the previous reports by others demonstrating that spontaneously hypertensive rats show elevated HSP70 expression in response to heat stress, it was of interest to examine whether restraint-induced HSP70 expression was affected by chronic hypertension. Therefore, we examined blood pressure and HSP70 mRNA expression in unrestrained and restrained 6 month old SHR and control rats. We found that under non-stress conditions, systolic pressure of SHR averaged about 160 mm Hg, similar to that seen in our Fischer 344 rats subjected to restraint (see Figure 1). Restraint resulted in an elevation in blood pressure to about 180 mm Hg in the SHR. Despite the significant differences in blood pressure, no differences were observed in either basal or restraint-induced HSP70 expression of SHR and control rats (Xu et al., 1995). Thus, HSP70 expression appears to depend on acute changes in blood pressure regardless of the baseline blood pressure level seen in the absence of stress.

Role of HSF1 in Mediating the Response to Hypertension

Given the pivotal role of HSF1 in mediating HSP induction in response to stress, and the huge induction of HSP70 and HSP27 mRNA in vessels during hypertension, we assumed that demonstrating that HSF1 mediates the response would be a straightforward matter. However, this proved to be more difficult than anticipated. Examination of DNA binding activity in aortic extracts from restrained rats revealed surprisingly low levels of binding to the HSE. Nonetheless, as illustrated in the left panel of Figure 3, compared to unstressed animals in which DNA binding activity was virtually undetectable, DNA binding activity increased markedly in restrained animals. The kinetics of the response were found to be consistent with that seen for mRNA induction; maximum DNA binding activity was seen at 30 min, and attenuated with longer time periods of time. Furthermore, each of the hypertensive agents shown to induce HSP70 mRNA expression in the aorta, likewise caused an increase in DNA binding activity (Fig. B, right panel) (Xu et al., 1996). That the binding activity was specific and comprised of HSF1 was verified through competition studies with cold HSE oligonucleotides and nonspecific competitors, and use of anti-HSF1 antibodies which caused a "supershift" in the mobility of the DNA-binding complexes. Importantly, the magnitude of the increase in DNA binding activity seen with hypertension was similar to that seen with heat stress, suggesting that the low level of DNA binding activity seen in this tissue reflected low levels of HSF protein.

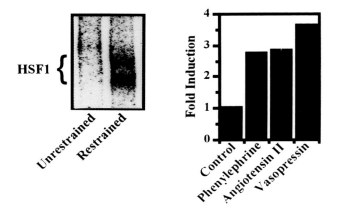

Figure 3. Restraint and hypertensive agents elevate HSE-binding activity in vessel extracts. DNA binding was assessed using a radiolabeled oligonucleotide containing a consensus HSE binding element. Doses of the vasoactive agents are the same as noted in Figure 2.

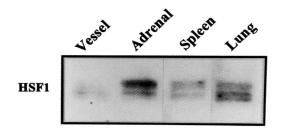

Figure 4. Western analysis of HSF1 protein expression in various rat tissues. Protein was detected in tissues of unstressed rats using an anti-HSF1 antibody .

Analysis of HSF1 protein by Western analysis showed this to be the case (Figure 4). Comparison of HSF1 expression in different tissues revealed that vessels contained significantly less HSF1 than any of the other tissue examined. Nonetheless, examination of HSF1 protein in extracts of rats exposed to restraint for varying lengths of time indicated a time-dependent shift in the mobility of HSF1 protein, indicative of hyperphosphorylation (Xu et al., 1996). These findings suggest that, as for heat and other classical stressors capable of eliciting the heat shock response, restraint-induced HSP70 expression is mediated through activation of HSF1.

Age-related decline in restraint-induced HSP70

Restraint-induced HSP70 and HSP27 expression was found to be attenuated in aged vessels (Udelsman et al., 1993). However, the magnitude of the decline in this response

106

was found to be much greater than that occurring in other tissues with other stresses (5 to 10-fold decline comparing 24 month and 6 month old Fischer 344 rats), and greater than that which could be accounted for by a two-fold reduction in HSF1 DNA binding activity. This suggested that other host factors are important in controlling the response to restraint and these too are affected by aging. We began to address these possibilities using several approaches.

In view of the relationship we had established between blood pressure and aortic HSP expression, we compared the effect of restraint on blood pressure in young and old rats. In contrast to young rats, which respond to restraint with an acute elevation in blood pressure, in most aged rats we observed little change in blood pressure (Xu et al., 1995). Therefore, we examined whether aged rats were capable of responding to hypertension-inducing agents. The effects of phenylephrine and vasopressin on blood pressure and HSP70 expression were examined. At the doses tested, both agents had a lesser effect on blood pressure in old rats compared to young rats. However, based on the dose-response relationship we had established for the induction of hypertension, it would be expected that the rise in blood pressure seen in the aged rats would be sufficient to induce HSP70 expression, and this is precisely what we observed. This direct correlation between the magnitude of the hypertensive response in old and young animals and the associated induction of HSP70 expression during restraint strengthens the relationship between acute hypertension and HSP70 expression.

The cause for this impaired hypertensive response in aged rats during restraint is unclear, but it is important to emphasize that it is not because the animals do not view restraint as stressful. Measurement of adrenocorticotropic hormone and glucocorticoid levels (Udelsman et al., 1993) revealed similar elevations in old and young rats. The differential responsiveness, could however, reflect changes in the sensitivity of adrenoreceptors to their ligands, or changes in peripheral arterioles which in turn serve to modulate systemic blood pressure. Age-related alterations in alpha adrenoreceptor-mediated events have been observed by others (Nielson et al., 1992). Further support for this hypothesis is provided by studies in which we transplanted aortas of old rats into young rats and aortas of young rats into old animals, and after allowing ample time for recovery from the surgery monitored the transplanted vessels' response to restraint. We observed that transplantation of young vessels to old rats leads to diminished HSP induction in the transplanted tissue in response to restraint, whereas transplantation of old vessels into young rats leads to a restoration of the response to restraint in the transplanted tissue. Thus, the age of the donated aorta was less important in determining its responsiveness to restraint than the host environment in which it was placed. Age-related differences in responsiveness of the peripheral vasculature could account for our findings with transplanted vessels.

SUMMARY AND CONCLUSIONS

Many factors, ranging from physical exertion to drug toxicity, noise, or emotional stress, lead to a rise in blood pressure that under certain circumstances can lead to severe damage to the vessel wall or even rupture. The induction of HSP70 expression during acute hypertension suggests a likely role for HSP70 in the host's defense to such hemodynamic stress. Precisely what that role is remains to be determined. However, an age-associated decline in the ability to express heat shock proteins in vessels as well as the heart is likely to contribute to the increased vulnerability to stress that accompanies aging. The recent development of transgenic mice containing elevated expression of HSP70 in cardiac tissue provides a unique opportunity to test the influence of HSP70 expression on age-related changes in heart function (Plumier et al., 1995; Marber et al., 1995). Further extension of such models to produce elevated HSP70 expression in vessels would likewise allow the assessment of the contribution of HSP70 expression to stress vulnerability of vessels during the aging process.

REFERENCES

Baler R, Dahl G, Voellmy R. Activation of human heat shock genes is accompanied by oligomerization, modification, and rapid translocation of heat shock transcraipton factor Hsf1. Mol Cell Biol 1993;13:2486-2496.

Blake MJ, Udelsman R, Feulner GJ, Norton DD, Holbrook NJ. Stress-induced heat shock protein 70 expression in adrenal cortex: an adrenocorticotropic hormone-sensitive, age-dependent response. Proc Natl Acad Sci USA 1991;88:9873-9877.

Blake MJ, Buckley DJ, Buckley AR. Dopaminergic regulationof heat shock protein-70 expression in adrenal gland and aorta. Endocrinology 1993;132:1063-1070.

Blake MJ, Buckley AR, Buckley DJ, LaVoi KP, Bartlett T. Neural and endocrine mechanisms of cocaine-induced 70 kDa heat shock protein expression in aorta and adrenal gland. J Pharm Exp Ther 1994;268:522-529.

Blake MJ, Klevay LM, Halas ES, Bode AM. Blood pressure and heat shock protein expression in response to acute and chronic stress. Hypertension 1995;25:539-544.

Bongrazio M, Comini L, Giuseppina G, Bachetti T, Ferrari R. Hypertension, aging and myocardial synthesis of heat-shock protein 72. Hypertension 1994;24:620-624.

Choi HS, Lin Z, Li B, Liu AYC. Age-dependent decrease in the heat-inducible DNA sequence-specific binding activity in human diploid fibroblasts. J Biol Chem 1990;265:18005-18011.

Craig EA, Weissman JS, Horwich AL. Heat shock proteins and chaperones. Cell 1994;78:365-372.

Crow MR, Boluyt MO, Lakatta EG. "The molecular and cellular biology of aging in the cardiovascular system" In Cellular Aging and Cell Death, Nikki J. Holbrook, George R Martin, Richard A Lockshin, Ed. New York: Wiley-Liss, 1996:81-107.

Deguchi Y, Negoro S, Kishimoto S. Age-related changes of heat shock protein gene transcription in human peripheral blood mononuclear cells. Biochem Biophys Res Commun 1988;157:580-584.

Effros RB, Zhu X, Walford RL. Stress response of senescent T lymphocytes: Reduced hsp70 is independent of the proliferative block. J Gerontol 1994;49:B65-B70.

Faassen AE, O'Leary JJ, Rodysill KJ, Bergh N, Hallgren HM. Diminished heat-shock protein synthesis following mitogen stimulation of lymphocytes from aged donors. Exp Cell Res 1989;183:326-334.

Fargnoli J, Kunisada T, Fornace AJ, Schneider EL, Holbrook NJ. Decreased expression of heat shock protein

70 mRNA and protein after heat treatment in cells of aged rats. Proc Natl Acad Sci USA 1990;87:846-850.

Fawcett TW, Sylvester SL, Sarge KD, Morimoto RI, Holbrook NJ. Effects of neurohormonal stress and aging on the activation of mammalian heat shock factor 1. J Biol Chem 1994;269:32272-32278.

Gaia G, Comini L, Pasini E, Tomelleri G, Agnoletti L, Ferrari R. Heat shock protein 72 in cardiac and skeletal muscles during hypertension. Molecular and Cellular Biochemistry 1995;146:1-6.

Hamet P, Malo D, Hashimoto T, and Tremblay J. Heat stress genes in hypertension. J Hypertension 1990;8:S47-S52.

Hamet P, Tremblay J, Pang SC, Walter SV, Wen Y-1. Primary versus secondary events in hypertension. Can J Physiol Pharmacol 1985;63:380-386.

Heydari AR, Wu B, Takahashi R, Strong R, Richardson A. Expression of heat shock protein 70 is altered by age and diet at the level of transcription. Mol Cell Biol 1993;13:2909-2918.

Isoyama S, Ito N, Komatsu M, Nitta Y, Abe K, Aoki M, Takishima T. Responses to hemodynamic stress in the aged heart. Jpn Heart J 1994;35:403-418.

Kregel KC, Moseley PL, Skidmore R, Gutierrez JA, Guerriero V, Jr. HSP70 accumulation in tissues of heat-stressed rats is blunted with advancing age. J Appl Physiol 1995;97:1673-1678.

Knowlton AA. The role of heat shock protein in the heart. J Mol Cell Cardiol 1995;27:121-131.

Kunes J, Poirier M, Tremblay J, Hamet P. Expression of hsp70 gene in lymphocytes from normotensive and hypertensive humans. Acta Physiol Scand 1992;146:307-311.

Lakatta EG. Cardiovascular regulatory mechanisms in advanced age. Physiol Rev 1993;73:413-467.

Liu AY, Lin Z, Choi H, Sorhage F, Li B. Attenuated induction of heat shock gene expression in aging diploid fibroblasts. J Biol Chem 1989;264:12037-12045

Luce MC, Cristofalo VJ. Reduction in heat shock gene expression correlates with increased thermosensitivity in senescent human fibroblasts. Exp Cell Res 1992;202:9-16.

Lukashev ME, Kliimanskaja IV, Postnov YV. Synthesis of heat shock proteins in cultured fibroblasts from normotensive and spontaneously hypertensive rat embryos. J Hyperten 1991;suppl 6:S182-183.

Marber MS, Mestril R, Chi SH, Sayen MR, Yellon DM, Dillmann WH. Overexpression of the rat inducible 70-kD heat stress protein in a transgenic mouse increases the resistance of the heart to ischemic injury. J Clin Invest 1995;95:1446-1456.

Martin GR, Danner DB, Holbrook NJ. Aging - causes and defenses. Annu Rev Med 1993;44:419-429.

McMurtry JP, Wexler BC. Hypersensitivity of spontaneously hypertensive rats (SHR) to heat, ether, and immobilization. Endocrinology 1981;108:1730-1736.

Moalic JM, Bauters C, Himbert D, Bercovici J, Mouas C, Guicheney P, Baudoin-Legros M, Rappaport L, Emanoil-Ravier R, Mezger V, Swynghedauw B. Phenylephrine, vasopressin and angiotensin II as determinants of proto-oncogene and heat-shock protein gene expression in adult rat heart and aorta. J Hypertension 1989;7:195-201.

Morimoto RI. Cells in stress: transcriptional activation of heat shock genes. Science 1993;259:1409-1410.

Morimoto RI, Tissieres A, and Georgopoulous C. Eds. *The Biology of Heat Shock Proteins and Molecular Chaperones.* Cold Spring Harbor, NY: Cold Spring Harbor Press, 1994.

Nielson H, Hasendam JM, Pilegaard HK, Aalkjaer C, Mortensen FV. Age-dependent changes in alpha-adrenoreceptor-mediated contractility of isolated human resistance arteries. Am J Physiol 1992;263:H1190-H1196.

Nitta Y, Abe K, Aoki M, Ohno I, Isoyama S. Diminished heat shock protein 70 mRNA indiuction in aged rat hearts after ischemia. Am J Physiol (Heart Circ Physiol)1994;H1795-1803.

Pahlavani MA, Denny M, Moore SA, Weindruch R, Richardson A. The expression of heat shock protein 70 decreases with age in lymphocytes from rats and rhesus monkeys. Exp Cell Res 1995;218:310-318.

Pardue S, Groshan K, Raese JD, Morrison-Bogorad M. Hsp70 mRNA induction is reduced in neurons of aged rat hippocampus after thermal stress. Neurobiol Aging 1992;13:661-672.

Pare WP, Glavin GB. Restraint stress in biomedical research: A review. Neurosci Biobehav Rev 1986;10:339-370

Plumier JC, Ross BM, Currie RW, Angelidis CE, Kazlaris H, Kollias G, Pagoulatos GN. Transgenic mice expressing the human heat shock protein 70 have improved post-ischemic myocardial recovery. J Clin Invest 1995;95:1854-1860.

Richardson A, Holbrook NJ. " Aging and the cellular response to stress: reduction in the heat shock response". In Cellular Aging and Cell Death, Nikki J. Holbrook, George R. Martin, and Richard A. Lockshin, eds. New York, NY: Wiley-Liss, 1996.

Shock NW, Greulich RC, Andres RA, Arenberg D, Costa PT, Jr, Lakatta EG, Tobin JD. Normal human aging. The Baltimore Longitudinal Study of Aging, vol 84. Washington, DC: US Government Printing Office, 1984;p 2450.

Sistonen L, Sarge KD, Morimoto RI. Human heat shock factors 1 and 2 are differentially activated and can synergistically induce hsp70 gene transcription. Mol Cell Biol 1994;14:2087-2099.

Stout RW. Ageing and atherosclerosis. Age Ageing 1987;16:65-72.

Udelsman R, Blake MJ, Stagg CA, Li D, Putney DJ, Holbrook NJ. Vascular heat shock protein expression in response to stress. Endocrine and autonomic regulation of this age-dependent response. J Clin Invest 1993;91:465-473.

Udelsman R, Blake MJ, Holbrook NJ. Molecular response to surgical stress: Specific and simultaneous heat shock protein induction in the adrenal cortex, aorta and vena cava. Surgery 1991;110:1125-1131.

Udelsman R, Li DG, Stagg CA, Holbrook NJ. Aortic co-transplantation between young and old rats: Effect upon the heat shock protein 70 stress response. J Gerontol 1995;50A:B187-192.

Wei JY, Gersh BJ. Heart disease in the elderly. Curr Probl Cardiol 1987;12:1-65.

Wei JY. Age and cardiovascular system. N Engl J Med 1992;327:1735-1739.

Welch WJ. Heat shock proteins functioning as molecular chaperones: their roles in normal and stressed cells. Philos Trans R Soc Lond 1993;339:327-333.

Xu Q, Li D, Holbrook NJ, Udelsman R. Acute hypertension induces heat shock protein 70 expression in rat aorta. Circulation 1995;92:1223-1229.

Xu Q, Fawcett TW, Udelsman R, Holbrook NJ. Activation of heat shock transcription factor 1 in rat aorta in response to high blood pressure. Hypertension 1996; in press.

7

TUMOR NECROSIS FACTOR-α AND THE MYOCARDIAL STRESS RESPONSE

A. A Knowlton, Masayuki Nakano, and Douglas L. Mann
Cardiology Section, Department of Medicine, Veterans Administration Medical Center and Baylor College of Medicine, Houston Texas 77030

INTRODUCTION

The ability of the myocardium to successfully compensate for and adapt to stress, such as a superimposed hemodynamic overload and/or myocardial ischemia/infarction, ultimately determines whether the heart will decompensate and fail, or whether instead it will maintain preserved function. As shown in Figure 1, the adult heart adapts to a superimposed environmental stress by at least three interrelated and integrated mechanisms: cardiac hypertrophy, cardiac remodeling and cardiac repair. However, while it is becoming increasingly clear that cell types residing within the mammalian myocardium both produce and respond to stress by synthesizing a variety of soluble protein factors that are capable of interacting in an autocrine or paracrine fashion, the molecules that mediate and integrate the myocardial response to environmental stress, both at the level of the intact myocyte and for the ventricle as a whole, remain poorly understood.

Tumor necrosis factor-alpha (TNF-α) is a pro-inflammatory cytokine that was originally discovered as a protein with necrotizing effects in certain transplantable mouse tumors,[7,37] is now recognized as a cytokine with pleiotropic biological capacities. Besides its cytostatic and cytotoxic effects on certain tumor cells, TNF-α influences growth, differentiation, and/or function of virtually every cell type investigated, including cardiac myocytes.[15,62] Moreover, TNF-α is thought to be part of an integral network of interactive signals that orchestrate inflammatory and immunological events. Relevant to this discussion is the repeated observation that elevated levels of TNF-α are detected peripherally in virtually all forms of cardiac injury, including but not limited to acute viral myocarditis,[28,53] cardiac allograft rejection,[1,46] myocardial infarction,[4,30] unstable angina,[29] myocardial reperfusion injury [18,23], hypertrophic cardiomyopathy,[29] and end-stage congestive heart failure.[10,24] Although the consistent expression of TNF-α in these destructive pathophysiological constructs has led to the suggestion that TNF-α might be deleterious, an alternative hypothesis is that TNF-α

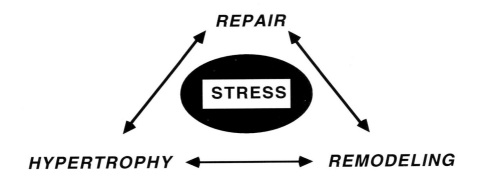

Figure 1 Myocardial Homeostasis. The adult heart adapts to superimposed environmental stress by at least three interrelated and integrated mechanisms: cardiac hypertrophy, cardiac remodeling and cardiac repair.

might play a beneficial "adaptive" role in these conditions.

Accordingly, the purpose of this brief review will be to highlight recent experimental material which delineates the role of TNF-α in the heart under normal and pathophysiological conditions. Two themes will emerge from this discussion: first, the short-term expression of TNF-α within the heart may provide the heart with an adaptive response to stress; second, the long term expression of TNF-α may be maladaptive by producing cardiac decompensation.

TNF-A AS AN IMMEDIATE EARLY HOMEOSTATIC STRESS RESPONSE GENE IN THE HEART

As noted above TNF-α is expressed in a virtually all forms of cardiac injury. The observation that TNF-α expression is not linked to a specific form of cardiac injury, but is instead observed in virtually *all* forms of injury, suggests the interesting possibility that TNF-α may serve as a "homeostatic stress response" gene in the heart.

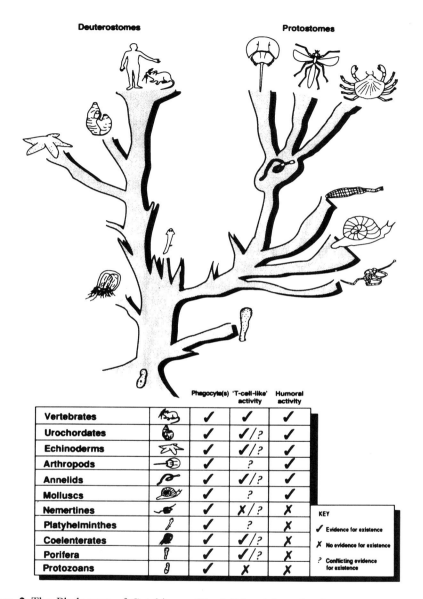

Deuterostomes   **Protostomes**

		Phagocyte(s)	'T-cell-like' activity	Humoral activity
Vertebrates		✓	✓	✓
Urochordates		✓	✓ / ?	✓
Echinoderms		✓	✓ / ?	✓
Arthropods		✓	?	✓
Annelids		✓	✓ / ?	✓
Molluscs		✓	?	✓
Nemertines		✓	✗ / ?	✗
Platyhelminthes		✓	?	✗
Coelenterates		✓	✓ / ?	✗
Porifera		✓	✓ / ?	✗
Protozoans		✓	✗	✗

KEY
✓ Evidence for existence
✗ No evidence for existence
? Conflicting evidence for existence

Figure 2 The Phylogeny of Cytokines. The left-hand branch of the tree shows the development of animals that gave rise to vertebrates (deuterostomes), whereas the right hand branch includes most of the classic invertebrates (protostomes). TNF-α like activity has been detected throughout subphyla of the animal kingdom, and is present in both protostome (annelids) and deuterostome invertebrates (echinoderms). (Reproduced with permission *Immunology Today.* [5])

113

The following lines of evidence support this point of view.

The first line in evidence in support for an important homeostatic role for TNF-α stems from the observation that this proinflammatory cytokine has been conserved by nature throughout the animal kingdom. Figure 2 shows a stylized tree that depicts the relationship between the various phyla and subphyla of the animal kingdom. The left-hand branch of the tree shows the development of animals that gave rise to vertebrates (deuterostomes), whereas the right hand branch includes most of the classic invertebrates (protostomes). The finding that TNF-α like activity is present in both protostome (annelids)[5,42] and deuterostome invertebrates (echinoderms)[5,42], suggests that TNF-α came into existence sometime before the split of the two major animal phyla occurred. This time line dates the origin of TNF-α to the onset of the Cambrian period. Thus, the observation that TNF-α has been conserved by nature for nearly 600,000 million years, suggests that expression of this protein may confer a survival benefit to the host.

A second line of evidence in support of the homeostatic role for TNF-α in the heart is implicit in the recent finding that TNF-α mRNA is expressed rapidly in the heart following certain forms of stress. As shown in Figure 3A, TNF-α mRNA is not detectable experimentally in naive (unstressed) hearts. However, TNF-α mRNA is expressed de novo in the heart within 30 minutes after a stressful stimulus (endotoxin provocation). As shown in Figure 3C, TNF-α mRNA levels returned rapidly towards baseline levels once the stressful stimulus is removed, thus suggesting that TNF-α gene expression is tightly regulated in the heart. Figure 4 shows that whereas TNF-α protein (detected as TNF-α bioactivity by L929 bioassay) was not detectable in the myocardial superfusates (insert) from unstressed hearts, there was a striking increase in the elaboration of biologically active TNF-α in the superfusates from the endotoxin stimulated hearts (Figure 3, and insert). TNF-α bioactivity, which was evident as early as 60 - 75 minutes following endotoxin stimulation, continued to increase throughout the course of endotoxin stimulation. Although the coordinated expression of TNF-α mRNA and protein in the heart argues for a transcriptional control mechanism for cytokine biosynthesis, the presence of an AT-rich region in the 3' untranslated region of the TNF-α gene suggests an alternative mechanism. That is, these sequences (TTATTTAT[6]), which are common in the 3'-untranslated regions of a variety of inflammatory cytokines, have been shown to promote mRNA instability.[6,51] Accordingly, it is not known whether TNF-α biosynthesis occurs in the heart, either wholly or in part, as a result of post-transcriptional stabilization of TNF-α mRNA levels. Thus, in summary Figures 3 and 4 illustrate three important points with respect to TNF-α gene expression in the heart. First, neither TNF-α mRNA nor TNF-α protein appear to be constitutively expressed in the unstressed adult mammalian heart.[13,21] Second, both TNF-α mRNA and protein are rapidly synthesized by the heart in responseto an appropriate stressful stimulus.[13,21] Third, once TNF-α mRNA biosynthesis is initiated, myocardial TNF-α mRNA levels return rapidly towards baseline following removal of the inciting stress[21]. Taken together, the rapidity with which TNF-α mRNA is expressed in response to a stressful stimulus and the rapidity with TNF-α mRNA is degraded following removal of the stressful stimulus, suggests that TNF-α may serve as a "immediate early stress response gene in the heart."

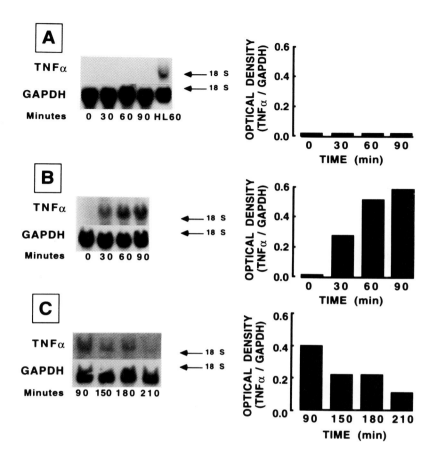

Figure 3: Myocardial TNF-α gene expression in vitro. TNF-α gene expression was assessed by Northern blot analysis in freshly isolated hearts perfused for various times with diluent or endotoxin (125 μg/ml); the expression of glyceraldehyde-3-phosphate dehydrogenase (GAPDH) mRNA was used as an internal control. Panel 3A shows the Northern blot analysis for TNF-α mRNA levels following diluent administration (0 - 180 minutes); mRNA isolated from endotoxin-stimulated (125 μg/ml for 180 minutes) HLA60 cells was used as positive control, and was processed along with the mRNA from the diluent stimulated hearts under identical conditions. Panel 3B shows the time course for the appearance of TNF-α mRNA following the administration of endotoxin; Panel 3C shows the time course for the decrease in TNF-α mRNA levels following 90 minutes of stimulation with endotoxin (125 μg/ml). The graphs accompanying Panels 3A- 3C show the relative optical density of the hybridization signal for TNF-α, normalized to the hybridization signal for GAPDH. (Reproduced with permission *J. Clin. Invest.* [21])

TNF RECEPTORS IN THE HEART

The biological effects of TNF-α are initiated by the binding of TNF-α to two distinct cell surface receptors with approximate molecular masses of 55 kDa (TNFR1) and 75 kDa (TNFR2). While both TNF receptor species have been cloned in

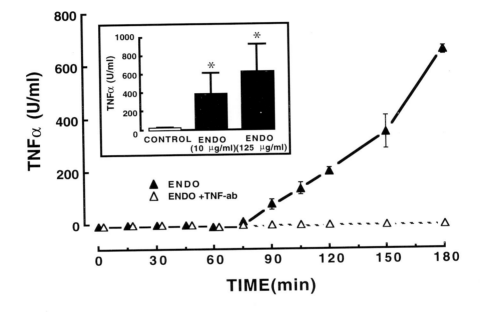

Figure 4: TNF-α Protein Synthesis in the Heart. Freshly excised cat hearts were perfused for 180 minutes with diluent, 10 μg/ml or 125 μg/ml of endotoxin. TNF-α bioactivity (L929 cytotoxicity assay was assessed in the myocardial superfusates starting immediately after endotoxin stimulation (time 0). The large panel shows the time course of appearance of TNF-α bioactivity (closed triangles) for a representative heart treated with endotoxin (125 μg/ml); TNF-α bioactivity was completely neutralized at each time point by an anti-TNF-α antibody (open triangles). The insert of this figure, depicts the values obtained for group datafor hearts perfused (180 minutes) with diluent (open bar, n = 5 hearts), 10 μg/ml endotoxin (solid bar, n=5 hearts) or 125 μg/ml endotoxin (solid bar, n=3 hearts). (ENDO = endotoxin; * = p < 0.05 compared to diluent treated hearts). (Reproduced with permission, *J. Clin. Invest.*[21])

man,[14,25,47,52] and while both TNF receptors are thought to be widely expressed in mammalian cells[45,60] the presence of TNF receptors in the heart has only recently been reported.[58] Studies in non-failing human myocardium have identified the presence of both types of TNF receptors; moreover, both receptor subtypes have been immunolocalized to the adult human cardiac myocyte, thus providing a potential signaling pathway for TNF-α in the heart.[58] Intracellular signaling occurs as a result of TNF-α-induced cross-linking of the receptors. Both the TNFR1 and TNFR2 receptor share homology in their extracellular domains, where each contain a characteristic repeated cysteine consensus motif. In contrast, the intracellular domains of TNFR1 and TNFR2 are different, suggesting that each receptor has distinct modes of signaling and cellular function. The signaling pathways that are coupled to TNFR1 have been well characterized, and include activation of a phosphatidylcholine specific phospholipase C,[49], activation of phospholipase A$_2$,[19] and activation of neutral sphingomyelinase.[61] In contrast, the signaling pathways that are coupled to TNFR2 are not known.[20] Unfortunately, very little is known with respect to which of the above pathways are activated in cardiac myocytes following stimulation with TNF-α.

TNF-A INDUCED HOMEOSTATIC EFFECTS IN THE HEART

While the potential salutary effects of TNF-α in the heart remain largely unknown at present, the expression of low concentrations of TNF-α for relatively brief periods of time may provide the heart with a short-term adaptive response to stress. Recent studies from our laboratory support this point of view. As shown in Figures 5 - 7, stimulating cultured cardiac myocytes with TNF-α provokes increased HSP 72 expression in adult cardiac myocytes. Given that HSP 72 is thought to protect the heart against environmental injury,[27,41] the findings with respect to TNF-α may have direct relevance to the homeostatic role that is played by this cytokine. As shown in Figure 5, continuous stimulation of cardiac myocytes with a single concentration of TNF-α (200 U/ml) showed that increased HSP 72 levels were apparent as early as 3 hours following cytokine stimulation, peaked by approximately 6 - 12 hours after stimulation, and then returned toward baseline by 48 hours of stimulation. Thus, TNF-α may provide the heart with an adaptive response to stress; however, as illustrated in Figure 5 this adaptive response is lost by 24 hours.

To determine whether cross-linking of TNFR1 and/or TNFR2 was responsible for HSP 72 expression in adult cardiac myocytes, we stimulated the cells with mutatedTNF-α ligands (TNF mutants) that have double point mutations in their TNF receptor binding domains,[26] such that they bind with a high degree of specificity to either humanTNFR1 (corresponding mutant = TNFM1[26]) or to TNFR2 (corresponding mutant = TNFM2[26]). The myocyte cultures were stimulated continuously for 12 hours either with 2 - 20 ng/ml (0.1 - 1.0 nM) of TNFM1 or 2 - 20 ng/ml (0.1 - 1.0 nM) of TNFM2. To determine whether TNFR2 modulated the effects of TNFR1, we simultaneously stimulated the myocytes with TNFM1 (2 ng/ml) and TNFM2 (2 ng/ml). As shown in Figure 6, stimulation of the myocytes with TNFα mutants that bind selectively to the t ype 1 TNF receptor produced an increase in HSP 72 expression that was equivalent to or greater than the maximal level of expression that was obtained with wild-type TNFα (200 U/ml). In contrast, there was no significant difference in HSP 72 expression in the myocyte cultures stimulated with 2 - 20 ng/ml TNFM2. The observation that the level of HSP 72 expression obtained with 20 ng/ml TNFM1 was greater than with wild-type TNFα alone, suggested that TNFR2 might supply a co-factor that negatively modulated signal transduction through TNFR1. To explore this possibility we examined HSP 72 expression after stimulating the cells simultaneously with TNFM1(2 ng/ml) and TNFM2 (2 ng/ml). As shown in the right hand portion of

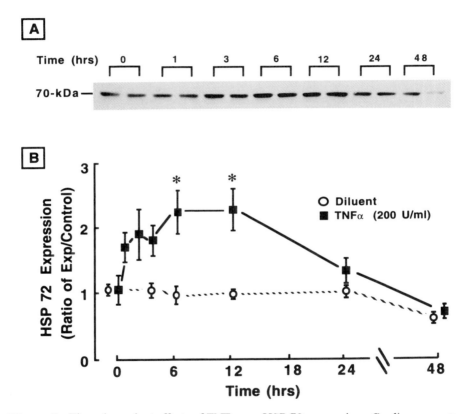

Figure 5: Time-dependent effects of TNF-α on HSP 72 expression. Cardiac myocytes were continuously stimulated for 0 - 48 hours with either diluent or 200 U/ml of TNF-α. The cells were harvested and analyzed by Western blotting (panel A) and competitive ELISA (panel B). The data shown in Panel A depict the level of HSP 72 expression by Western blotting from two separate myocyte cultures at each of the time points indicated. The data in panel B are shown as the fold-change from baseline values (time 0) for HSP 72 expression in the diluent and TNF-α stimulated cultures. (* = p < 0.05 compared to control values) (Reproduced with permission the *American Physiological Society*[33])

Figure 6, the level of HSP 72 expression following simultaneous stimulation with both TNF mutants was not significantly different from HSP 72 levels obtained in diluent treated myocytes, thus suggesting that TNFR2 negatively modulated the level of HSP 72 expression transduced by TNFR1.

Figure 7 shows that the *degree* of cytokine important is important. That is, whereas concentrations $\leq$ 10 U/ml TNF-α had no effect on HSP 72 expression, cytokine concentrations $\geq$ 50 U/ml produced significant increases in HSP 72 expression. Interestingly, extremely high (pathophysiological) concentrations of TNF-α (1000 U/ml) resulted in HSP 72 levels that were significantly less than those obtained with lower (200 U/ml) concentrations of TNF-α, although the resultant levels of HSP 72 expression were still significantly greater than values obtained at baseline. The specificity of the TNF-α-induced effects on HSP 72 expression was demonstrated by the studies in which a neutralizing polyclonal antibody against TNF-α completely blocked the cytokine-induced increase in HSP 72 expression, as well as by the studies wherein "TNF-α conditioned" medium failed to stimulate increased HSP 72 expression in isolated cardiac myocytes. Thus, the adaptive response of TNF-α may be less evident when TNF-α is expressed at extremely high levels, such as may occur in pathophysiological conditions. In addition to the effects of TNF-α on increased HSP 72 expression, the short-term expression of myocardial TNF-α may provide the heart with a panoply of additional homeostatic responses to environmental stress, including increased regional myocardial blood flow and increased resistance to ischemic induced arrhythmias through the generation of nitric oxide,[39,48] increased free radical scavenging through increased expression of manganese superoxide dismutase,[34] and protection against injury induced by oxidative stress.[32]

MALADAPTIVE EFFECTS INDUCED BY TNF-A IN THE HEART

Although there is increasing evidence that short-term expression of TNF-α may provide the heart with an adaptive response to stress, as shown in Table 1 there is also a large body of evidence which suggests that overexpression of TNF-α may produce frankly maladaptive effects in the heart, including but not limited to left ventricular (LV) dysfunction, pulmonary edema, LV remodelling, and cardiomyopathy. The following discussion will highlight recent advances in our understanding of how TNF-α regulates cardiac function.

Effect of TNF-α on Myocardial Function: The observation that TNF-α was capable of modulating LV function first became apparent following a series of experimental studies which showed that direct injections of TNF-α would produce hypotension, metabolic acidosis, hemoconcentration and death within minutes, thus mimicking the cardiac/hemodynamic response seen during endotoxin-induced septic shock [59]. Further, injections of antibodies raised against TNF-α were subsequently shown to attenuate the hemodynamic collapse seen in endotoxin shock. With respect to the potential mechanisms for the TNF-α induced cardiac decompensation, the current literature suggests that TNF-α produces both *immediate* and *delayed* effects on

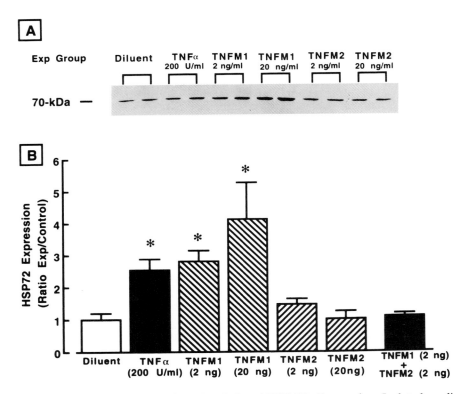

Figure 6: TNF Receptors and TNFα- Induced HSP 72 Expression. Isolated cardiac myocytes were stimulated with mutated TNFα ligands (TNF mutants) that have a high degree of specificity to either human TNFR1 (corresponding mutant = TNFM1) or to TNFR2 (corresponding mutant = TNFM2). Cardiac myocytes were continuously stimulated for 12 hours with a TNFM1 (2 - 20 ng/ml) or TNFM2 (2 - 20 ng/ml) or a combination of TNFM1 (2 ng/ml) and TNFM2 (2 ng/ml). The cells were harvested and analyzed qualitatively and quantitatively, respectively, by Western blotting (panel A) and competitive ELISA (panel B), as described in the methods. Panel A depicts the level of HSP 72 expression from two separate myocyte cultures for each concentration of TNF mutant tested. The data shown for each item in Panel B depict the ratio of the level of HSP 72 expression in cardiac myocytes cultures stimulated with 200 U/ml TNFα; TNFM1 (2, 20 ng/ml); TNFM2 (2,20 ng/ml) for each concentration; and TNFM1 and TNFM2 compared to values obtained in diluent treated myocytes. (* = p < 0.05 compared to control values) (Reproduced with permission the *American Physiological Society*[33])

TABLE 1
THE POTENTIAL UNTOWARD EFFECTS OF TNF-α IN HEART FAILURE

- Produces Left Ventricular Dysfunction in Humans[57]
- Produces Pulmonary edema in Humans[31]
- Produces Cardiomyopathy in Humans[17]
- Promotes Left Ventricular Remodeling Experimentally[35,40]
- Produces Abnormalities in Myocardial Metabolism Experimentally[50]
- Produces Anorexia and Cachexia Experimentally [38,54,55]
- Produces β-receptor Uncoupling from Adenylate Cyclase Experimentally[8]
- Produces Abnormalities of Mitochondrial Energetics[22,56]

myocardial contractility. That is, important early studies in neonatal cardiac myocytes showed that although continuous exposure (72 hours) to TNF-α did not affect baseline contractile function, it did blunt the positive inotropic response to isoproterenol in a fashion that was completely reversible.[8,15,16] Delayed effects of TNF-α have also been observed in dogs in vivo, wherein a single infusion of TNF-α resulted in abnormalities of systolic function within the first 24 hours of infusion.[11,35,40] However, it is possible that earlier effects of TNF-α might have been observed if the animals were studied at earlier time points. More recent studies in the adult heart have suggested that TNF-α also has immediate effects on contractility.[11,12,62] As a case in point, a study in which thin strips of myocardial tissue from Syrian hamsters [12] were exposed to graded concentrations of TNF-α showed an immediate (2-3 minutes) concentration-dependent decrease in myocardial contractility, which was completely reversible upon removal of this cytokine. This study was confirmed by a recent study in isolated adult feline cardiac myocytes, which showed that the negative inotropic effects of TNF-α were the direct result alterations in intracellular calcium homeostasis.[62] In this study treatment with "pathological" concentrations of TNF-α ($\geq$ 200 U/ml) produced a 20 - 30 % decrease in the extent of cell shortening and a 40% decrease in peak levels of intracellular calcium; moreover, whole cell patch-clamp studies suggested that the decrease in intracellular calcium was not the result of changes in the voltage sensitive inward calcium current. Of note, a recent in vivo canine study, in which LV function was examined at early time points (2 hrs) also suggests that TNF-α has short term effects on contractility which were similar to those recently observed in vitro.[11] Thus, in summary, the literature suggests that TNF-α can produce *immediate* and *delayed* negative inotropic effects in the adult heart. These findings suggest that TNF-α may produce negative inotropic effects by activating different signaling pathways, each of which are sufficient to modulate myocardial contractility, albeit with different time courses.

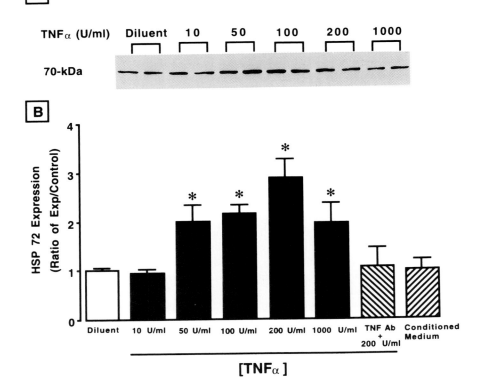

Figure 7: Concentration-dependent effects of TNF-α on HSP 72 expression. Myocyte cultures were stimulated with diluent or 10 - 1000 U/ml TNF-α for 12 hours, harvested and analyzed qualitatively and quantitatively, respectively, by Western blotting (panel A) and competitive ELISA (panel B). The data shown in Panel B depict the level of HSP 72 expression, expressed as a fold-change from control values, for myocyte cultures stimulated with diluent (open bar) and 10 - 1000 U/ml TNF-α (solid bars). The specificity of TNF-α-induced effects was determined in two separate control experiments: first, an anti-TNF-α antibody was used to neutralize the effects of TNF-α (left-hand hatched bar); second, "conditioned medium" from TNF-α and diluent treated cultures was applied to the freshly isolated cardiac myocytes (right hand hatched bar) for 12 hours. (* = p < 0.05 compared to control values) (Reproduced with permission the *American Physiological Society*[33])

Signaling Pathways for the Negative Inotropic Effects of TNF-α. Many cytokines, including TNF-α, are thought to exert their effects by increasing the *inducible* expression of an enzyme termed nitric oxide synthase (iNOS). On the other hand, the constitutive form of NOS (cNOS), which releases NO for short periods of time in response to receptor or physical stimulation and which is calcium/calmodulin dependent, is not thought to be regulated by cytokines.[44] Recent studies have shown that both cNOS and iNOS are expressed in rat cardiac myocytes;[2,3,48] moreover, iNOS activity has recently been described in human myocardial tissue.[9] Recent work by Smith and colleagues[3] suggests that treatment of adult cardiac myocytes ($\geq$ 24 hrs) with culture medium "conditioned" by activated macrophages (but not TNF-α per se), produced a defect in isoproterenol-stimulated contractile function, that was mediated by NO. A second mechanism for the negative inotropic effects of TNF-α, as suggested by findings of Smith and colleagues,[3] is that NO leads to a defect in ß-adrenergic stimulated generation of cAMP. However, the mechanism linking increased NO production to a G-protein mediated defect in ß-adrenergic signaling is unclear. Finally, a very recent report suggests that TNF-α stimulation (72 hours) in neonatal myocytes results in a decrease in basal and α_1-adrenoceptor-induced formation of the calcium mobilizing second messenger inositol trisphosphate (IP_3); however, the functional implications of this finding were not addressed in this study.[43]

With respect to the mechanism for the immediate effects of TNF-α, one recent study provided indirect evidence in support of the point of view that TNF-α-induced contractile dysfunction resulted from "enhanced activity of a constitutive nitric oxide synthase (cNOS) in the myocardium."[12] However, these findings with respect to induction of cNOS activity by TNF-α have not been confirmed by other laboratories.[44,62] Further, as noted above, the direct induction of cNOS by cytokines is unprecedented.[36] Thus, the signaling pathways responsible for the immediate negative inotropic effects of TNF-α remain unknown. This statement notwithstanding, a recent study in isolated contracting feline cardiac myocytes has shown that activation of TNFR1 is responsible for mediating the negative inotropic effects of TNF-α.[58] Given, as noted above, that at least three major signaling pathways are known to be coupled to activation of TNFR1, future studies may identify the molecular mechanisms that are responsible for the immediate negative inotropic effects of TNF-α.

CONCLUSION

In this brief review we have summarized clinical and experimental material which suggest that TNF-α, a pro-inflammatory cytokine that is elaborated in a variety of cardiac disease states, has different effects on cardiac structure and function, depending both upon the duration and degree of cytokine expression in the heart. That is, short-term expression of TNF-α may be beneficial by providing the heart with an adaptive homeostatic response to stress. Moreover, since TNF-α is produced and secreted by cardiac myocytes in response to stressful stimuli, TNF-α may play an important role in integrating the various components of the stress response, such as cardiac hypertrophy, cardiac remodeling and cardiac repair (Figure 1). This statement notwithstanding, the short-term beneficial effects of TNF-α may be lost if myocardial

TNF-α expression either becomes sustained and/or excessive, in which case the salutary effects of TNF-α may be contravened by the know deleterious effects of pathological elevations of TNF-α. Therefore, in order to maximize the potential portfolio of beneficial responses conferred by TNF-α in the heart, it will become increasingly important in future studies to delineate the mechanisms that regulate normal and abnormal TNF-α expression in the heart.

ACKNOWLEDGEMENTS

The authors acknowledge the secretarial assistance of Jana Grana and the past and present guidance and support of Dr. Andrew I. Schafer. The research reviewed herein was supported, in part, by research funds from the Department of Veterans Affairs and the N.I.H. (P50 HL-O6H,DLM, and R29 HL 52910,AAK).

REFERENCES

1. Carswell EA, Old LJ, Kassel RL, Green S, Fiore N, Williamson B: An endotoxin-induced serum factor that causes necrosis of tumors. *Proc Natl Acad Sci USA* 1975;72:3666-3670
2. Old LJ: Tumor necrosis factor (TNF). *Science* 1985;230:630-632
3. Yokoyama T, Vaca L, Rossen RD, Durante W, Hazarika P, Mann DL: Cellular basis for the negative inotropic effects of tumor necrosis factor-alpha in the adult mammalian heart. *J Clin Invest* 1993;92:2303-2312
4. Gulick TS, Chung MK, Pieper SJ, Lange LG, Schreiner GF: Interleukin 1 and tumor necrosis factor inhibit cardiac myocyte β-adrenergic responsiveness. *Proc Natl Acad Sci USA* 1989;86:6753-6757
5. Smith SC, Allen PM: Neutralization of endogenous tumor necrosis factor ameliorates the severity of myosin-induced myocarditis. *Circ Res* 1992;70:856-863
6. Matsumori A, Yamada T, Kawai C: Immunomodulating therapy in viral myocarditis: Effects of tumour necrosis factor, interleukin 2 and anti-interleukin-2 receptor antibody in an animal model. *Eur Heart J* 1991;12:203-205
7. Arbustini E, Grasso M, Diegoli M, Bramerio M, Foglieni AS, Albertario M, Matinelli L, Gavazzi A, Goggi C, Campana C, Vigano M: Expression of tumor necrosis factor in human acute cardiac rejection: an immunohistochemical and immunoblotting study. *Am J Pathol* 1991;139:709-715
8. Sakobar A, Horton JD, Bowler K, Manning R, Meager A, Dark JH: Raised levels of tumor-necrosis factor alpha (TNFα) in cardiac transplant patients. *Clin Transplantation* 1993;7:459-466
9. Maury CPJ, Teppo AM: Circulating tumour necrosis factor-α (cachectin) in myocardial infarction. *J Intern Med* 1989;225:333-336
10. Basaran Y, Basaran MM, Babacan KF, Ener B, Okay T, Gok H, Ozdemir M: Serum tumor necrosis factor levels in acute myocardial infarction and unstable angina pectoris. *J Vascular Diseases* 1993;332-337
11. Matsumori A, Yamada T, Suzuki H, Matoba Y, Sasayama S: Increased circulating cytokines in patients with myocarditis and cardiomyopathy. *Br Heart J* 1994;72:561-566
12. Lefer AM, Tsao P, Aoki N, Palladino MA, Jr. Mediation of cardioprotection by transforming growth factor-β. *Science* 1990;249:61-64
13. Herskowitz A, Choi S, Ansari AA, Wesselingh S: Cytokine mRNA expression in postischemic/reperfused myocardium. *Am J Pathol* 1995;146:419-428
14. Levine B, Kalman J, Mayer L, Fillit HM, Packer M: Elevated circulating levels of tumor necrosis factor in severe chronic heart failure. *N Engl J Med* 1990;223:236-241
15. Dutka DP, Elborn JS, Delamere F, Shale DJ, Morris GK: Tumour necrosis factor-alpha in severe congestive cardiac failure. *Br Heart J* 1993;70:141-143
16. Raftos DA, Cooper EL, Habicht GS, Beck G: Invertebrate cytokines: tunicate cell proliferation stimulated by an interleukin 1-like molecule. *Proc Natl Acad Sci U S A* 1991;88:9518-9522
17. Beck G, Habicht GS: Primitive cytokines: harbingers of vertebrate defense. *Immunol Today*

1991;12:180-183

18. Caput D, Beutler B, Hartog K, Thayer R, Brown-Shimer S, Cerami A: Identification of a common nucleotide sequence in the 3'-untranslated region of mRNA molecules specifying inflammatory mediators. *Proc Natl Acad Sci USA* 1986;83:1670-1674

19. Shaw G, Kamen R: A conserved AU sequence from the 3' untranslated region of GM-CSF mRNA mediates selective mRNA degradation. *Cell* 1986;46:659-667

20. Giroir BP, Johnson JH, Brown T, Allen GL, Beutler B: The tissue distribution of tumor necrosis factor biosynthesis during endotoxemia. *J Clin Invest* 1992;90:693-698

21. Kapadia S, Lee JR, Torre-Amione G, Birdsall HH, Ma TS, Mann DL: Tumor necrosis factor gene and protein expression in adult feline myocardium after endotoxin administration. *J Clin Invest* 1995;96:1042-1052

22. Schall TJ, Lewis M, Koller KJ, Lee A, Rice GC, Wong GHW, Gatanaga T, Granger GA, Lentz R, Raab H, Kohr WJ, Goeddel DV: Molecular cloning and expression of a receptor for human tumor necrosis factor. *Cell* 1990;61:361-370

23. Smith CA, Davis T, Anderson D, Solam L, Beckmann MP, Jerzy R, Dower SK, Cosman D, Goodwin RG: A receptor for tumor necrosis factor defines an unusual family of cellular and viral proteins. *Science* 1990;248:1019-1023

24. Gray PW, Barret K, Chantry D, Turner M, Feldmann M: Cloning of human necrosis factor (TNF) receptor cDNA and expression of recombinant soluble TNF-binding protein. *Proc Natl Acad Sci USA* 1990;87:7380-7384

25. Loetscher H, Pan YCE, Lahm HW, Gentz R, Brockhaus M, Tabuchi H, Lesslauer W: Molecular cloning and expression of the human 55 kd tumor necrosis factor receptor. *Cell* 1990;61:352-359

26. Rothe J, Gehr G, Loetscher H, Lesslauer W: Tumor necrosis factor receptors - structure and function. *Immunol Res* 1992;11:81-90

27. Vilcek J, Lee TH: Tumor necrosis factor. New insights into the molecular mechanisms of its multiple actions. *J Biol Chem* 1991;266:7313-7316

28. Torre-Amione G, Kapadia S, Lee J, Bies RD, Lebovitz R, Mann DL: Expression and functional significance of tumor necrosis factor receptors in human myocardium. *Circulation* 1995;92:1487-1493

29. Schutze S, Potthoff K, Machleidt T, Berkovic D, Wiegmann K, Kronke M: TNF activates NF-kB by phosphatidylcholine-specific phospholipase C-induced "acidic" sphingomyelin breakdown. *Cell* 1992;71:765-776

30. Hoeck WG, Ramesha CS, Chang DJ, Fan N, Heller RA: Cytoplasmic Phospholipase-A2 Activity and Gene Expression Are Stimulated by Tumor Necrosis Factor - Dexamethasone Blocks the Induced Synthesis. *Proc Natl Acad Sci USA* 1993;90:4475-4479

31. Wiegmann K, Schutze S, Machleidt T, Witte D, Kronke M: Functional dichotomy of neutral and acidic sphingomyelinases in tumor necrosis factor signaling. *Cell* 1994;78:1005-1015

32. Hsu H, Xiong J, Goeddel DV: The TNF receptor 1-associated protein TRADD signals cell death and NF-kB activation. *Cell* 1995;81:495-504

33. Marber MS, Mestril R, Chi SH, Sayen R, Yellon DM, Dillmann WH: Overexpression of the rat inducible 70-kd heat stress protein in a transgenic mouse increases the resistance of the heart to ischemic injury. *J Clin Invest* 1995;95:1446-1456

34. Plumier JCL, Ross BM, Currie RW, Angelides CE, Kazlaris H, Kollias G, Pagoulatos GN: Transgenic mice expressing the human heat shock protein 70 have improved post-ischemic myocardial recovery. *J Clin Invest* 1995;95:1854-1860

35. Loetscher H, Stueber D, Banner D, Mackay F, Lesslauer W: Human tumor necrosis factor α (TNFα) mutants with exclusive specificity for the 55-kDa or 75 kDA TNF receptors. *J Biol Chem* 1993;268:26350-26357

36. Schulz R, Nava E, Moncada S: Induction and potential biological relevance of a Ca^{2+}-independent nitric oxide synthase in the myocardium. *Brit J Pharmacol* 1992;105:575-580

37. Pabla R, Curtis MJ: Effects of NO modulation on cardiac arrhythmias in the rat isolated heart. *Circ Res* 1995;77:984-992

38. Nakata T, Suzuki K, Fujii J, Ishikawa M, Taniguchi N: Induction and Release of Manganese Superoxide Dismutase from Mitochondria of Human Umbilical Vein Endothelial Cells by Tumor Necrosis Factor-alpha and Interleukin-1 alpha. *Int J Cancer* 1993;55:646-650

39. Nakano M, Knowlton AA, Lee-Jackson D, Mann DL: Tumor necrosis factor-α protects against hypoxic injury in adult cardiac myocytes: the role of heat shock protein 70. *Circulation* 1994;90:I-467(Abstract)

40. Tracey KJ, Beutler B, Lowry SF, Merryweather J, Wolpe S, Milsark IW, Hariri RJ, Fahey TJ, III, Zentella A, Albert JD, Shires GT: Shock and tissue injury induced by recombinant human cachectin. *Science*

1986;234:470-474

41. Chung MK, Gulick TS, Rotondo RE, Schreiner GF, Lange LG: Mechanism of action of cytokine inhibition of β-adrenergic agonist stimulation of cyclic AMP in rat cardiac myocytes: impairment of signal transduction. *Circ Res* 1990;67:753-763

42. Gulick TS, Pieper JS, Murphy MA, Lange LG, Schreiner GF: A new method for assessment of cultured cardiac myocyte contractility detects immune factor-mediated inhibition of β-adrenergic responses. *Circulation* 1991;84:313-321

43. Natanson C, Eichenholz PW, Danner RL, Eichacker W, Hoffman D, Kuo SM, Banks TJ, MacViottie TJ, Parrillo JE: Endotoxin and tumor necrosis factor challenges in dogs simulate the cardiovascular profile of human septic shock. *J Exp Med* 1989;169:823-832

44. Pagani FD, Baker LS, Hsi C, Knox M, Fink MP, Visner MS: Left ventricular systolic and diastolic dysfunction after infusion of tumor necrosis factor-α in conscious dogs. *J Clin Invest* 1992;90:389-398

45. Eichenholz PW, Eichacker PQ, Hoffman WD, Banks SM, Parrillo JE, Danner RL, Natanson C: Tumor necrosis factor challenges in canines: patterns of cardiovascular dysfunction. *Am J Physiol* 1992;263:H668-H675

46. Finkel MS, Oddis CV, Jacob TD, Watkins SC, Hattler BG, Simmons RL: Negative inotropic effects of cytokines on the heart mediated by nitric oxide. *Science* 1992;257:387-389

47. Roberts AB, Vodovotz Y, Roche NS, Sporn MB, Nathan CF: Role of nitric oxide in antagonistic effects of transforming growth factor-β and interleukin-1β on the beating rate of cultured myocytes. *Mol Endocrinol* 1992;6:1921-1930

48. Balligand JL, Kelly RA, Marsden PA, Smith TW, Michel T: Control of cardiac muscle cell function by an endogenous nitric oxide signaling system. *Proc Natl Acad Sci USA* 1993;90:347-351

49. Balligand JL, Ungureanu D, Kelly RA, Kobzik L, Pimental D, Michel T, Smith TW: Abnormal contractile function due to induction of nitric oxide synthesis in rat cardiac myocytes follows exposure to activated macrophage-conditioned medium. *J Clin Invest* 1993;91:2314-2319

50. De Belder AJ, Radomski MW, Why HJF, Richardson PJ, Bucknall CA, Salas E, Martin JF, Moncada S: Nitric oxide synthase activities in human myocardium. *Lancet* 1993;341:84-86

51. Reithmann C, Werdan K: Tumor necrosis factor α decreases inositol phosphate formation and phosphatidylinositol-bisphosphate (PIP₂) synthesis in raat cardiomyocytes. *Naunyn-Schmiedeberg's Archiv Pharmacol* 1994;349:175-182

52. Nathan CF: Nitric oxide as a secretory product of mammalian cells. *FASEB J* 1992;6:3051-3064

53. Suffredini AF, Fromm RE, Parker MM, Brenner M, Kovacs JA, Wesley RA, Parrillo JE: The cardiovascular response of normal humans to the administration of endotoxin. *N Engl J Med* 1989;321:280-287

54. Millar AB, Singer M, Meager A, Foley NM, Johnson NM, Rook GA: Tumor necrosis factor in bronchopulmonary secretions of patients with adult respiratory distress syndrome. *Lancet* 1989;2:712-713

55. Hegewisch S, Weh HJ, Hossfeld DK: TNF-induced cardiomyopathy. *Lancet* 1990;2:294-295

56. Semb H, Peterson J, Tavernier J, Olivecrona T: Multiple effects of tumor necrosis factor on lipoprotein lipase in vivo. *J Biol Chem* 1987;262:8390-8394

57. Oliff A, Defeo-Jones D, Boyer M, Martinez D, Kiefer D, Vuocolo G, Wolfe A, Socher SH: Tumors secreting human TNF/Cachectin induce cachexia in mice. *Cell* 1987;50:555-563

58. Spiegelman BM, Hotamisligil GS: Through thick and thin: wasting, obesity, and TNFα. *Cell* 1993;73:625-627

59. Socher SH, Friedman A, Martinez D: Recombinant human tumor necrosis factor induces reductions in food intake and body weight in mice. *J Exp Med* 1988;167:1957-1962

60. Lancaster, Jr., Laster SM, Gooding LR: Inhibition of target cell mitochondrial electron transfer by tumor necrosis factor. *FEBS Lett* 1989;248:169-174

61. Stadler J, Bentz BG, Harbrecht BG, Disilvio M, Curran RD, Billiar TR, Hoffman RA, Simmons RL: Tumor necrosis factor alpha inhibits hepatocyte mitochondrial respiration. *Ann Surg* 1992;216:539-546

62. Nakano M, Knowlton AA, Yokoyama T, Lesslauer W, Mann DL: Tumor necrosis factor-α induced expression of heat shock protein 72 in adult feline cardiac myocytes. *Am J Physiol* 1995;(In Press)

8

ROLE OF SMALL HEAT SHOCK PROTEINS
IN THE CARDIOVASCULAR SYSTEM

Hari S. Sharma
Erasmus University
Rotterdam, The Netherlands

and

Joachim Stahl
Max Delbrück Center for Molecular Medicine
Berlin, Germany

ABSTRACT

There are five different small heat shock proteins (sHSPs), *HSP27, B-crystallin, HSP20, HSP32* and *ubiquitin*, that occur at relatively high levels in heart tissues which therefore can be considered important for the cardiovascular system. The properties of the three structurally related sHSPs, *HSP27, B-crystallin* and *HSP20*, and their location in developing and differentiated heart tissues, in particular in cardiomyocytes, support their participation in heart muscle contraction, in which way, however, is in detail not yet elucidated. The functional role of these sHSPs is most likely influenced and regulated by phosphorylation via the MAPKAP kinase signalling system in correlation with stress-dependent protein kinases as well as by interactions with other important cardiac proteins as actin desmin, and vimentin. A fourth small heat shock protein, *HSP32*, is the enzyme hemoxygenase 1 (HO-1), part of the intracellular oxidoreductase system. It is induced in the cardiovascular system by various kinds of oxidative stress. High levels of HSP32 contribute to cardioprotection by maintaining and regulating the intracellular glutathione level. Finally, the role of the smallest heat shock protein, *ubiquitin*, and its possible importance for degradation and removal of molecularly damaged proteins is discussed in some detail. Altogether, these sHSPs are expressed in considerable amounts in heart tissues of many animals and elevated levels can be induced under stress and pathophysiological conditions. The cardioprotective functions of these proteins may contribute in different ways also to cardiac recovery from certain pathological states.

INTRODUCTION

Stressful conditions caused by heat, heavy metals, irradiation, drugs or other non-physiological circumstances can damage living cells by destabilizing and subsequently denaturing endogenous proteins, bringing about inactivation of enzymes and disorder in cell metabolism. To cope for such disturbances and to renature the proteins concerned, living cells have developed stress response systems that contribute to maintenance of basic cellular functions in the tissue [Kampinga et al., 1995]. Thus, upon onset of unfavourable conditions in cell environment, at first endogenous stress proteins fulfill protective functions by renaturing proteins and, after some induction period, new stress proteins get synthesized in order to enhance the protective cellular potential. In general, stress proteins are heat inducible and hence referred to as heat shock proteins (HSPs). Induction of HSP gene expression is caused via activation of heat shock transcription factors that bind to heat shock elements located in the 5' end promoter region of specific HSP genes [Morimoto et al., 1994], subsequently leading to transcription of these genes and HSP synthesis. So, occurrence of heat shock proteins is generally accepted to imply a basis for self-preservation of cells and organisms against various kinds of stress and high levels of heat shock proteins therefore mean high protective potential of cells.

During the last couple of years the cardioprotective role of stress protein HSP70 has been convincingly proven. Besides the endogenous levels of HSC70 (heat shock cognate protein 70), in particular the inducible HSP70 contributes considerably to cardioprotection against stress, locally caused by hypoxia, ischemia and reperfusion induced injury [Iwaki et al., 1993, Mestril et al., 1994, Heads et al., 1995], or whole body stress caused by heat [Currie et al., 1988, Donnelly et al., 1992, Hutter et al., 1994]. Transgenic animals overexpressing human HSP70 [Plumier et al., 1995] or rat HSP70 [Marber et al., 1995] showed increased resistance of the heart to ischemic injury. The cardioprotective role of the inducible HSP70 was also proven in studies using Langendorff heart preparations as a model of cardiac ischemia [Currie et al., 1990, Amrani et al., 1993].

For small heat shock proteins (sHSPs), a cardioprotective role has not been published yet, but data from Dillmann's group in San Diego, Ca. presented at the Cold Spring Harbor Meeting in May 1996 [Martin et al., 1996] suggest a clear correlation between high levels of HSP27 and αB-crystallin and a high protective potential of cardiomyocytes against ischemic injury. Earlier analyses of heart tissue from a great number of vertebrates, including human heart biopsies, have suggested that at least some sHSPs play important roles in the cardiovascular system, since elevated levels of these proteins were detected. When separating human ventricular tissue by high-resolution two-dimensional gel electrophoresis the mixture of total proteins of heart tissue showed nearly 10.000 different moieties [Thiede et al., 1996], only 50 of which have been identified and characterized on a molecular basis. Besides the known major heart proteins - such as actin, desmin, myoglobin and myosin - and functionally important enzymes, like ATP-synthase or creatine kinase, 2-D positions of multiple forms of stress proteins HSP27 and α-crystallin moieties have been elucidated.

The heterogeneous group of sHSPs summarized within this chapter, contributes in different ways to protection of the cardiovascular system. While the function of ubiquitin, the smallest stress protein known so far, is obviously to facilitate degradation of denatured proteins, the modes of action of the other sHSPs in the heart and their possible roles in cardioprotection are not yet well understood. With regard to small stress proteins HSP27 and α-crystallin, the reader is recommended to consult the reviews by Arrigo and Landry [1994) on sHSPs and of Yellon and Latchman (1992), Knowlton (1995), and Mestril and Dillmann (1995) on HSPs in the cardiovascular system.

Here, we describe the so far known general structural parameters and functional properties of small stress proteins and their importance for the cardiovascular system. In particular, the recent data on location of the small stress proteins HSP27 and αB-crystallin in cardiomyocytes will be discussed in relation to the different sarcomeric zones involved in heart muscle contraction.

SMALL HEAT SHOCK PROTEINS HSP27, B-CRYSTALLIN AND HSP20

Induction, Properties and Occurrence of HSP27

The genes coding for small heat shock protein 27 (also designated as HSP25 or HSP28, but in this text referred to as HSP27) from a multitude of species have been characterized earlier [for review see Arrigo and Landry, 1994] and even complete phylogenic trees have been developed [deJong et al., 1993, and Plesofsky-Vig et al., 1992]. HSP27 genes from several higher vertebrates have been sequenced: human [Hickey et al., 1986, Carper et al., 1990], rat [Uoshima et al., 1993] and mouse [Gaestel et al., 1993, Frohli et al., 1993]; and always one single active gene has been found besides up to two pseudogenes. The transcribed region of human HSP27 gene consists of three exons, the promoter region contains two TATA boxes, GC-rich SP1 binding elements, two structures with consensus sequences called heat shock elements (HSE) for binding of heat shock factors (HSF) and a semi-palindromic motif of an estrogen receptor (ERE) [Gaestel et al., 1993], which has been used as a suitable means to induce HSP27 expression in various cells [reviewed in Benndorf and Bielka, 1996].

Sequencing data from 6 different vertebrate species, demonstrated HSP27 to belong to highly conserved proteins of strong homology in the N-terminal and central regions and some amino acid deviations near the C-terminus. Related domains occur also in two other sHSPs, namely αB-crystallin and HSP20 (see below). The molecular weights of the monomeric HSP27 molecules range from 21671 for chicken [Miron et al., 1991], 22327 for human HSP27 [Hickey et al., 1986], 23014 for mouse [Gaestel et al., 1989] and 23419 for hamster [Lavoie et al. 1990]. With regard to secondary structure arrangements of HSP27, predictions of Walsh et al., 1991, suggest predominance of ß-sheet conformation with less than 5% α-helix structures. For the observed interactions with membranes and also with other proteins, amphiphilic alpha-helixes with high hydrophobic moment seem to be of major importance [Plesofsky-Vig et al., 1990].

As to the tertiary structure of HSP27 (as well as for αB-crystallin and HSP20) their tendency to associate to multimeric complexes is most remarkable [Zantema et al., 1992]. For instance, *in vitro* studies with recombinant murine HSP27 have demonstrated compact globular homopolymeric structures [Behlke et al., 1991] that are similar to αB-crystallin. In contrast, when analyzing "native" HSP27 isolated from Ehrlich ascites tumor cells, highly associated complexes forming ring-like particles with diameters of about 16 nm most likely consisting of four stacked rings each containing eight HSP27 molecules could be demonstrated by electron microscopy and subsequent image processing [Behlke et al., 1995]. From this supramolecular arrangement of HSP27 similarities to multimeric structures of other known chaperones like HSP60 or TCP-1 can be deduced. *In vivo*, also heteropolymers between different small stress proteins and, in addition, with other cellular proteins can be formed and may fulfill protective functions under stress conditions.

The small stress protein HSP27 has been shown to occur in relatively high concentrations in heart tissue of various species including rat [Wilkinson and Pollard, 1993, Maulik et al., 1993, Das et al., 1993, Lu and Das, 1993, Kato et al., 1994 , Maulik et al., 1994, Inaguma et al., 1995], mouse [Klemenz et al., 1993, Gernold et al., 1993], turkey [Miron et al., 1991], pig [Andres et al., 1993] and man [Kato et al., 1992, Offhauss, unpublished]. The amounts of HSP27 in heart tissues of various species were determined on a quantitative basis and values between 700 and 2000 ng/mg extracted protein were measured (compare Table 1).

Table 1:
Quantitative determination of HSP27 in heart tissue from different vertebrates: Method A: Heart tissue was sonicated in 50 mM Tris-HCl, pH 7.5, 5 mM EDTA and the amount of HSP27 was determined by an enzyme immunoassay (Inaguma et al., 1993). *Method B:* Heart tissue was extracted by Laemmli sample buffer, incubated for 5 min at 95°C and the amount of HSP27 determined on immunoblots using HSP27 antibodies [Klemenz et al., 1993, Offhauss, unpublished].

Organ	HSP 27 (ng/mg protein	Method	Reference
Rat heart	700 - 750	A	Inaguma et al., 1995
Human heart	1 700	A	Kato et al., 1992
Human heart	1 000	B	Offhauss, unpublished*)
Mouse heart	ca 2 000	B	Klemenz et al., 1993**)

*) average from biopsies after heart transplantation
    (means of values between 500 and 2 500 ng/mg protein)
**) calculated from immunoblots of Fig. 1 in Klemenz et al., 1993.

Induction, properties and occurrence of B-crystallin

The small stress protein αB-crystallin, first identified as a major protein in the eye-lens, has a primary structure closely related to HSP27. αB-crystallin is encoded by a single-copy gene located in humans on chromosome 11. Human [Dubin et al., 1990] and rat αB-crystallin [Srinavasan and Bhat, 1994] genes have a high degree of similarity in several regions, as discussed in detail in the latter paper and the amino acid sequences of αB-crystallin show common major domains with HSP27 [Arrigo and Landry, 1994]. αB-crystallin can be modified *in vivo* with O-linked N-acetyl-glucosamine as well as by calcium-activated transglutaminase crosslinking the crystallins to other cellular proteins [deJong et al., 1993]. In general, alpha-crystallins have, similar to HSP27, protease-inhibitory activity that has been shown with elastase [Merck et al., 1993]. This activity may be of importance also for heart metabolism, because it can be expected to compete with ubiquitin, a protease of obvious importance for cardiomyocytes as will be discussed later on. αB-crystallin is also reported to become reversibly phosphorylated in two or three Ser residues [for review see deJong et al., 1993], the significance of these modifications is, however, not understood yet.

Among the nonocular tissues αB-crystallin is found in highest concentration in heart tissue of different species, as demonstrated for rat heart [Iwaki et al., 1989 and 1990, Chiesa et al., 1990, Chiesi et al., 1990, Longoni et al., 1990, Iwaki et al., 1990, Kato et al., 1991, Bhat et al., 1991, Chepelinski et al., 1991, Srinavasan et al., 1992 and 1994, Bennardini et al., 1992, Chiesi and Bennardini, 1992, Srinavasan and Bhat, 1994], mouse heart [Dubin et al., 1990, Gernold et al., 1993, Klemenz et al., 1993, Gopal-Srivastava and Piatigorsky, 1994], and for human heart [Bhat et al., 1991], Lowe et al., 1992, Kato et al., 1992, Leach et al., 1994, Groenen et al., 1994, Knecht et al. 1994, Thiede et al., 1996]. From quantitative analyses it is evident that especially tissues rich in muscle cells contain, in addition to the high levels of HSP27, also relatively high amounts of αB-crystallin. So, Kato et al., 1991, found levels of αB-crystallin to amount to about 3 μg/mg extractable protein in human heart, 4 μg/mg in bovine and about 1 μg/mg in porcine heart. Klemenz et al., 1993, analyzed αB-crystallin in different mouse tissues in a semi-quantitative way, and compared 18 different organs with maximal values of about 2 μg/mg protein in heart tissue and up to 20 μg αB-crystallin/mg protein in soleus muscle. Inaguma et al., 1995, determined αB-crystallin levels in normal and heat stressed rats. Again, highest endogenous values were found in soleus muscle reaching up to 30 μg αB-crystallin/mg detergent-free extracted protein which, however, did not increase upon heat stress. In rat heart, heat shock for 20 min at 42°C only slightly increased the baseline value of 3.6 μg αB-crystallin/mg. Interestingly, the other rat tissues tested responded quite differently to whole body heat stress with regard to αB-crystallin induction. In contrast to αB-crystallin, the closely related αA-crystallin, occurring in high concentrations in eye lenses, is not present in heart tissue as shown in studies by Chepelinsky et al., 1991, and Srinavasan et al., 1992.

Small Stress Protein HSP20

Another small stress protein, designated as HSP20, was recently isolated from human and rat skeletal muscle [Kato et al., 1994]. It reveals amino acid sequences closely related to both, HSP27 and α-crystallins. Quantitative values were determined in different rat tissues, and for heart about 1 μg/mg and for diaphragm about 2 μg/mg extracted protein were estimated, compared to tongue with 1.5 μg/mg, and bladder of up to 2 μg/mg protein, while in spleen, lung, kidney or liver almost zero levels and in soleus muscle maximal values of more than 10 μg/mg were detected.

Phosphorylation of HSP27

For more than ten years HSP27 is known to be the main phosphoprotein in a variety of cells in response to cell stimuli as growth factors, serum as well as various stressors. Upon two-dimensional electrophoresis, two phosphorylated isoforms were found in many vertebrate cells and three in humans [see Arrigo and Landry, 1994]. Phosphorylation sites of human small HSP27 have been detected in Ser-15, Ser-78 and Ser-82 and in rodent HSP27 Ser-15 and Ser-82 (here human Ser-78 is replaced by an Asp residue [Gaestel et al., 1989, 1991, Lavoie et al., 1990]. Although the functional significance of phosphorylation of HSP27 is not fully elucidated yet, it obviously affects the size of the high molecular weight aggregate structure of sHSPs. All phosphorylation sites have Arg-X-X-Ser as a common consensus sequence that is phosphorylated *in vitro* and *in vivo* as well [Stokoe et al., 1992a].

The kinetics of HSP27 induction and phosphorylation have been summarized and thoroughly discussed by Arrigo and Landry, 1994. From the data illustrated therein it can be clearly deduced that the general cellular heat shock response may consist of two phases: an initial, short-term phase, characterized by phosphorylation of endogenously present HSP27 - starting within minutes, reaching maximal values after half an hour and then declining, and a second, long-term phase, in which new HSP27 protein is being formed - starting after about 3 hours of recovery from stress at 37°C, reaching maximal concentrations around 10 hours and then declining within days back to normal levels. Such kind of stress response seems to be typical for heat shock as well as for general stress response most likely operative in cardiomyocytes. So, TNF-α, a multipotent cytokine, is known as an inducer of HSP27 phosphorylation and, in addition, was shown [Sharma et al., 1996b] to induce in cardiac myocytes HSP27 mRNA levels by 2-4-fold, as will be discussed later on.

HSP27 is phosphorylated most efficiently by MAPKAP kinase-2, a protein kinase purified to homogeneity from rabbit skeletal muscle [Stokoe et al., 1992b]. The enzyme is a member of a signal cascade that is activated for instance by various growth factors, TNF-α, as well as during mitosis. In addition, there are kinase activities described that are capable of phosphorylating HSP27, so in Ehrlich ascites tumor cells [Benndorf et al., 1992], Chinese hamster cells [Zhou et al., 1993], MRC-5 fibroblasts [Guesdon et al., 1993], HL60 cells [Zu et al., 1994] and HeLa cells [Huot et al., 1995]. HSP27 kinase(s) can be activated by phosphorylation through enzymes participating in the MAP kinase signal transduction pathway, as proven for ERK1 and ERK2 [Engel et al., 1995] and the reactivating kinase RK38 [Freshney et al., 1994, Rouse et al., 1994]. For the cardiovascular system, the HSP27 phosphorylation cascade is most likely of special importance in view of the complicated isoform pattern that has been found in human heart biopsies upon high-performance 2-D separation [Thiede et al., 1996], although direct data on the location of HSP27 kinase(s) in the two-dimensional protein map of the cardiac system are still missing.

132

The *in-vivo* HSP27 phosphorylation status is also regulated by specific phosphatases. Thus, by using specific phosphatase inhibitors, Cairns et al., 1994, have demonstrated that *in-vivo* HSP27 dephosphoryation is obviously achieved by PP2A (protein phosphatase 2A). Another phosphatase that is activated by okadaic acid and oxyradicals may also play a role in HSP27 regulation [Guy et al., 1993].

Intracellular localization of HSP27 and B-crystallin

The constitutively expressed small stress protein HSP27 has been repeatedly described in different cell types to be located in the cytoplasm and often found located in somewhat higher concentration in the perinuclear zone. Upon heat shock or other stresses, several reports have demonstrated by immunofluorescence and electron microscopy, HSP27 and αB-crystallin to translocate into the nucleus. This location is, however, reversed to cytoplasm during recovery from stress [Arrigo et al., 1988], for discussion compare Arrigo and Landry, 1994]. Temporary nuclear location of sHSPs is presumably connected with protein renaturation within the nucleus, in favour with the hypothesis of Kampinga et al., 1995, as discussed in the introduction to this chapter. Additional data supporting a chaperoning activity have been reported for HSP27 [Jakob et al., 1993] and for αB-crystallin [Horwitz, 1992, Jakob et al., 1993, Groenen et al., 1994], however, only in *in vitro*-systems up to now.

Myocardial occurrence of HSP27, B-crystallin and HSP20

With regard to possible cardioprotection, interactions between small stress proteins and components forming cytoskeleton and myofibrils, require special interest. High levels of HSP27, αB-crystallin and also HSP20 in heart tissue point to functional importance of these small stress proteins for heart function. An inhibitor of actin polymerization (IAP) isolated by Miron et al., 1988 and 1991, from vinculin-rich extract of turkey gizzard muscle turned out to be the small stress protein HSP27. The protein was shown to bind specifically to the plus-end of F-actin filaments and in this way to stop actin polymerization. Further, it was shown to depolymerize actin, a fact also confirmed by Rahman et al., 1995, for the yeast small stress protein HSP26. The data were confirmed later on by Benndorf et al., 1994, in a kinetic and electron microscopic *in vitro*-study using HSP27 isolated from Ehrlich ascites tumor cells. In this study, unphosphorylated HSP27 was proven to inhibit actin polymerization by acting as a barbed-end capping protein. *In vivo*-experiments of Bitar et al., 1991, have shown HSP27 to associate with smooth muscle cells and microinjection of anti-HSP27 antibodies to inhibit bombesin- and kinase-C-induced sustained muscle contraction in mouse cells. Additional evidence for correlations between HSP27 and actin filament dynamics comes from *in vivo*-experiments, in which HSP27 was overexpressed in Chinese hamster fibroblasts and as a consequence, microfilament disruption was demonstrated to be partially prevented [Lavoie et al., 1993a, 1993b]. HSP27 used, during actin polymerization, to maximally accumulate at the leading edge, the most active actin polymerizing region, that is characterized by a rapid reorganization of microfilament network [Lavoie et al., 1993b]. In addition, Lavoie et al., 1995, have proven HSP27 to stabilize the microfilament network in rodent cells. By using Chinese hamster cell mutants overexpressing either wild-type or a nonphosphorylatable human HSP27, Huot et al., 1996, demonstrated in a most recent study that phosphorylation of HSP27 is causally related to regulation of microfilament dynamics following oxidative stress and that phosphorylated HSP27 confers resistance against actin fragmentation. Although the cardiac system is possibly protected in a somewhat more complex way against oxidative stress than the experimental system of the above authors, the relative high levels of HSP27 expressed in cardiomyocytes would support a quick cardiac response to stress by HSP27 phosphorylation and subsequent improved cardiac muscle protection, a hypothesis worthwhile to be proven in corresponding experimental systems.

The related cardiac sHSP, αB-crystallin, was shown to associate with intermediate filaments in the eye-lens [Fitzgerald and Graham, 1991]. In addition, αB-crystallin inhibits assembly of vimentin *in vitro* [Nicholl and Quinlan, 1994]. For heart, αB-crystallin was found to interact specifically with actin and desmin, two major cardiac proteins [Chiesi et al., 1990, Longoni et al., 1990]. It was further proven that αB-crystallin prevents aggregation of actin filaments at acidic pH [Bennardini et al., 1992] and it was described to localize at the Z-line in cardiomyocytes [Longoni et al., 1990; Bennardini et al., 1992].

Localization of HSP27 and B-crystallin in the developing embryo

From various studies the levels of HSP27 and αB-crystallin are known to be subject to quite dramatic changes in different phases of cell growth and differentiation. Using mouse models, for embryonic carcinoma cells and for embryonal stem cells it has been demonstrated that with differentiation HSP27 levels rise steadily [Stahl et al., 1993]. Analyzing the distributions of HSP27 and αB-crystallin during embryonal mouse development [Gernold et al., 1993], there are, in parallel to a continuous increase in HSP27 levels, considerable changes in localization of this protein through days 13-20 of embryogenesis and, most remarkably, HSP27 accumulates preferentially in various muscle tissues. The most striking structural alterations during this period concern HSP27 localization in the developing mouse heart pointing to an important role of this protein for heart differentiation. In a study on rat embryos, Wilkinson and Pollard, 1993, have described HSP27 to be localized preferentially in the developing myocardium of day 10.5-, 11.5- and 12.5-embryos, closely correlated with muscle fiber differentiation and associated with cytoskeletal proteins.

Very recently, the distribution of HSP27 in developing rat heart was analyzed by electron microscopy of cryosections through different cell types in various regions of heart tissue at high magnification [Lutsch et al., 1995, Hoch et al., 1996a,b]. Tissue sections through the left ventricle, revealing particularly high HSP27 contents - of day 20 rat embryos of gestation - show a strong cytoplasmic labeling of HSP27 mainly in undifferentiated cardiomyocytes. In developing myofibrils of this cell type there is weak labeling, and nuclei and mitochondria are not labeled at all. In fully differentiated cardiomyocytes, HSP27 labeling is rather weak and cannot be attributed to distinct intracellular compartments. Using antibodies directed against αB-crystallin, a very similar distribution in heart probes of the different developmental stages was observed, only the labeling density in the latter samples occurred to be slightly reduced in comparison to HSP27 intensity.

Localization of HSP27 and B-crystallin in adult heart tissue

Localization of small stress proteins has been studied also in adult heart muscle cells. Electron microscopic analysis of ventricular tissue revealed in sarcomeres of myofibrils double-labeling by anti-HSP27 (labeled by 10 nm gold particles) and anti-αB-crystallin antibodies (labeled by 15 nm gold particles) suggesting colocalization of both sHSPs [Lutsch et al., 1995, Hoch et al., 1996a,b]. Whether this colocalization is due to homo- or heterooligomeric complexes of both sHSPs, however, remains to be demonstrated. Analyzing heart tissue from 12 days old rats electron microscopic images show, in comparison to embryonal rat heart reduced labeling density of HSP27 in cardiomyocytes, which, at this postnatal stage already largely belong to the differentiated cell type. Accordingly by Western blot analysis a simultaneous decrease in the HSP27 level is observed in cardiomyocytes from prenatal to postnatal stages. In cardiomyocytes of heart tissue from adult rats a rather sparse labeling pattern for HSP27 is observed and the few gold particles in the region of myofibrils were seen mainly in connection with the I-band.

Using the immunofluorescence technique to characterize HSP27 location (compare Fig. 1 taken from [Hoch et al., 1996a], with permission) in isolated neonatal cardiomyocytes (day 1) still bearing large amounts of undifferentiated cardiomyocytes, HSP27 staining was found in flattened areas of the cell in myofibrillar structures (Fig. 1A) and colocalization with the I-band of myofibrils could be demonstrated. In heart tissue of neonatal rats, HSP27 antibodies lead to a clearly cross-striated staining pattern (arrowheads in Fig. 1A) which is similar to staining observed for sarcomeres in myofibrils. In comparison, isolated adult cardiomyocytes show a regular staining pattern throughout the whole cell with striations oriented perpendicularly to the longitudinal axis of the rod-shaped cells corresponding to the staining of sarcomeres in myofibrils (Fig. 1B). By double-labeling of cryosections with anti-HSP27 and anti-α-sarcomeric actin antibodies, HSP27 staining was confirmed to occur at the level of the I-band in myofibrils and in strongly stained cells also at the M-line demonstrating that both structures overlap and therefore HSP27 and actin colocalize [Hoch et al., 1996a,b]. In parallel experiments, also double-staining of HSP27 and αB-crystallin in myofilaments was proven in the same regions of sarcomeres, that means at the I-band of myofibrils.

For comparison, semi-thin cryosections through isolated perfused rat hearts after normothermic perfusion for 210 min were double-labeled with HSP27 and actin antibodies and subsequently analyzed by fluorescence microscopy. A labeled left ventricular cardiomyocyte demonstrates a striking similarity in the stained bands (Fig. 1C,D). Because the bands stained by actin antibodies represent the I-bands of sarcomeres and the stained regions are split into two parts by the unlabeled Z-line, it is

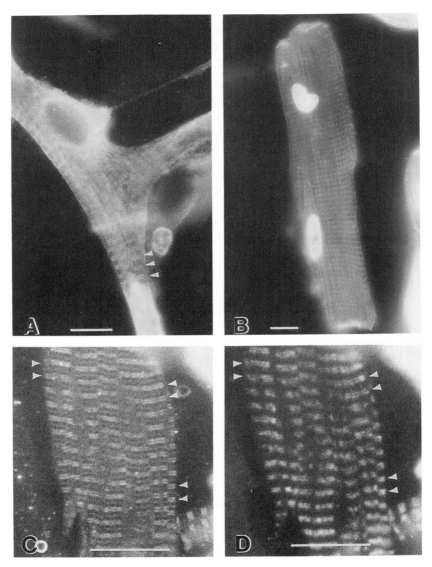

Figure 1: Immunofluorescence micrographs of isolated rat cardiomyocytes (A,B) and isolated perfused rat hearts (C,D) (taken from Hoch et al., 1996a). Bars 10 μm. Isolated neonatal rat cardiomyocyte (A) and adult rat cardiomyocyte (B), labeled with primary HSP27 and DTAF-labeled secondary antibodies. Nuclei are stained by DAPI (4',6-diamidino-2-phenylindole). C,D: Semithin cryosection of left ventricular cardiomyocyte from isolated perfused rat heart double-labeled with HSP27 (C) and actin antibody (D), visualized by DTAF-(C) and Cy3-labeled secondary antibodies (D). Arrowheads in A, C and D point to doublets of HSP27 and doublets of actin staining.

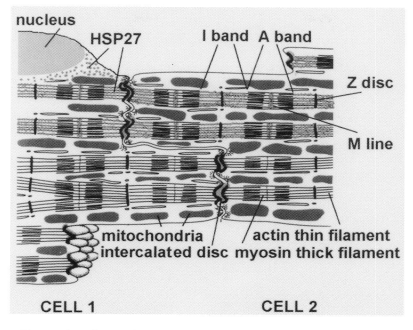

Figure 1b: Schema of HSP27 localization in cardiomyocytes. Dark dots represent HSP27 (designed by R.Benndorf on the basis of Figure 11-22, page 625, from the Molecular Biology of the Cell, second edition, ed. by Alberts, B., Bray, D., Lewis,J., Raff,M., Roberts,K., Watson,J.D., Garland Publishing Inc., New York and London, 1989).

herewith proven that HSP27 is located at the I-band of myofibrils (see arrowheads in Fig. 1C,D). In some cases, additional staining of HSP27 at the level of the M-line is observed. The schematic drawing in fig.1b illustrates the location of HSP27 in relation to the known structures of cardiomyocytes.

Summarizing the immunfluorescence data on HSP27 and αB-crystallin localization in ventricular tissue of adult rats, there are significant differences to prenatal stages, because HSP27 staining was observed not only in cardiomyocytes, but also in endothelial cells and in smooth muscle cells surrounding blood vessels, cell types in which the presence of αB-crystallin could not be demonstrated. This points to cell type-specific abundance and functions of both small stress proteins in the myocardium. In view of the available literature, HSP27 seems to play a regulatory role in the process of differentiation of certain tissues, in particular muscle tissues including cardiomyocytes in the developing heart. Later on, when the whole organ has fully differentiated, moderate levels of HSP27 obviously suffice for maintaining regular heart function. In which way HSP27 fulfills important functions in metabolism of the adult heart is, however, not yet elucidated and still a matter of discussion. Studies on the localization of small stress proteins strongly point to a regulatory role in muscle contraction. Further data are needed either on the phosphorylation status and the association status of small stress proteins one with another, with actin and with actin binding proteins, in particular vinculin, a protein occurring in particularly large amounts in heart tissue. It is by no means questionable that small HSPs play an important role, at least for cardioprotection, since under stress conditions the stress response system signals within seconds to minutes sHSP phosphorylation and within few hours induction of new HSP27-mRNA, possibly just to guarantee maintenance of a certain HSP27 level. It will be important to learn in future studies what role phosphorylation of small stress protein does play in heart function and in which way this process coincides with the intracellular MAPKAP kinase signal transduction pathway.

HSP32 (Heme Oxygenase-1, HO-1)

Enzymic activity and induction of heme oxygenase

The heme oxygenase (HO) system (heme hydrogen donor:oxygen oxidoreductase, EC 1.14.99.3] consists of two isozymes, heme oxygenase-1 (HO-1) and heme oxygenase-2 (HO-2). It generates the putative cellular messenger carbon monoxide (CO) in mammalian cells [Maines, 1988, and Trakshel and Maines, 1989]. Both HO-1 and HO-2 catalyze the cleavage of heme b (Fe-protoporphyrin-IX) at the a-meso carbon bridge to form the antioxidant biliverdin IXa, iron and CO [Maines, 1988, Trakshel and Maines, 1989, Prabhakar et al., 1995, Vile et al., 1994]. Though CO is known as a highly toxic combustion product, its endogenous production in tissue may have important physiological functions particularly in regulating the cardiovascular system. The CO produced in the body is believed to modulate blood flow under normal and pathophysiological conditions [Prabhakar et al., 1995, Ewing et al., 1995, Morita et al., 1995, Christodoulides et al., 1995]. Furthermore, CO has been suggested to be a neurotransmitter in the brain [Stevens and Wang, 1993]. Both forms of heme oxygenase, HO-1 and HO-2, are products of two different genes [Cruse and Maines, 1988, Shibahara et al., 1993] and they differ markedly in their tissue distribution and molecular properties [Maines, 1988, Raju and Maines, 1994]. Whereas HO-2 is a constitutively expressed and non-inducible gene product, HO-1 is induced by several noxious conditions including oxidative stress [Ewing and Maines, 1991, Maines et al., 1986, Keyse et al., 1990].

Originally, HO-1 was identified as a metal inducible enzyme in the cell. Being a heat inducible protein, it is now also referred to as heat shock protein-32 (HSP32) and regarded as a member of HSP family. In the following text, HO-1 will also be referred as HSP32. Binding of a transcription factor to a heat shock element sequence in the promotor region of HSP32 gene is regarded as the responsible cellular event for heat shock response in various species [Mueller et al., 1987]. Unlike c-jun oncogene, whose expression is induced by UVC (254 nm) radiation, HSP32 gene is not induced by UVC radiation, but strongly induced by oxidizing agents such as UVA [H320-380 nm) radiation or hydrogen peroxide [Keyse and Tyrrell, 1989]. In addition to oxidative stress, the HSP32 gene is induced by phorbol esters, heavy metals, and sodium arsenite [Keyse and Tyrrell, 1989].

Although the induction of the HSP32 gene by the above mentioned agents was originally observed in cultured skin fibroblasts, this now holds true to different species and different cell types [Tyrrell et al., 1993]. The induction is clearly related to the cellular redox state since lowering of cellular glutathione levels strongly enhances HSP32 mRNA accumulation [Lautier et al., 1992]. For these reasons enhanced expression of HSP32 gene appears to be a fairly sensitive marker of oxidative stress and may be applied as a diagnostic tool such as in cardiovascular system. It may be mentioned here that the promotor region of human HSP32 gene contains the binding sites for transcription factors NFκB and AP-2 [Lavrovsky et al., 1994]. The presence of regulatory sequences for binding of NFκB and AP-2, whose activation is associated with immediate response of the cell to an injury, may underly the role for HSP32 in defense mechanisms against tissue injury [Tyrrell et al., 1993, Lavrovsky et al., 1994, Takeda et al., 1994].

HSP32 as an indirect blood flow regulator

Carbon monoxide is produced endogenously by various cell types as a byproduct of heme catabolism through the HO system. CO is the diatomic gas molecule that shares some of the physicochemical properties of another physiological messenger called endothelium-derived relaxing factor or nitric oxide (NO). CO, like NO has the ability to bind to the iron atom of the heme moiety associated with soluble guanyl cyclase, thereby activating this enzyme and raising intracellular levels of cyclic guanosine 3',5'-monophosphate (cGMP) [Morita et al., 1995, Christodoulides et al., 1995]. It is believed that enhanced intracellular levels of cGMP regulate blood vessel tone and blood flow by inhibiting the smooth muscle contraction and platelet aggregation. Vascular smooth muscle cells (VSMC) have both constitutive and inducible HO activity and when exposed to hypoxia, enhanced transcription and translation of HSP32 have been observed in these cells. Enhanced HSP32 expression in hypoxic VSMC leads to drastically increased amounts of CO resulting in elevated levels of cGMP and consequently relaxing the blood vessel [Morita et al., 1995].

Myocardial expression of HSP32 in response to different stimuli

Elevated ambient temperature (42°C) for 20 min have been reported to induce significantly HSP32 mRNA expression in various organs including rat hearts [Raju and Maines, 1994]. Maximum induction was observed 1 h after hyperthermia and reached a value 20-40 times as high as in normothermic rats. Using an *in vitro* nuclear run-on assay, Raju and Maines, 1994, verified that hyperthermia-induced expression of HSP32 was a result of enhanced transcription of the HSP32 gene and not due to decreased RNA degradation. Furthermore, the increase in HSP32 mRNA transcription was accompanied by an increase in binding of nuclear factor(s) to the heat shock element in the promotor region of HSP32 gene. Using Western blot analysis it could be confirmed that hyperthermia for 6 h led to increased levels of HSP32 protein in heart and kidney of rats resulting in enhanced activity of this detoxifying enzyme in the hyperthermic tissue.

To assess the role of HSPs including HSP32 in the heart, Katayose et al., 1993, have examined the expression of HSP32 in rats subjected to hypoxia or pulmonary artery banding, both of which produce severe right ventricular pressure overload. They found that at 3 days after hypoxia HSP32 mRNA levels were elevated by four-fold, whereas HSP70 mRNA levels remained unchanged. Pulmonary artery banding markedly and immediately (within 6 h) increased HSP32 mRNA levels in both ventricles indicating its important role in cardioprotection against oxidative stress, since bile pigments, the products of heme catabolism are shown to act as radical scavangers [Maines, 1988].

Expression of HSP32 in porcine stunned myocardium

A period of reversible cardiac dysfunction can occur after brief episodes of coronary occlusion and ischemia. It is a reversible decrease in force of systolic contraction, a phenomenon that is called "stunning". Hence, stunned myocardium is defined as hypo-contractile reperfused myocardium with delayed but complete recovery of function following a brief period of ischemia. Among the cellular organelles whose altered function might account for contractile dysfunction are the sarcoplasmic reticulum, the contractile filaments and the sarcolemma [Sharma et al., 1993]. We have shown that brief periods of coronary artery occlusion followed by reperfusion in anaesthetized pigs produce prolonged regional cardiac dysfunction (stunning) associated with altered expression of a number of genes. Recently, we have reported on a coordinated expression pattern of HSP32 and ubiquitin in the porcine model in which the left anterior descending coronary artery (LAD) was occluded for 10 min and reperfused for 30 min (group I) and after a second occlusion of 10 min, reperfused for either 30 min (group II) or 90 min (group III) or 210 min (group IV) [Sharma et al., 1996c] (see Fig. 2). Myocardial tissue from LAD (stunned) and left circumflex coronary artery (LCx, control) perfused regions were collected in liquid nitrogen and analyzed for the expression of HSP32. Northern blot analysis revealed that a single mRNA species of 1.8 kb encoding HSP32 was expressed in the porcine heart. The steady state mRNA levels of HSP32 were significantly enhanced by repetitive coronary artery occlusion and reperfusion, i.e in the stunned myocardium as compared to the control (Fig 2). The time course of induction of the HSP32 gene showed maximal mRNA levels after two cycles of 10 min ischemia and 30 min of reperfusion. Thereafter, expression in the stunned

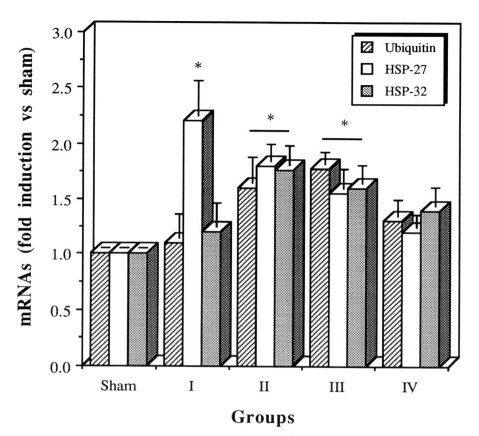

Figure 2: Northern blot analysis of HSP27, HSP32 and ubiquitin expression in stunned and normal myocardium. Bar graph showing quantitative analysis of the small HSP genes. Total RNA extracted from stunned and control (sham animal) tissue at various time points of reperfusion was subjected to Northern hybridization with respective radiolabeled cDNA probes. Hybridization signals from mRNA bands of HSPs as well as from GAPDH blots were quantitated by video densitometry and normalized. Values are expressed as mean of fold induction vs sham $\pm$ SEM (n = 4). *P<0.05 vs sham.

myocardial tissue declined but remained slightly elevated as compared to control. These results indicate that the HO-1 gene increased with ischemia, but significant myocardial accumulation of mRNA occurred only during the reperfusion phase. Several reports have established that HSP32 activity is induced by a number of stimuli e.g. heavy metals [Maines et al., 1988, Trakshel and Maines, 1989], heat shock [Shibahara et al., 1987, Ewing et al., 1994], ultraviolet A (UVA) radiation [Keyse et al., 1990, Lautier et al., 1992] and hydrogen peroxide [Keyse et al., 1990]. Induction of HSP32 in human skin fibroblasts by UVA irradiation has been shown to lead to an increased level of intracellular ferritin, an iron storage protein that has been implicated in cellular protection against oxidative stress [Keyse et al., 1990]. Earlier we have reported that myocardial ischemia followed by reperfusion resulted in enhanced expression of heat shock proteins, HSP70 and HSP27 [Sharma et al., 1994 and 1996b, Andres et al., 1993]. Similar to other heat shock proteins, human HSP32 gene contains a heat shock element (HSE) in its promotor region [Tyrrell et al., 1993, Lavrovsky et al., 1994]. It is likely that also the porcine HO-1 gene contains the HSE region that responds to the ischemic episode, whereby, binding to heat shock factor eventually activates HSP32 mRNA transcription. Additionally, the heme oxygenase system may function as a defense pathway of the tissue against oxidative stress as bilirubin, produced via this system may act as a physiological antioxidant. The bile pigments that were thought to be biologically inert, are now known to possess potent antioxidant activity [Stocker et al., 1987]. It is plausible that the HO system plays an important role during cardiac adaptation to ischemia and reperfusion and participates in the cellular defense mechanisms by which the myocardium regains its function after the ischemic episode. The HO system has been implicated in endogenous CO generation. Though, we did not measure the production of CO, it is presumed that the induced expression HSP32 may generate enhanced levels of CO during the reperfusion phase, which in turn may modulate the myocardial vascular tone. These results suggest that the myocardial adaptive response to ischemia involves the induction of HSP32, which may be indicative for the existence of a pathophysiologically important defense mechanism by which generation of biologically active products of heme metabolism is accelerated.

Oxygen-free radicals induce HSP32 in reperfused rat myocardium

Recently, we have examined in a rat model whether an ischemic stress can induce HSP32 in the heart [Maulik et al., 1996]. Isolated perfused rat hearts were subjected to either 5 min or 20 min of global normothermic ischemia followed by 30, 45 and 60 min of reperfusion in each case. Hearts were snap-frozen in liquid nitrogen and processed for the expression analysis for HSP32 using Northern blot and immunohistochemistry. HSP32 mRNA expression was not induced by ischemia alone. However, induction was obvious even after 15 min of reperfusion and a more than four-fold increase occured in the postischemic myocardium during persisting reperfusion. These results indicate that myocardial HSP32 induction was a function of the duration of reperfusion after ischemia. To examine whether induction of HSP32 was due to the development of oxidative stress associated with the reperfusion of ischemic myocardium, a group of hearts were pre-perfused for 15 min in the presence of SOD (50 U/ml) and catalase (50 U/ml) prior to ischemia and reperfusion. This induction of HSP32 was blocked by pre-perfusing the hearts with oxygen-free radical scavengers, superoxide dismutase (SOD) and catalase. HSP32 was also induced in the hearts by perfusing them with oxygen-free radical generating substances like, hydrogen peroxide. This induction was also blocked by SOD and catalase. So, obviously, oxygen-free radicals being produced during the reperfusion trigger the expression of HSP32 in the reperfused myocardium [Maulik, et al., 1996]. The results further indicate that, unlike other HSPs, HSP32 is not inducible by acute ischemic insult, but it is the oxidative stress developed during reperfusion of the ischemic heart that is responsible for its expression.

HSP32 has been shown to be induced by oxygen-free radicals in mammalian cells that include brain and skin [Keyse and Tyrrell, 1989, Keyse et al., 1990, Maines and Kappas, 1977, Vile and Tyrrell, 1993]. HSPs are induced in both eukaryotic and prokaryotic cells in response to a variety of stresses whereas, HSP32 mRNA, on the other hand was not inducible in rat liver even after 60 min of ischemia while appreciable amounts of HSP32 were detectable after 4 h of reperfusion of the ischemic liver [Tacchini et al., 1993]. HSP32 mRNA was induced in rat kidney after 6 h of reperfusion following 30 min of ischemic insult [Maines et al., 1993]. Similar to these findings our study also demonstrates that in rat heart, HSP32 is not induced by ischemia and is inducible only after reperfusion.

Numerous evidences support reperfusion of ischemic myocardium to be associated with the reduction of antioxidants and generation of oxygen-free radicals that play a role in the pathogenesis of ischemic reperfusion injury [Das and Engelman, 1989, Kukreja and Hess, 1993]. Presence of both hydroxyl radical OH• and singlet oxygen ($^1O2$) has been documented in the ischemic reperfused myocardium [Das et al., 1989]. Both $^1O2$ and OH• have been implicated in the induction of HSP32 expression [Basu-Modak and Tyrrell, 1993]. The fact that expression of HSP32 can be induced directly by oxygen-derived free radicals [Keyse and Tyrrell, 1989, Keyse et al, 1990, Maines and Kappas, 1977, Vile and Tyrrell, 1993] or the depletion of glutathione [Ewing and Maines 1993] raises the interesting possibility that oxidative stress developed during reperfusion potentiates HSP32 induction. Inhibition of induction by SOD plus catalase conclusively demonstrate the involvement of oxygen-free radicals in the process of induction. This is further supported by the induction of HSP32 mRNA in the heart by OH• radicals. The progressive increase in HSP32 transcription as a function of duration of reperfusion further suggests that induction of the mRNA is an adaptive phenomenon occurring in response to tissue injury.

Another intriguing hypothesis could be that HSP32 is being induced by cytokines. Cytokines such as interleukin-1 (IL-1), IL-8 and TNF-α are known to be induced by ischemia/reperfusion during cardiac bypass surgery [Kalfin et al., 1993]. Results of a recent study suggest that HSP32 induction may be a reaction to cytokines [Rizzardini et al., 1993]. Marked induction of HSP32 was observed in mouse liver within 2 h after injecting the animal with TNF-α or IL-1. Treatment of mice with IL-1 stimulated transcription of the HSP32 gene by 4-fold suggesting cytokine-induced upregulation of HSP32 at the transcriptional level.

Myocardial localization of HSP32

To examine the location of HSP32 in the myocardium, immunohistochemical localization was performed [Maulik et al., 1996] by analysis of paraffin-embedded 5μm-sections on polylysine-coated glass slides. After quenching of the endogenous peroxidase by 3% hydrogen peroxide, sections were incubated with HO-1 antibody, processed for color development by using 3-amino-9-ethylcarbonate (ACE), counterstained with hematoxylin and subsequently visualized under the microscope. HO-1 protein was localized in cardiomyocytes and in the interstitium: Immunoreactive HO-1 was also found in the perivascular region (mainly fibroblasts) around blood vessels. The presence of HO-1 in cardiomyocytes indicates that these cells possess an endogenous protective mechanism by which bile pigments are produced that act as radical scavengers, particularly during the reperfusion phase after ischemia. The perivascular existence of HO-1 may be attributed to its role in regulating the vascular tone by generating carbon monoxide as a result of haem metabolism. Therefore, it is conceivable that HO-1 plays an important role in improving cardiac function after ischemia by dilating coronary arteries with carbon monoxide via endothelium independent mechanism. As stated earlier, HO-1 gene induction in hearts during the reperfusion phase after ischemia and in the OH• generating system of perfused hearts may be one of the protective mechanisms against oxidative stress.

Possible role of HSP32 in cytoprotection

The role of HSP32 in cellular protection remains controversial. According to a recent study HSP32 could not protect human cells against oxidative stress [Nutter et al., 1994]. In another study, HSP32 was found to mediate an adaptive response to oxidative stress in human skin fibroblasts [Vile et al., 1994]. The authors showed that human skin fibroblasts, preirradiated by UVA, have increased levels of HSP32 and sustain less membrane damage during a subsequent exposure to UVA radiation than cells that had not been preirradiated. Pretreating cells with HSP32 antisense oligonucleotides inhibited the irradiation-dependent induction of the HSP32 enzyme and abolished the protective effect of preirradiation implicating HSP32 as the initial inducible mediator of the adaptive process. At least three plausible mechansims may be put forward to support the beneficial role of HSP32. Firstly, induction of HSP32 could increase the cellular capacity to generate biliverdin and bilirubin, potent antioxidants capable of scavenging peroxy radicals and inhibit lipid peroxidation [Stocker et al., 1987]. Secondly, induction of HSP32 is coupled to the synthesis of ferritin [Nutter et al., 1994], a proven cytoprotective antioxidant [Balla et al., 1992]. Thirdly, the processes of HSP32 activation and bilirubin formation generate CO, a potential chemical messenger that leads to generation of cGMP [Verma et al., 1993]. Activation of cGMP is likely to potentiate the activation of a signal transduction pathway leading to generation of diacylglycerol and protein kinase C.

Ubiquitin

Location and function of ubiquitin
Ubiquitin is a highly conserved 76-residue protein found in all eukaryotic cells [Rechsteiner, 1991, Jentsch, 1992]. It can covalently bind to a wide variety of proteins in nucleus, cytosol and cytoskeleton of many cells including cardiomyocytes [Hilenski et al., 1992]. Immunohistochemically, ubiquitin has been localized as ubiquitin conjugates at Z-bands and at intercalated discs in cardiomyocytes [Hilenski et al., 1992]. In cultured cardiomyocytes, immunoreactive ubiquitin conjugates were found in the nucleus as aggregates and in the cytoplasm as striated pattern indicative of Z-bands. The physiological siginificance of such a ubiquitination of different proteins in different cellular compartments is largely unknown. It is very likely that ubiquitin conjugation plays an important role in regulating protein turnover and/or stability of vital proteins in the heart.

Ischemia as a potent inducer for ubiquitin

We have examined the expression pattern of ubiquitin in the heart in relation to ischemia and reperfusion [Andres et al., 1993; Sharma et al., 1996b]. Total cellular RNA isolated from the stunned as well as the control myocardium was observed to hybridize to multiple mRNA bands (at least three major mRNA species) encoding ubiquitin (monomer and polymers). Dot-blot hybridization and scanning densitometry was performed in order to evaluate the expression pattern of ubiquitin in the porcine heart subjected to ischemia and reperfusion (Fig. 2). Densitometric analysis of blots revealed a significant increase in the levels of mRNAs encoding ubiquitin in the stunned myocardium of groups II and III as compared to their respective controls (Fig. 2). Earlier, we have reported the organ distribution of ubiquitin mRNAs and shown that porcine hearts express multiple mRNAs encoding ubiquitin [Andres et al., 1993]. Enhanced expression of mRNAs encoding ubiquitin during ischemia and reperfusion points towards the rapid production of this vital protein needed for the ATP-dependent proteolysis, particularly after ischemia when a number of proteins got denatured and/or structurally altered. Induction of the ubiquitin gene in different cells *in vitro* in response to stress and heat has been shown earlier by different groups [Hershko and Ciechanover, 1992, Jentsch, 1992, Brand et al., 1992]. In the brain, enhanced levels of ubiquitin-protein conjugates have been found after five minutes of cerebral ischemia [Hayashi et al., 1992]. In addition to clearance (by proteolysis) of structurally altered proteins during ischemia and reperfusion, ubiquitin may also contribute to various cellular events including cell cycle and differentiation, pointing to other important roles for ubiquitin [Hershko and Ciechanover, 1992, Hayashi et al., 1992, Rechsteiner, 1991, Welch, 1992].

145

Ubiquitin expression as a sign of molecular damage

Enhanced expression of mRNA encoding polyubiquitin during reperfusion after brief periods of repetitive ischemia may reflect the increased requirement for ubiquitin in response to the intracellular accumulation of partially damaged proteins. The induction of the ubiquitin multigene family after heat shock and following treatment with iron has been observed in cultured mammalian cells [Parag et al., 1987, Uney et al., 1993]. It is believed that stress conditions in cultured cells lead to accumulation of irreversibly injured proteins [Ananthan et al., 1986], an increase in cytosolic calcium concentration [Kiang et al., 1992] and expression of several heat shock proteins including ubiquitin [Hodgin et al., 1992]. Increased expression of ubiquitin mRNAs has also been observed in acidotic skeletal muscle [Greiber et al., 1991] and in epidermal tumors [Finch et al., 1992, Kanayama et al., 1991]. In our experimental model, the increased steady state of mRNA encoding polyubiquitin was associated with the transient formation of new ubiquitin-protein conjugates. Increased amounts of ubiquitin-protein conjugates together with acceleration of proteolysis after heat shock was also observed in cultured mammalian cells [Parag et al., 1987, Carlson et al., 1987]. Hence, upregulation of genes encoding ubiquitin and heat shock proteins indicate the activation of the so-called heat shock response, which is universally present among all living species and represents a model of inducible genomic response.

Expression of sHSPs in Relation to TNF-α

Dysfunction of the coronary endothelium as well as injury to cardiac muscle cells are the consequences of myocardial ischemia and reperfusion. A number of factors including various cytokines like TNF-α are released in the postischemic myocardium [Maury and Tempo, 1989, Lefer et al., 1990, and Herskowitz et al. 1995]. These ischemia induced cytokines may mimic the local cellular injury and may contribute in altering the molecular phenotype of the postischemic myocardium. Increase in local expression as well as in circulation of TNF-α has been reported in experimental animals and in patients with myocardial ischemia and infarction [Maury and Tempo, 1989, Herskowitz et al., 1995]. In a recent study, pretreatment of rat hearts with TNF-α was found to be protective against ischemia and reperfusion injury [Eddy et al., 1992]. However, in the normal heart, TNF-α may exert negative inotropic effects by directly altering intracellular calcium homeostasis in a concentration and time dependent manner [Yokoyama et al., 1993]. Biological effects of TNF-α in the target cell are initiated by its binding to high affinity cell surface receptors [Tartaglia et al., 1991, Wiegmann et al., 1992, Heller and Kronke, 1994]. TNF receptors are expressed on the membranes of virtually all somatic cell types [Wiegmann et al., 1992, Tartaglia et al., 1991]. TNF receptors channel signals to cytoplasm and nucleus, and thereby initiate profound alterations in the metabolic pathway and nuclear transcription [Rothe et al., 1992]. Two immunologically distinct TNF receptors of apparent molecular masses of 55 kDa and 75 kDa have been identified and characterized [Tartaglia et al., 1991, Wiegmann et al., 1992]. Many studies have demonstrated that TNF-α induces phosphorylation of a stress protein of about 28 kDa in different cell types [Löw-Friedrich et al., 1992, Kaur et al., 1989, Vietor and Vilcek, 1994, Mehlen et al., 1995] and this phosphorylation results from stimulation of G protein coupled signal transduction involving the mitogen activated protein (MAP) kinase cascade [Reithmann et al., 1991, Engel et al., 1995].

We have shown earlier that perfusion of spontaneously contracting cultures of cardiomyocytes with a high dose of TNF-α (10,000 units/ml) led to arrhythmias with time and complete cessation of spontaneous contractions followed by severe loss of myocyte inotropy [Weisensee et al., 1993]. More recently, we have reported that TNF-α as well as interleukins (IL-2, IL-3, IL-6) induce the formation of stress proteins in cultured cardiomyocytes [Löw-Friedrich et al., 1992, Sharma et al., 1996 b, c]. Heat shock proteins participate in cellular defense mechanisms and enable cells to survive and recover from stressful conditions [Welch, 1992, Schlesinger, 1990, Ciocca et al., 1993, Heads et al., 1995]. It is believed that the heart has its own endogenous system(s) for protecting itself against ischemia-reperfusion injury and a number of HSPs that may act as chaperones in saving vital cellular proteins from degradation have been proposed [Mestril and Dillmann, 1990, Schlesinger, 1990, Andres et al., 1993, Ciocca et al., 1993, Iwaki et al. 1993, Sharma et al., 1993, Heads et al., 1995, Knowlton, 1995].

We hypothesize that TNF-α stimulates cytoprotective mechanisms in cardiomyocytes, and such mechanisms can be examined by investigating the expression pattern of various stress protein genes. To get insight into endogenous cytoprotective mechanisms, we developed an *in vitro* model based on cultured cardiomyocytes treated with TNF-α at which we examined gene expression of several heat shock proteins (HSP27, HSP70 and ubiquitin) [Sharma et al., 1996b]. Cardiomyocytes were isolated from the hearts of 18 days old fetal mice by enzymatic dissociation and grown in minimum essential medium containing 10% fetal calf serum. Spontaneously contractile cells were serum deprived for 24 h and treated with TNF-α (25 ng/ml = 1,500 units/ml) for 1, 2, 4, 6, 8, 12, and 24 h. After each incubation, cells were processed for the extraction of total proteins for Western blot or for total RNA by Northern blot analyses. TNF-α induced arrhythmias and cessation of spontaneous contractions in concentration and time dependent manner. Steady state (ubiquitin) or undetectable mRNA levels (HSP27, HSP70) were drastically induced as compared to untreated control cells by TNF-α being maximal between 6-8 h of stimulation and thereafter, the expression of these stress genes declined. By Western blot analysis, we found increased multiple bands of ubiquitin-protein conjugates in TNF-α treated cells whereas no significant change in HSP27 protein accumulation until 12 h was observed as compared to control. 24 h of TNF-α incubation resulted in partial cellular necrosis. We have shown that TNF-α is a potent inducer of heat shock protein genes in cardiomyocytes. Induction of genes conferring resistance to the cytotoxic property of TNF-α may provide a means of cardiomyocytes for self-defense under pathophysiological conditions. Hence, the induced expression of cytoprotective molecules such as stress proteins (HSP27, HSP70 and ubiquitin) in response to TNF-α may activate protective and/or repair mechanisms in cardiomyocytes for making them more resistant toward a subsequent challenge such as ischemia. It appears that TNF-α on the one hand mimics cellular injury in the heart and at the same time it stimulates synthesis of vital proteins like HSPs and MnSOD making it a very interesting and relevant cytokine for the cardiovascular system. Furthermore, the ubiquitin system could play an important role in cytosolic degradation of damaged proteins in TNF-α treated cardiomyocytes where HSPs may counteract the proteolytic events and preserve many vital proteins.

References

Amrani M, Allen NJ, O'Shea J, Corbett J, Dunn J, Tadjikarimi J, Theodoropoulos S, Pepper J, Yacoub MH. Role of catalase and heat shock protein on recovery of endothelial and mechanical function. Cardioscience 1993; 4: 193-198

Ananthan J, Goldberg A, Voellmy R. Abnormal proteins serve as eukaryotic stress signals and trigger the activation of heat shock genes. Science 1986; 232: 522-524

Andres J, Sharma HS, Knoll R, Stahl J, Sassen LM, Verdouw PD, Schaper W. Expression of heat shock proteins in the normal and stunned porcine myocardium. Cardiovasc Res 1993; 27: 1421-1429

Arrigo AP, Suhan JP, Welch WJ. Dynamic changes in the structure and intracellular locale of the mammalian low-molecular-weight heat shock protein. Mol Cell Biol 1988; 8: 5059-5071

Arrigo AP, Landry J. "Expression and function of the low-molecular-weight heat shock proteins." In: *The biology of heat shock proteins and molecular chaperones"*, Morimoto RI, Tissieres A; Georgopoulus C; ed. Cold Spring Harbor Laboratory Press, 1994.

Balla G, Jacob HS, Balla J, Rosenberg M, Nath K, Apple F, Eaton JW, Vercellotti GM: Ferritin: a cytoprotective antioxidant strategem of endothelium. J Biol Chem 1992; 267: 18148-18152

Basu-Modak S, Tyrrell RM: Singlet: A primary effector in the ultraviolet A near-visible light induction of the heme oxygenase gene. Cancer Res 1993; 53: 4505-4510

Behlke J, Lutsch G, Gaestel M, Bielka H: Supramolecular structure of the recombinant murine small heat shock protein HSP27. FEBS Lett. 1991; 288: 119-122

Behlke J, Dube P, van Heel M, Wieske M, Hayess K, Benndorf R, Lutsch G: Supramolecular structure of the small heat shock protein hsp25. Progr. Colloid Polym. Sci. 1995; 99: 87-93.

Bennardini F; Wrzosek A; Chiesi M. Alpha B-crystallin in cardiac tissue. Association with actin and desmin filaments. Circ-Res. 1992; 71: 288-294

Benndorf R, Hayess K, Stahl J, Bielka H. Cell-free phosphorylation of the murine small heat shock protein hsp25 by an endogenous kinase from Ehrlich ascites tumor cells. Biochim Biophys Acta 1992; 1136: 203-207

Benndorf R, Hayess K, Ryazantsev S, Wieske M, Behlke J, Lutsch G. Phosphorylation and supramolecular organization of murine small heat shock protein HSP25 abolish its actin polymerization-inhibiting activity. J Biol Chem 1994; 269: 20780-20784

Benndorf R, Bielka H. Cellular stress response: stress proteins - physiology and implications for cancer. Recent Results in Cancer Res 1996; 143: 129-144

Bhat SP, Nagieni CN. Alpha-B subunit of lens-specific alpha-B crystallin is present in other ocular and non-ocular tissues. Biochem Biophys Res Commun 1988; 158: 319-325

Bhat SP, Horwitz J, Srinivasan A, Ding L. Alpha B-crystallin exists as an independent protein in the heart and in the lens. Eur J Biochem 1991; 202: 775-781

Bitar KN, Kaminski MS, Hailat H, Cease KB, Strahler JR. Hsp27 is a mediator of sustained smooth muscle contraction in response to bombesin. Biochem Biophys Res Commun 1991; 181: 1192-1200

Brand T, Sharma HS, Fleischmann KE, Duncker DJ, McFalls EO, Verdouw PD and Schaper, W. Proto-oncogene expression in porcine myocardium subjected to ischemia and reperfusion. Circ. Res. 1992; 71: 1351-1360

Cairns J, Qin SX, Philp R,Tan YH, Guy GR. Dephosphorylation of the small heat shock protein hsp27 *in vivo* by protein phosphatase 2A. J Biol Chem 1994; 269: 9176-9183

Carlson N, Rogers S, Rechsteiner M. Microinjection of ubiquitin: changes in protein degradation in HeLacells subjected to heat-shock. J Cell Biol 1987; 104: 547-555

Carper SW, Rocheleau TA, Storm FK. cDNA sequence of a human heat shock protein HSP25. Nucl Acids Res 1990; 18: 1637

Chepelinsky AB, Pitigorsky J, Pisano MM, Dubin RA, Wistow G, Limjoco TI, Klement JF, Jaworski CJ. Lens protein gene expression: alpha-crystallins and MIP. Lens Eye Toxic Res 1991; 8: 319-344

Chiesa R, McDermott J, Mann E, Spector A. The apparent molecular size of native alpha-crystallin B in non-lenticular tissues. FEBS-Lett. 1990; 268: 222-226

Chiesi M, Longoni S, Limbruno U. Cardiac alpha-crystallin. III. Involvement during heart ischemia. Mol Cell Biochem 1990; 97: 129-136

Chiesi M, Bennardini F. Determination of alpha B crystallin aggregation: a new alternative method to assess ischemic damage of the heart. Basic Res Cardiol 1992; 87: 38-46

Christodoulides N, Durante W, Kroll MH, Schafer AI. Vascular smooth muscle cell heme oxygenases generate guanylyl cyclase-stimulatory carbon monoxide. Circulation 1995; 91: 2306-2309

Ciocca DR, Oesterreich S, Chamness GC, McGuire WL, Fuqua SA. Biological and clinical implications of heat shock protein 27,000 (Hsp27): a review. [Review]. J Natl Cancer Inst 1993; 85: 1558-1570

Cruse I, Maines MD. Evidence suggesting that the two forms of heme oxygenase are products of different genes. J Biol Chem 1988; 263: 3348-3353

Currie RW, Karmazyn M, Kloc M, Mailer K. Heat-shock response is associated with enhanced postischemic ventricular recovery. Circ Res 1988; 63: 543-549

Currie RW, Ross BM, Davis TA. Induction of the heat shock response in rats modulates heart rate, creatine kinase and protein synthesis after a subsequent hyperthermic treatment. Cardiovasc Res. 1990; 24: 87-93

Das DK, George A, Liu X, Rao P: Detection of hydroxyl radical in the mitochondria of ischemic-reperfused myocardium by trapping with salicylate. Biochem Biophys Res Commun 1989; 165: 1004-1008

Das DK, Engelman RM : Mechanism of free radical generation in ischemic and reperfused myocardium. In : Oxygen Radicals : Systemic Events and Disease Processes (Das DK, Essman WB eds). 1989; Karger, Basel, Switzerland, pp 97-131

Das DK, Engelman RM, Kimura Y: Molecular adaptation of cellular defences following preconditioning of the heart by repeated ischaemia. Cardiovasc Res 1993; 27: 578-584

DeJong WW, Leunissen JAM, Voorter C. Evolution of the -crystallin/small heat-shock protein family. Mol Biol Evol 1993; 10: 103-126

Donnelly TJ, Sievers RE, Vissern FL, Welch WJ, Wolfe CL. Heat shock protein induction in rat hearts. A role for improved myocardial salvage after ischemia and reperfusion? Circulation 1992; 85: 769-778

Dubin RA, Wawrousek EF, Piatigorsky J. Expression of the murine alpha B-crystallin gene is not restricted to the lens. Mol Cell Biol 1989; 9: 1083-1091

Dubin RA, Ally AH, Chung S, Piatigorsky J. Human B-crystallin gene and preferential promoter function in lens. Genomics 1990; 7: 594-601

Eddy LJ, Goeddel DV, Wong GH: Tumor necrosis factor- pretreatment is protective in a rat model of myocardial ischemia-reperfusion injury. Biochem Biophys Res Comm 1992; 184: 1056-1059

Engel K, Ahlers A, Brach MA; Herrmann F; Gaestel M. MAPKAP kinase 2 is activated by heat shock and TNF: *In vivo* phosphorylation of small heat shock protein results from stimulation of the MAP kinase cascade. J Cell Biochem 1995; 57: 321-330

Ewing JF, Maines MD: Rapid induction of heme oxygenase 1 mRNA and protein by hyperthermia in rat brain: heme oxygenase 2 is not a heat shock protein. Proc Natl Acad Sci (USA) 1991; 88: 5364-5368

Ewing JF, Maines MD: Glutathione depletion induces heme oxygenase 1 (HSP 32) mRNA and protein in rat brain. J Neurochem 1993; 60: 1512-1519

Ewing, J.F., Raju, V.S., and Maines, M.D.: Induction of heart heme oxygenase-1 (HSP32) by hyperthermia: possible role in stress-mediated elevation of cyclic 3':5'-guanosine monophosphate. J Pharmacol Exp Therap 1994; 271: 408-414

Finch J, John T, Krieg P, et al. Overexpression of three ubiquitin genes in mouse epidermal tumors is associated with enhanced cellular proliferation and stress. Cell Growth and Differentiation 1992;3:269-278

Fitzgerald PG; Graham D. Ultrastructural localization of alpha A-crystallin to the bovine lens fiber cell cytoskeleton. Curr Eye Res 1991; 10: 417-436

Freshney NW, Rawlinson L, Guesdon F, Jones E, Cowley S, Hsuan J, Saklatvala J. Interleukin-1 activates a novel protein kinase cascade that results in the phosphorylation of HSP27. Cell 1994; 78: 1039-1049

Frohli E, Aoyama A, Klemenz R. Cloning of the mouse hsp25 gene and an extremely condserved hsp25 pseudogene. Gene 1993; 128: 273-277

Gaestel M, Gross B, Benndorf R, Strauss M, Schunck WH, Kraft R, Otto A, Böhm H, Stahl J, Drabsch H, Bielka H. Molecular cloning, sequencing and expression in Escherichia coli of the 25kDa growth-related protein of Ehrlich ascites tumor and its homology to mammalian stress proteins. Eur J Biochem 1989; 179: 209-213

Gaestel M, Schroder W, Benndorf R, Lippmann C, Buchner K, Hucho F, ErdmannVA, Bielka H. Identification of the phosphorylation sites of the murine small heat shock protein hsp25. J Biol Chem 1991; 266: 14721-14724

Gaestel M, Gotthardt R, Mueller T. Structure and organisation of a murine gene encoding small heat shock protein hsp25. Gene 1993; 128: 279-283

Gernold M, Knauf U, Gaestel M, Stahl J, Kloetzel PM. Development and tissue-specific distribution of mouse small heat shock protein hsp25. Dev Genet 1993; 14: 103-111

Gopal-Srivastava R, Piatigorsky J. Identification of a lens-specific regulatory region (LSR) of the murine alpha B-crystallin gene. Nucl Acids Res 1994; 22: 1281-1286

Greiber S, Medina R, Goldberg A, Mitch W. Mechanisms for accelerated muscle proteolysis in metabolic acidosis: increased mRNA for ubiquitin and subunit of the ATP-dependent protease (Abstract). Clin Res 1991; 39: 359A.

Groenen PJ, Merck KB, deJong WW, Bloemendal-H. Structure and modifications of the junior chaperone alpha-crystallin. From lens transparency to molecular pathology. Eur J Biochem 1994; 225: 1-19

Guesdon F, Freshney N, Waller RJ, Rawlinson L, Saklatvala J. Interleukin 1 and tumor necrosis factor stimulate two novel protein kinases that phosphorylate the heat shock protein hsp27 and beta-casein. J Biol Chem 1993; 268: 4236-4243

Guy GR, Cairns J, Ng SB, Tan YH. Inactivation of a redox- sensitive protein phosphatase during the early events of tumor necrosis factor/interleukin-1 signal transduction. J Biol Chem 1993; 268: 2141-2148

Hayashi T, Takeda K, Matsuda M: Post-transient ischemia increase in ubiquitin conjugates in the early reperfusion. NeuroReport 1992; 3: 519-520

Heads RJ, Yellon DM, Latchman DS. Differential cytoprotection against heat stress or hypoxia following expression of specific stress protein genes in myogenic cells. J Mol Cell Cardiol 1995; 27: 1669-1678

Heller RA, Kronke M: Tumor necrosis factor receptor-mediated signaling pathways. [Review] J Cell Biol 1994; 126: 5-12

Hershko A, Ciechanover A. The ubiquitin system for protein degradation. Annu Rev Biochem 1992, 61: 761-807

Herskowitz A, Choi S, Ansari AA, Wesselingh S: Cytokine mRNA expression in postischemic/reperfused myocardium. Am J Pathol 1995; 146: 419-428

Hickey E, Brandon SE, Potter R, Stein G, Stein J, Weber LA. Sequence and organization of genes encoding the human 27 kDa heat shock protein. Nucl Acids Res 1986; 14: 4126-4145 [published erratum appears in Nucl Acids Res 1986, 24: 8230]

Hickey E, Brandon SE, Sadis S, Smale G, Weber LA. Molecular cloning of sequences encoding the human heat-shock proteins and their expression during hyperthermia. Gene 1986; 43: 147-154

Hilenski LL, Terracio L, Haas AL, Borg TK. Immunolocalization of ubiquitin conjugates at Z-bands and intercalated discs of rat cardiomyocytes *in vitro* and *in vivo*. J. Histochem Cytochem 1992; 40: 1037-1042

Hoch B, Lutsch G, Schlegel W-P, Stahl J, Wallukat G, Bartel S, Krause EG, Benndorf R, Karczewski P. HSP25 in isolated perfused rat hearts: Localization and response to hyperthermia. Mol Cell Biochem 1996a; in press

Hoch B, Lutsch G, Vetter R, Schlegel W-P, Bartel S, Stahl J, Wallukat G, Krause EG, Karczewski P, Benndorf R. Expression and subcellular location of small mammalian heat shock protein HSP25 in rat heart. Cold Spring Harbor Meeting on "*Molecular chaperones and the heat response*", 1996b, May 1 - May 5, Cold Spring Harbor Press, New York:, Abstract p. 129.

Hodgins R, Ellison K, Ellison M. Expression of a ubiquitin derivative that conjugates to protein irreversible produces phenotypes consistent with a ubiquitin deficiency. J Biol Chem 1992; 267: 8807-8812

Horwitz-J. -crystallin can function as a molecular chaperone. Proc Natl Acad Sci 1992; 89: 10449-10453

Huot J, Lambert H, Lavoie JN, Guimond A, Houle F, Landry J. Characterization of 45-kDa/54-kDa HSP27 kinase, a stress-sensitive kinase which may activate the phosphorylation-dependent protective function of mammalian 27-kDa heat-shock protein HSP27. Eur J Biochem 1995; 227: 416-427

Huot J, Houle F, Spitz DR, Landry J. HSP27 phosphorylation-mediated resistance against actin fragmantation and cell death induced by oxidative stress. Cancer Res 1996; 56: 273-279

Hutter MM, Sievers RE, Barbosa V, Wolfe CL. Heat-shock protein induction in rat hearts. A direct correlation between the amount of heat-shock protein induced and the degree of myocardial protection. Circulation 1994; 89: 355-360

Inaguma Y, Hasegawa K, Goto S, Ito H, Kato-K. Induction of the synthesis of hsp27 and alpha B crystallin in tissues of heat-stressed rats and its suppression by ethanol or an alpha 1-adrenergic antagonist. J Biochem Tokyo 1995; 117: 1238-1243

Iwaki T, Kume-Iwaki A, Liem RK, Goldman JE. Alpha B-crystallin is expressed in non-lenticular tissues and accumulates in Alexander's disease brain. Cell 1989; 57: 71-78

Iwaki T, Kume-Iwaki A, Goldman JE. Cellular distribution of alpha B-crystallin in non-lenticular tissues. J Histochem Cytochem 1990; 38: 31-39

Iwaki K, Chi SH, Dillmann WH, Mestril R. Induction of HSP70 in cultured rat neonatal cardiomyocytes by hypoxia and metabolic stress. Circulation 1993; 87: 2023-2032

Jakob U, Gaestel M, Engel K, Buchner J. Small heat shock proteins are molecular chaperones. J Biol Chem 1993; 268: 1517-1520

Jentsch S. Ubiquitin-dependent protein degradation: a cellular perspective. Trends in Cell Biol 1992; 2: 98-103

Johnson RA, Lavesa M, Askari B, Abraham NG, Nasjletti A: A heme oxygenase product, presumably carbon monoxide, mediates a vasodepressor function in rats. Hypertension 1995; 25: 166-169

Kalfin RE, Engelman RM, Rousou JA, Flack JE, Deaton DW, Kreutzer DL, Das DK: Induction of interleukin-8 expression during cardio-pulmonary bypass. Circulation 1993; 88 (part II): 401-406

Kampinga HH, Brunsting JF, Stege GJJ, Burgman WJJ, Konings AWT. Thermal protein denaturation and protein aggregation in cells made thermotolerant by various chemicals: Role of heat shock proteins. Exp Cell Res 1995; 219, 536-546

Kanayama H, Tanaka K, Aki M, et al. Changes in expression of proteasome and ubiquitin genes in human renal cancer cells. Cancer Res 1991; 51: 6677-6685

Katayose D, Isoyama S, Fujita H, Shibahara S: Separate regulation of heme oxygenase and heat shock protein 70 mRNA expression in the rat heart by hemodynamic stress. Biochem Biophys Res Comm 1993; 191: 587-594

Kato K, Shinohara H, Kurobe N, Inaguma Y, Shimizu K, Ohshima K. Tissue distribution and developmental profiles of immunoreactive alpha B crystallin in the rat determined with a sensitive immunoassay system. Biochim Biophys Acta 1991; 1074: 201-208

Kato K, Shinohara H, Goto S, Inaguma Y, Morishita R, Asano T. Copurification of small heat shock protein with alpha B crystallin from human skeletal muscle. J Biol Chem 1992; 267: 7718-7725

Kato K, Goto S, Inaguma Y, Hasegawa K, Morishita R, Asano T. Purification and characterization of a 20-kDa protein that is highly homologous to alpha B crystallin. J Biol Chem 1994; 269: 15302-15309

Kaur P, Welch WJ, Saklatvala J. Interleukin 1 and tumour necrosis factor increase phosphorylation of the small heat shock protein. Effects in fibroblasts, Hep G2 and U937 cells. FEBS Lett 1989; 258: 269-273

Keyse SM, Tyrrell RM : Heme oxygenase is the major 32 KDa stress protein induced in human skin fibroblasts by UVA radiation, hydrogen peroxide and sodium arsenite. Proc Natl Acad Sci 1989; 86: 99-103

Keyse SM, Applegate LA, Tromvoukis Y, Tyrrell RM. Oxidant stress leads to transcriptional activation of the human heme oxygenase gene in cultured skin fibroblast. Mol Cell Biol 1990; 10: 4967-4969

Kiang J, Koenig M, Smallridge R. Heat shock increases cytosolic free Ca 2+ concentration via Na+ Ca2+ exchange in human epidermoid A 431 cells. Am J Physiol 1992; 263: C30-C38

Klemenz R, Frohli E, Steiger RH, Schafer R, Aoyama A. Alpha B-crystallin is a small heat shock protein. Proc Nat Acad Sci USA 1991; 88: 3652-3656

Klemenz R, Andres AC, Frohli E, Schafer R, Aoyama A. Expression of the murine small heat shock proteins hsp 25 and alpha B crystallin in the absence of stress. J Cell Biol 1993; 120: 639-645

Knecht M, Regitz-Zagrosek V, Pleissner KP, Jungblut P, Steffen C, Hildebrandt A, Fleck E. Characterization of myocardial protein composition in dilated cardiomyopathy by two-dimensional gel electrophoresis. Eur Heart J 1994; 15 Suppl D: 37-44

Knowlton AA. The role of heat shock proteins in the heart. J Mol Cell Cardiol 1995; 27: 121-131

Kukreja RC, Hess ML. Oxygen radicals, neutrophil-derived oxidants, and myocardial reperfusion injury. In: (Das DK ed) : Pathophysiology of Reperfusion Injury. CRC Press, Boca Raton, 1993; pp 221-241.

Lautier D, Luscher P, Tyrrell RM. Endogenous glutathione levels modulate both constitutive and UVA radiation/hydrogen peroxide inducible expression of the human heme oxygenase gene. Carcinogenesis. 1992; 13. 227-232

Lavoie JN, Chretien P, Landry J. Sequence of the Chinese hamster small heat shock protein HSP27. Nucl Acids Res 1990; 18: 1637

Lavoie JN, Gingras-Breton G,Tanguay RM, Landry J. Induction of chinese hamster HSP27 gene expression in mouse cells confers resistance to heat shock. J Biol Chem 1993a; 268: 3420-3429

Lavoie JN, Hickey E, Weber LA, Landry J. Modulation of actin microfilament dynamics and fluid phase pinocytosis by phosphorylation of heat shock protein 27. J Biol Chem 1993b; 268: 24210-24214

Lavoie JN, Lambert H,Hickey E, Weber LA, Landry J. Modulation of cellular thermoresistance and actin filament stability accompanies phosphorylation-induced changes in the oligomeric structure of heat shock protein 27. Mol Cell Biol 1995; 15: 505-516

Lavrovsky Y, Schwartzman ML, Levere RD, Kappas A, Abraham NG. Identification of binding sites for transcription factors NF-kappa B and AP-2 in the promoter region of the human heme oxygenase 1 gene. Proc Natl Acad Sci (USA) 1994; 91: 5987-5991

Leach IH, Tsang ML, Church RJ, Lowe J. Alpha-B crystallin in the normal human myocardium and cardiac conducting system. J Pathol 1994; 173: 255-260

Lefer AM, Tsao P, Aoki N, Palladino MJ: Mediation of cardioprotection by transforming growth factor-. Science 1990; 249: 61-64

Löw-Friedrich I, Weisensee D, Mitrou P, Schoeppe W: Cytokines induce stress protein formation in cultured cardiac myocytes. Basic Res Cardiol 1992; 87: 12-18

Longoni S, James P, Chiesi M. Cardiac alpha-crystallin. I. Isolation and identification [corrected and republished with original paging, article originally printed in Mol Cell Biochem 1990; 97:113-120, Mol Cell Biochem 1990; 99: 113-120

Longoni S, Lattonen S, Bullock G, Chiesi M. Cardiac alpha-crystallin. II. Intracellular localization. Mol Cell Biochem 1990; 97: 121-128

Lowe J, McDermott H, Pike I, Spendlove I, Landon M, Mayer RJ. alpha B crystallin expression in non-lenticular tissues and selective presence in ubiquitinated inclusion bodies in human disease. J Pathol 1992; 166: 61-68

Lu D, Das DK. Induction of differential heat shock gene expression in heart, lung, liver, brain and kidney by a sympathomimetic drug, amphetamine. Biochem Biophys Res Commun 1993; 192: 808-812

Lutsch G, Stahl J, Offhauß U, Schimke I. Localization of HSP-27 and B-crystallin in heart and kidney tissue by immunofluorescence and immunoelectron microscopy. Eur J Cell Biol 1995; 67 (suppl. 41): 25

Maines MD, Kappas A: Metals as regulators of heme oxygenase. Science 1977; 198: 1215-1221

Maines MD, Trakshel GM, Kutty RK. Characterization of two constitutive forms of rat liver microsomal heme oxygenase. Only one molecular species of the enzyme is inducible. J Biol Chem 1986; 261: 411-419

Maines MD. Heme oxygenase: function, multiplicity, regulatory mechanisms, and clinical applications. [Review]. FASEB J 1988; 2: 2557-2568

Maines MD, Mayer RD, Ewing JF, McCoubrey WK. Induction of kidney heme oxygenase-1 (HSP 32) mRNA and protein by ischemia/reperfusion: Possible role of heme as both promoter of tissue damage and regulator of HSP 32. J Pharmacol Exp Therap 1993; 264: 457- 462

Marber MS, Mestril R, Chi SH, Sayen MR, Yellon DM, Dillmann WH. Overexpression of the rat inducible 70-kD heat stress protein in a transgenic mouse increases the resistance of the heart to ischemic injury. J Clin Invest 1995; 95: 1446-1456

Martin JL, Mestril R, Hilal-Dandan R, Dillmann W. Small heat shock proteins and protection against ischemic injury in cardiomyocytes. Cold Spring Harbor Meeting on "Molecular chaperones and *the heat response*", 1996, May 1 - May 5, Cold Spring Harbor Press, New York:, Abstract p. 342.

Maulik N, Engelman RM, Wei Z, Lu D, Rousou JA, Das DK. Interleukin-1 alpha preconditioning reduces myocardial ischemia reperfusion injury. Circulation 1993; 88(5 Pt 2): II387-394

Maulik N, Wei Z, Liu X, Engelman RM, Rousou JA, Das DK. Improved postischemic ventricular functional recovery by amphetamine is linked with its ability to induce heat shock. Mol Cell Biochem 1994; 137: 17-24

Maulik N, Sharma HS, Das DK: Induction of heme oxygenage gene expression during the reperfusion of ischemic rat myocardium. J Mol Cell Cardiol 1996; 28: 1261-1270

Maury CP, Tempo AM. Circulating tumor necrosis factor- (cachectin) in myocardial infarction. Am J Pathol 139: 709-715, 1989.

Mehlen P, Mehlen A, Guillet D, Preville X, Arrigo AP. Tumor necrosis factor- induces changes in the phosphorylation, cellular localization, and oligomerization of human hsp27, a stress protein that confers cellular resistance to this cytokine. J Cell Biochem 1995; 58: 248-259

Mehlen P, Kretz-Remy C, Preville X, Arrigo AP. Human hsp27, *Drosphila* hsp27 and human B-crystallin expression-mediated increase in glutathione is essential for the protective activity of these proteins against

TNF--induced cell death. EMBO J 1996; 15: 2695-2706

Merck KB, Groenen PJ, Voorter CE, de-Haard-Hoekman WA, Horwitz J, Bloemendal H, de-Jong WW. Variation in the expression and/or phosphorylation of the human low molecular weight stress protein during *in vitro* cell differentiation. J Biol Chem 1993; 268: 1046-1052

Mestril R, Chi SH, Sayen MR, O'Reilly K, Dillmann WH. Expression of inducible stress protein 70 in rat heart myogenic cells confers protection against simulated ischemia-induced injury. J Clin Invest 1994; 93: 759-767

Mestril R, Dillmann WH. Heat shock proteins and protection against myocardial ischemia. J Mol Cell Cardiol 1995; 27: 45-52

Miron T, Wilchek M, Geiger B. Characterization of an inhibitor of actin polymerization in vinculin-rich fraction of turkey gizzard smooth muscle. Eur J Biochem 1988; 178: 543-553

Miron T, Vancompernolle-K, Vandekerckhove J, Wilchek M, Geiger B. A 25-kD inhibitor of actin polymerization is a low molecular mass heat shock protein. J Cell Biol 1991; 114: 255-261

Morimoto RI, Tissieres A; Georgopoulus C; *The Biology of Heat shock proteins and molecular chaperones*, Cold Spring Harbor Laboratory Press, 1994.

Morita T, Perrella MA, Lee ME, Kourembanas S. Smooth muscle cell-derived carbon monoxide is a regulator of vascular cGMP. Proc Natl Acad Sci (USA) 1995; 92: 1475-1479

Mueller HM, Taguchi H, Shibahara S. Nucleotide sequence and organization of thge rat heme oxygenase gene. J Biol Chem 1987; 262: 6795-6802

Neil TK, Abraham NG, Levere RD, and Kappas A: Differential heme oxygenase induction by stannous and stannic ions in the heart. J Cell Biochem 1995; 57: 409-414

Nicholl O, Quinlan RA. Chaperone activity of -crystallins modulates intermediate filament assembly. EMBO J 1994; 13, 945-953

Nutter LM, Sierra EE, Ngo NG. Heme oxygenase does not protect human cells against oxidant stress. J Lab Clin Med 1994; 123: 506-514.

Parag HA, Raboy B, Kulka R. Effect of heat shock on protein degradation in mammalian cells: involvement of the ubiquitin system. EMBO J 1987; 6: 55-61.

Plesofsky-Vig N, Brambl R. Gene sequence analysis of hsp30, a small heat shock protein of Neurospora crassa which associates with mitochondria. J Biol Chem 1990; 265: 15432-15440

Plesofsky-Vig N, Vig J; Brambl R. Phylogeny of the alpha-crystallin-related heat-shock proteins. J Mol Evol 1992; 35: 537-545

Plumier JC, Ross BM, Currie RW, Angelidis CE, Kazlaris H, Kollias G, Pagoulatos GN. Transgenic mice expressing the human heat shock protein 70 have improved post-ischemic myocardial recovery. J Clin Invest 1995; 95: 1854-1860

Prabhakar NR, Dinerman JL, Agani FH, Snyder SH. Carbon monoxide: a role in carotid body chemoreception. Proc Natl Acad Sci (USA) 1995; 92: 1994-1997

Rahman DR, Bentley NJ, Tuite MF. The Saccharomyces cerevisiae small heat shock protein Hsp26 inhibits actin polymerisation. Biochem Soc Trans 1995; 23: 77S

Raju VS, Maines MD. Coordinated expression and mechanism of induction of HSP32 (heme oxygenase-1) mRNA by hyperthermia in rat organs. Biochim Biophys Acta 1994; 1217: 273-280

Rechsteiner M. Natural substrates of the ubiquitin proteolytic pathway. Cell 1991; 66: 615-618

Reithmann C, Gierschik P, Werdan K, Jakobs KH. Tumor necrosis factor up-regulates Gi alpha and G beta proteins and adenylyl cyclase responsiveness in rat cardiomyocytes. Eur J Pharmacol 1991; 206: 53-60,

Rizzardini V, Terao M, Falciani F, Cantoni L. Cytokine induction of haem oxygenase mRNA in mouse liver. Biochem J 1993; 290: 343-347

Rothe J, Gehr G, Loetscher H, Lesslauer W. Tumor necrosis factor receptors--structure and function. [Review] Immunol Res 1992; 11: 81-90

Rouse J, Cohen P, Trigon S, Morange M, Alonso-Llamazares A, Zamanillo D, Hunt T, Nebrada AR. A novel kinase cascade triggered by stress and heat shock that stimulates MAPKAP kinase-2 and phosphorylation of the small heat shock proteins. Cell 1994; 78: 1027-1037

Schlesinger M: Heat shock proteins. J Biol Chem 1990; 265: 12111-12114

Sharma HS, Wünsch M, Brand T, Verdouw PD, Schaper W. Molecular biology of the coronary vascular and myocardial responses to ischemia. J Cardiovas Pharmacol 1992; 20: 23-31

Sharma HS, Snoeckx LH, Sassen LMA, Knoell R, Andres J, Verdouw PD, Schaper W. Expression and immunohistochemical localization of heat shock protein-70 in preconditioned porcine myocardium. Ann NY Acad Sci 1993; 723: 491-494

Sharma HS, Maulik N, Das DK, Gho BCG, Verdouw PD. Coordinated Expression of heme oxygenase-1 and ubiquitin in the porcine heart subjected to ischemia and reperfusion. Mol Cell Biochem 1996a; 157: 111-116

Sharma HS, Stahl J, Weisensee D, Loew-Friedrich I. Cytoprotective mechanisms in cultured cardiomyocytes. Mol Cell Biochem 1996b, (in press)

Sharma HS, Weisensee D, Löw-Friedrich I. Tumor necrosis factor- induced cytoprotective mechanisms in cardiomyocytes: Analysis by mRNA phenotyping. Ann NY Acad Sci 1996c (in press)

Shibahara S, Yoshizawa M, Suzuki H, Takeda K, Meguro K, Endo K. Functional analysis of cDNAs for two types of human heme oxygenase and evidence for their separate regulation. J Biochem 1993; 113: 214-218

Srinivasan AN, NagineniCN, Bhat SP. alpha A-crystallin is expressed in non-ocular tissues. J Biol Chem 1992; 267: 23337-23341

Srinivasan AN, Bhat SP. Complete structure and expression of the rat B-crystallin gene. DNA Cell Biol 1994; 13: 651-661

Stahl J, Wobus A, Ihrig S, Lutsch G, Bielka H. The small heat shock protein hsp25 is accumulated in P19 embryonal carcinoma cells and embryonic stem cells of line BLC6 during differentiation. Differentiation 1993; 51: 33-37

Stevens CF, Wang Y. Reversal of long-term potentiation of haem oxygenase. Nature 1993, 364, 147-149

Stocker R, Yamamoto Y, McDonagh AF, Glazer AN, Ames BN: Bilirubin is an antioxidant of possible physiologic significance. Science 1987: 235: 1043-1046

Stokoe D, Engel K, Campbell DG, Cohen P, Gaestel M. Identification of MAPKAP kinase 2 as a major enzyme responsible for the phopshorylation of the small mammalian heat shock proteins. FEBS Lett 1992a;

313: 307-313

Stokoe D, Campbell DG, Nakielny S, Hidaka H, Leevers SJ, Marshall C, Cohen P. MAPKAP kinase-2: A novel protein kinase activated by mitogen-activated protein kinase. EMBO J 1992b; 11: 3985-3994

Tacchini L, Schiaffonati L, Pappalardo C ,Gatti S,.Bernelli-Zazzera.
A: Expression of HSP 70, immediate-early response and heme oxygenase genes in ischemic-reperfused rat liver. Lab Invest 1993; 68: 465-471

Takeda K, Ishizawa S, Sato M, Yoshida T, Shibahara S. Identification of a cis-acting element that is responsible for cadmium-mediated induction of the human heme oxygenase gene. J Biol Chem 1994; 269: 22858-67

Tartaglia LA, Weber RF, Figari IS, Reynolds C, Palladino MJ, Goeddel DV. The two different receptors for tumor necrosis factor mediate distinct cellular responses. Proc Natl Acad Sci U S A 1991; 88: 9292-9296

Thiede B, Otto A, Zimny-Arndt U, Mueller EC, Jungblut P. Identification of human myocardial proteins separated by two-dimensional electrophoresis with matrix-assisted laser desorption/ionization mass spectrometry. Electrophoresis 1996; 17: 588-599

Trakshel GM, Maines MD. Multiplicity of heme oxygenase isozymes. HO-1 and HO-2 are different molecular species in rat and rabbit. J Biol Chem 1989; 264: 1323-1328

Tyrrell, RM, Applegate LA, Tromvoukis Y. The proximal promoter region of the human heme oxygenase gene contains elements involved in stimulation of transcriptional activity by a variety of agents including oxidants. Carcinogenesis 1993; 14: 761-765

Uney J, Anderton B, Thomas S. Changes in heat shock protein 70 and ubiquitin mRNA levels in C1300 N2A mouse neuroblastoma cells following treatment with iron. J Neurochem 1993; 60: 659-665.

Uoshima K, Handelman B, Cooper LF. Isolation and characterization of rat HSP27 gene. Biochem Biophys Res Commun 1993, 197:1388-1395

Verma A, Hirsh D, Glatt CE, Ronnett GV, Snyder SH. Carbon monoxide: A putative neutral messenger. Science 1993; 259: 381-383.

Vietor I, Vilcek J. Pathways of heat shock protein 28 phosphorylation by TNF in human fibroblasts. Lymphokine Cytokine Res 1994; 13, 315-323

Vile GF, Tyrrell RM. Oxidative stress resulting from ultraviolet A irradiation of human skin fibroblasts leads to a heme oxygenase-dependent increase in ferritin. J. Biol Chem 1993; 268 : 14678-14681

Vile GF, Basu-Modak S, Waltner C, Tyrrell RM. Heme oxygenase 1 mediates an adaptive response to oxidative stress in human skin fibroblasts. Proc Natl Acad Sci USA 1994; 91: 2607-2610

Walsh MT, Sen AC, Chakrabarti B. Micellar subunit assembly in a three-layer model of oligomeric -crystallin. J Biol Chem 1991; 266: 20079-20084

Weisensee D, Bereiter HJ, Schoeppe W, Löw-Friedrich I. Effects of cytokines on the contractility of cultured cardiac myocytes. Int J Immunopharmacol 1993; 15: 581-587

Welch W. Mammalian stress response: cell physiology, structure/function of stress proteins, and implications for medicine and disease. Physiol Rev 1992; 72:1063-1081

Wiegmann K, Schutze S, Kampen E, Himmler A, Machleidt T, and Kronke M. Human 55-kDa receptor for tumor necrosis factor coupled to signal transduction cascades. J Biol Chem 1992; 267: 17997-18001

Wilkinson JM, Pollard I. Immunohistochemical localisation of the 90, 70 and 25 kDa heat shock proteins in control and caffeine treated rat embryos. Annals Anatomy 1993; 175: 561-566

Wistow G. Domain structure and evolution in alpha-crystallins and small heat shock proteins. FEBS Lett. 1985; 181: 1-6

Yellon DM, DS Latchman. Stress proteins and myocardial protection. J Mol Cell Cardiol 1992; 24: 113-124

Yokoyama T, Vaca L, Rossen RD, Durante, W, Hazarika P, Mann DL: Cellular basis for the negative inotropic effects of tumor necrosis factor- in the adult mammalian heart. J Clin Invest 1993; 92: 2303-2012

Zantema A, Verlaan-De-Vries M, Maasdam D, Bol S, van-der-Eb A. Heat shock protein 27 and alpha B-crystallin can form a complex, which dissociates by heat shock. J Biol Chem 1992; 267: 12936-12941

Zhou M, Lambert H, Landry J. Transient activation of a distinct serine protein kinase is responsible for 27-kDa heat shock protein phosphorylation in mitogen- stimulated and heat-shocked cells. J Biol Chem 1993; 268: 35-43

Zu YL, Wu F, Gilchrist A, Ai YX, Labadia ME, Huang CK. The primary structure of a human MAP kinase activated protein kinase 2. Biochem Biophys Res Commun 1994; 200: 1118-1124

9

ROLE OF SMALL HSP GENE EXPRESSION IN MYOCARDIAL ISCHEMIA AND REPERFUSION

Dipak K. Das and Nilanjana Maulik

Cardiovascular Division, Department of Surgery, University of Connecticut School of Medicine, Farmington, CT, USA.

INTRODUCTION

All organisms whether prokaryotes or eukaryotes, respond to environmental stresses by rapidly inducing the expression of the genes for a number of stress-inducible proteins. Among them, heat shock proteins (HSPs) are ubiquitously present in almost all organisms including mammalian tissues. Most of the mammalian systems studied so far respond to stresses by inducing genes for highly conserved proteins encoding HSP 70 and HSP 90. mRNAs for these HSPs are also induced in mammalian tissues including hearts when subjected to a variety of stresses including heat shock, oxidative stress, hypoxia and ischemia. Genes of other HSPs are similarly induced when mammalian hearts are subjected to similar environmental stresses. Recently, genes encoding small heat shock proteins HSP 27, HSP 32 and ubiquitin have been found to be induced in the hearts in response to ischemia and reperfusion. The cells that survive after the ischemic insult exhibit a greater degree of tolerance against subsequent ischemia and reperfusion.

For eukaryotic cells, the heat shock response induced by environmental stress involves transcriptional activation mediated by the heat shock transcription factor (HSF) which is ubiquitously present in both the nucleus and cytoplasm. In response to stress, this HSF is rapidly activated and accumulated in the nucleus where it binds to the heat shock element (HSE).

The HSP 90 group is one of the most abundant cytoplasmic proteins present in most type of cells under normal conditions. This group may exist in two forms, HSP 90a and HSP 90 b [1]. The two forms differ slightly in molecular mass and have been identified in mammalian cells. They are encoded by distinct genes which are regulated differently during normal development. Also, they form transient associations with various regulatory and structural proteins including viral oncogene products having tyrosine kinase activity. This associative capacity of HSP 90 makes them as regulatory molecules. The additional accumulation may inhibit inappropriate activation of regulatory cascades during metabolic perturbations caused by stresses such as ischemia. HSP 90 has been recently found to be a component of most steroid receptors and take part in the transport and regulation of tyrosine kinases [2]. The common 90-kDa protein component of non-transformed "8S" steroid receptors is a heat shock protein [3].

The HSP 70 family are localized in cytoplasm, mitochondria and endoplasmic reticulum organelles. HSP 70 is of particular importance during a stress response to prevent protein aggregation, dissolution of protein aggregates and in renaturation of denatured proteins [4]. They are believed to participate in energy dependent processes such as disassembly of the clathrin coat of the vesicle and reversible binding of various abnormal proteins and translocation of proteins across membranes. The HSP 70 family of cytoplasmic origin appear to bind with nascent polypeptide chains associated with ribosomes during the process of elongation. It is speculated that HSP 70 proteins can reversibly interact with internal regions of preexisting proteins that are exposed resulting from stress-induced denaturation and facilitate correct refolding. These proteins accumulate in the nucleus primarily in association with the nucleoli, the location of ribosomal formation; it is of interest that ribosomal assembly is extremely sensitive to stress.

A number of studies have shown that heat shock pretreatment is associated with reduction of myocardial ischemia reperfusion injury. For example, heat shock resulted in significant infarct size reduction after prolonged coronary artery occlusion and reperfusion in the in vivo rat model [5]. Heat shock also ameliorated ischemia reperfusion injury in isolated rat heart [6]. Another recent study has demonstrated a direct correlation between the amount of heat-shock protein induced and the degree of myocardial protection [7]. A recent study from our own laboratory showed that heat shock using warm blood cardioplegia resulted in significant myocardial protection during the reperfusion of ischemic swine heart [8]. Interestingly, all of these studies also demonstrated the induction of the expression of HSP 70. Diverse stresses including ischemia, ischemic preconditioning, and oxidative stress can induce the expression of HSP 70 mRNA simultaneously providing significant cardioprotection. Based on these findings, it was assumed that the induction of HSP 70 play a significant role in myocardial protection. The results of two recent studies showed that hearts of transgenic mice overexpressing HSP 70 were more resistant to myocardial ischemia reperfusion injury [9,10].

While a great deal is known about HSP 70 and HSP 90 families, relatively little is known regarding the smaller HSPs such as ubiquitin, HSP 27 and HSP 32. The small HSPs have long been known to be associated with mRNA during stress in insect and plant cells. Many recent studies now implicate an important role of these small HSPs in the pathophysiology of many diseases including ischemia and reperfusion. It is likely that the small HSPs play a role in growth, signal transduction as well as cellular protection. This review will focus on the importance of the induction of small HSP genes in the ischemic reperfused hearts.

SMALL HSP GENES

The small HSP gene family includes the genes encoding HSP 22, 23, 26 and 27 and share homologies among themselves and with mammalian a-crystallin genes [11]. These HSP genes are independently expressed during the growth and development [12]. At mRNA level, transcription of HSP 26 was identified in several tissues [13]. Similar, but not identical, developmental profile was found for HSP 27 [14]. The activation of the small HSP genes at the beginning of the pupal stage was found to be regulated in part by ecdysone, a molting hormone [15]. It is believed that DNA sequences necessary for the regulation of small HSP genes during the growth and development are different from those involved in heat shock induction [16]. Ubiquitin, another small heat shock protein, binds to unfold proteins which are then be degraded during protein turnover in cells [17].

HSP 25/HSP 27

In contrast to HSP 70 and HSP 90 families, the multiplicity of small HSPs is variable between organisms. However, despite of the heterogeneity, these are grouped under the HSP 20 family. Multiple small HSPs were found in Drosophila [18], Dictyostelium [19], Xenopus [20], and most of the plants [21]. To the contrary, single small HSPs are found in yeasts (HSP 26), avians (HSP 24) or mammalian cells (HSP 27). Interestingly, in the C-terminal part of all the genes encoding these HSPs, a 36 amino acid residue sequence element is remarkably conserved.

Sequence analyses of the members of HSP 20 family revealed a single 35 to 37 amino acid residue conserved domain for all proteins [22]. Sequences for the mammalian HSP 25 to 27 were derived from a mouse cDNA clone [23] and from genomic clones of the human HSP 27 gene [24]. The human HSP 27 gene which contained two introns, was subsequently found in an 18-kb genomic fragment along with a pseudogene (Figure 1).

The precise function of HSP 27 remains unclear, but the primary function of this protein is believed to be in embryogenesis, growth regulation and differentiation [25]. Interestingly, during progressive differentiation of rat osteoblasts and

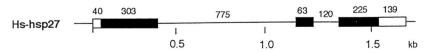

Figure 1 - Structure of HSP 27 gene (Nucl Acids Res 14:4127-4146, 1986). Length of exons and introns are indicated in base pairs and 5' and 3' untranslated sequences in open boxes.

promyelocytic leukemia cells, the HSP 27 mRNA expression was increased with corresponding downregulation of proliferation [26]. In both normal and neoplastic human B lymphocytes, HSP 27 serves as a marker for growth arrest [27]. Another striking feature of HSP 27 is that it is phosphorylated in response to stress [28,29]. Additionally, HSP 27 was showed to be involved in the modulation of actin microfilament dynamics [30] and smooth muscle contraction [31]. Transfection of Chinese hamster cells with the human HSP 27 gene inhibited the disappearance of microfilaments commonly observed after heat shock. A recent study described a role of HSP 27 in controlling the growth rate of endothelial cells in an estrogen-responsive manner [32].

Like HSP 70, an increase in HSP 27 expression was found to render the cells more resistant to hyperthermic injury [33]. Generally, after a heat shock, HSP is rapidly phosphorylated and then its synthesis is enhanced. Such enhancement not only conferred the cells resistant to subsequent heat stress, but also made them more resistant to oxidative stress [34]. TGFb$_1$ was found to inhibit DNA synthesis in mouse osteoblastic cells in parallel with the phosphorylation of HSP 27 [35] and that the effects of both events were abolished by catalase [36]. A recent study demonstrated that constitutively high expression of HSP 27 in immortalized human fibroblast cell line, KMST-6, made them susceptible to oxidative stress resulting in growth arrest, and further suggested that this mechanism could involve the phosphorylation of HSP 27 [37].

A number of studies from different laboratories demonstrated the induction of the expression of HSP 27 mRNA in the mammalian hearts after ischemia and reperfusion. For example, in a preconditioned pig heart model where the left anterior descending coronary artery was occluded for two periods of 10 min, separated by 30 min of reperfusion, a significant increase in HSP 27 mRNA level was found after the first occlusion which became 2- to 3- fold during 30 min of the first and second reperfusion periods [38]. During the prolonged reperfusion following the second occlusion, the HSP 27 mRNA levels in stunned tissue remained significantly raised. The authors also observed increased levels of HSP 27 mRNA in the adjacent non-stunned myocardium. This was significant during 30 min of the second reperfusion period as compared to sham operated animals. In another study using preconditioned isolated rat heart model where hearts were preconditioned either by 5 min of ischemia followed by 10 min of reperfusion (1 x PC) or repeating this process for four times (4 x PC), our own laboratory found the enhanced induction for the expression of HSP 27 mRNA only in the 4 X PC hearts (Figure 2) [39]. A similar kind of induction of HSP 27 gene expression was found when isolated rat hearts were subjected to oxidative stress induced by interleukin 1a (IL-1a) [40]. In biological system including heart, cytokines such as IL-1a and tissue necrosis factor (TNF) potentiate generation of oxygen free radicals. In this study, IL-1a induced the expression of HSP 27 mRNA within 2 hr and HSP protein after 48 hours. The hearts pretreated with IL-1a for 48 hours and then subjected to 30 min of ischemia followed by 30 min of reperfusion showed increased tolerance to ischemia reperfusion injury (Table I). In an another related study, heat shock was induced by injecting the pigs with amphetamine and after 40 hr, the isolated in situ pig hearts were subjected to 1 hr of LAD occlusion followed

162

by 1 hr of global hypothermic cardioplegic arrest and 1 hr of normothermic reperfusion [41]. Such heat shock was associated with the enhanced induction of the HSP 27 mRNA in the hearts in concert with the reduction of post-ischemic myocardial injury [42] (Figure 3). These hearts demonstrated increased tolerance to ischemia reperfusion injury (Table II).

Table I. Effect of Oxidative Stress Induced by Interleukin-1a (IL-1a) Pretreatment on the Post-Ischemic Ventricular Recovery

Rats were injected with recombinant IL-1a (30 mg/kg, ip); after 48 hr, they were sacrificed and isolated hearts perfused by Langendorff technique, were made ischemic for 30 min followed by 60 min of reperfusion. IL-1a developed the oxidative stress which was subsequently translated into the induction of antioxidant enzymes and induction of the expression of HSP 27 mRNA. *p < 0.05 compared to control.

| | | REPERFUSION | | |
		Baseline	30R	60R
LVDP	Control	159±5.9	76±10.9	63±10.9
(mm Hg)	IL-1	162±9.7	150±20	102±14*
LVdp/dtmax	Control	3055±277	1428±120	1388±277
(mm Hg/sec)	IL-1	3124±208	2583±276	2166±166*
Coronary flow	Control	7.4±0.22	3.7±0.27	2.9±0.58
(ml/min)	Il-1	7.3±0.25	5.8±0.57	5.2±0.43*
CK release	Control	4.0±2.1	85±2.3	110±5.8
(IU/L)	IL-1	3.9±1.6	64±3.2*	82±4.4*

In a very recent study, our laboratory has found that HSP 25/27 is a major potential substrate for MAPKAP kinase 2 in rat cardiac myocytes [43,44]. In this study, MAPKAP kinase 2 proteins were fractionated from cultured H9c2 cells, and then phosphorylated in vitro with an active recombinant mutant MAPKAP kinase 2 (T334A). Phosphorylated proteins were then separated on SDS-PAGE and analyzed by autoradiography. Protein phosphorylation analysis indicated that MAPKAP kinase 2 significantly stimulated the phosphorylation of the 25 kDa cytosolic protein derived from rat cardiac myocytes. Furthermore, myocardial HSP 25 isolated from cytosolic fraction of H9c2 cells using specific antibody, after immunoprecipitation, phosphorylation by the active recombinant MAPKAP kinase 2, separation by SDS-PAGE, and detection of the induced protein phosphorylation by autoradiography, revealed that myocardial HSP 25 was phosphorylated by MAPKAP kinase 2, and had a similar mobility on SDS-PAGE as the kinase-induced 25 kDa phosphoprotein derived

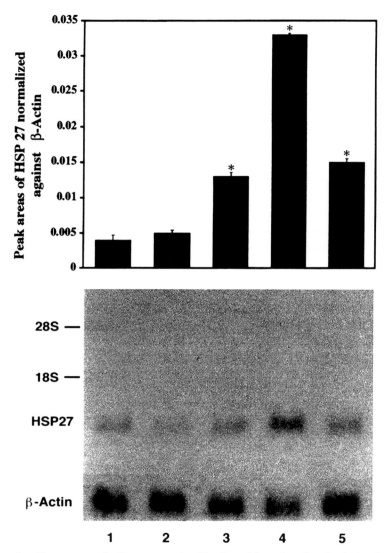

Figure 2 - Bottom panel : Representative Northern blots showing the induction for the expression of HSP 27 mRNAs obtained from control (1), 1xPC (2), 4xPC (3), heat shock (4) and oxidative stress (5) induced myocardium. (Das DK and Maulik N, In: Cell Biology of Trauma (Ed: J.J.Lemasters and C. Oliver, CRC Press, 1995, pp.193-211) . Top Panel : Denistometric scanning of the blots after normalization with b-actin.

from rat cardiac myocytes. This suggests that myocardial HSP 25/27 is a major substrate for MAPKAP kinase 2 in rat cardiac myocytes. Heat shock, oxidative stress and PMA - all stimulated the HSP 25 phosphorylation in the cardiac myocytes.

Table II. Effect of Amphetamine-induced Heat Shock on the Post-Ischemic Ventricular Recovery

Pigs were injected with amphetamine (3mg/kg, i.m) which raised their body temperatures to 42.5oC within 1 hr, maintained this temperature up to 2 hr, and then progressively came back to baseline levels. After 40 hr, pigs were sacrificed and isolated in situ hearts were subjected to 1 hr hypothermic cardioplegic arrest (Occl 60) followed by 1 hr of reperfusion (R-60).   Amphetamine-induced heat shock induced the expression of HSP 27 mRNA within 2 hr in all the vital organs including heart (Biochem Biophys Res Commun 192: 808-812, 1993 ; Mol Cell Biochem 137: 17-24, 1994) *p < 0.05 compared to control.

		REPERFUSION		
		Baseline	Occl 60	R-60
LVDP	Control	190±20	99±11	98±6.6
(mm Hg)	Heat shock	226±18	137±20	137±14*
LVdp/dtmax	Control	2100±270	945±110	935±58*
(mm Hg/sec)	Heat shock	2400±60	1370±170	1250±136*
Coronary flow	Control	107±8.6	102±6.9	86±9
(ml/min)	Heat shock	116±10.4	98±6.5	100±11.3
Segment	Control	100	0	10±0.9
shortening (%)	Heat shock	100	10±5	46 ±7

There is some evidence that HSP 27 may function as a molecular chaperone [46]. For example, HSP 27 has been localized in different intracellular compartments. It is able to bind other proteins thereby affecting the protein assembly, and has been found to participate in protein degradation. More importantly, HSP 27 possesses a serine protease-like active site that is instrumental in regulating Drosophila development. Evidences also exist to show that HSP 27 may prevent aggregation and promote functional refolding of denatured proteins, because the expression of HSP 25/HSP 27 was found to be associated with an ATP-dependent increase in refolding of denatured substrate proteins, and prevent protein aggregation in in vitro systems.

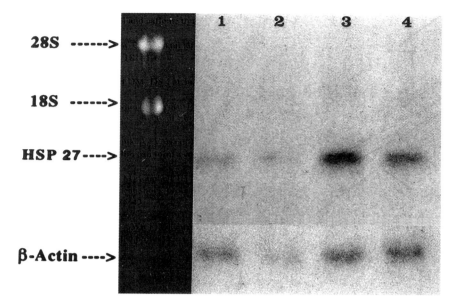

28S ------>

18S ------>

HSP 27 ---->

β-Actin ---->

1   2   3   4

Figure 3 - Northern blot analysis of RNA obtained from pig hearts that were treated for 3 hr either with a single dose of amphetamine or saline (control). (Maulik et al : Mol. Cell Biochem 137: 17-24, 1994).Ten microgram of total RNA from pig heart was subjected to 1% agarose-formaldehyde gel electrophoresis, transferred to Gene Screen plus membrane, and hybridized with HSP 27 cDNA probe. Reprobing of the same membrane revealed the transcripts of b-actin, which served as control. The positions of the 28S and 18S ribosomal RNA bands after staining with ethidium bromide are indicated on the left. Lane 1 and 2 : control; lane 3 and 4 : heat shock.

In summary, it is tempting to speculate that HSP 27 may be an important component of the signal transduction pathway that regulates the adaptive modification of the myocardial cells after subjecting to a variety of stresses including ischemia and reperfusion. In view of the existing evidences that myocardial protection by ischemic preconditioning/adaptation involves rapid intracellular changes triggered by signal transduction and late molecular changes mediated by gene expression [43,45], HSP 27 seems to play an important role in preconditioning/adaptation.

HSP 32 (HEME OXYGENASE)

Heme oxygenase isoenzymes catalyze the initial step for heme degradation by oxidatively cleaving the a-meso carbon bridge to produce the bile pigment, biliverdin which is subsequently reduced to bilirubin. The bile pigments that were thought to be biologically inert, are now known to possess potent antioxidant activity. Formation of bilirubin from the oxidative degradation of heme is catalyzed by two microsomal enzymes in sequence heme oxygenase and biliverdin reductase [47]. Heme oxygenase comprises two isoenzymes, heme oxygenase-I and heme oxygenase-II of which the former is known to be regulated by various endogenous as well as exogenous factors such as hemoglobin, metals and oxygen free radicals [48,49].

The two isoenzymes are also different gene products that differ in their tissue distribution, biochemical properties and transcription regulation [50]. Microsomal heme oxygenase comprises two isoenzymes, heme oxygenase 1 and heme oxygenase 2. While the former isoenzyme is induced in response to a stress, the later is the constitutive and non-inducible form. Heme oxygenase-I has recently been identified as HSP 32, and oxygen free radicals have been found to be one of its inducers in mammalian cells that include brain and skin [51,52]. HSPs are induced in both eukaryotic and prokaryotic cells in response to a variety of agents including oxidative stress as well as transition elements and heavy metals such as iron, aluminum, cobalt,

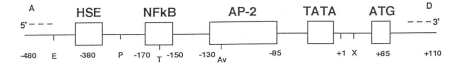

Figure 4 - Schematic representation of the HO-1 gene upstream region. Presence of AP-2 and NF-kB transcription sites in the HO-1 promoter region is shown in the figure. Restriction sites are indicated by E : Eco47III; P : Pst I, T : EcoT141; Av : AVa 1; X : XhoI. (Proc. Natl. Acad. Sci. 91:5989, 1994)

zinc, ozone, ischemia/ reperfusion, cytokines and heat stress. HSP 27, HSP 70 as well as HSP 90 mRNAs have been shown to be induced in mammalian heart during ischemia [38,39,53]. Heme oxygenase (HSP 32) mRNA, on the other hand was not inducible in rat liver even after 60 min of ischemia while appreciable amount of heme oxygenase was detectable after 4 hr of reperfusion of the ischemic liver [54]. Heme oxygenase-I mRNA was induced in rat kidney after 6 hr of reperfusion following a 30 min ischemic insult [55]. Similar to these findings our study also demonstrate that in rat heart, hemeoxygenase-I is not induced by ischemia and is inducible only after reperfusion of ischemic myocardium.

Recently heme oxygenase-I isoenzyme has been found to be synonymous with heat shock protein 32 (HSP 32) based on the fact that heme oxygenase-1 was found to be transcriptionally controlled by heat shock [56]. Highly coordinated 20-40 fold increases in the level of 1.8 kb mRNA within a short period of time (@ 1 hr) make the HSP 32 distinct from other HSPs. HO-1 heme contains a AP-2 binding site in the proximal part of the transcription site in HO-1 promoter region close to the NFkB site [57] (Figure 4).

A recent study [58] has demonstrated the myocardial expression of both HO-1 and HO-2 at both the transcription and protein levels under normal conditions. They also showed that heat stress can induce only HO-1 and not HO-2 in the heart. By using immunohistochemistry, HO-1 expression was found in the atrioventricular bundle in the heart of the heat-stressed hearts. In another recent study, Balla et al [59] have demonstrated the induction of heme oxygenase in pulmonary endothelial cells by hemoglobin. In the present study, we found predominant expression of HO-1 in the perivascular region with significantly less localization in cardiomyocytes. Interestingly, ischemia/reperfusion-induced expression of HO-1 primarily occurred in the interstitial spaces with light to moderate expression in the myocytes in contrast to the OH.-induced expression which showed homogenous cytoplasmic localization of HO-1 in the cardiomyocytes. The differential localization of the HO-1 expression may suggest extracellular nature of the oxidants generation in the ischemic reperfused myocardium.

The results of a recent study from our own laboratory demonstrated that heme oxygenase mRNA is not induced in the heart during ischemia, but is induced during reperfusion, and the induction of the expression is a function of the duration of reperfusion time [60]. This induction of heme oxygenase mRNA is inhibited by the scavengers of oxygen free radicals, SOD and catalase, suggesting that oxygen free radicals generated during the reperfusion of ischemic myocardium is instrumental for the expression of heme oxygenase gene (Figure 5). The results further indicate that unlike other HSPs, heme oxygenase is inducible by oxidative stress developed during reperfusion of the ischemic heart is responsible for its expression. This is further supported by the induction of HO-1 mRNA in heart by OH. radicals (Figure 6). The progressive increase in the heme oxygenase transcript as a function of the duration of reperfusion further suggests that the induction of heme oxygenase mRNA is an adaptive phenomenon and the induction occurs in response to tissue injury.

The role of heme oxygenase in cellular protection remains controversial. In a recent study heme oxygenase could not protect human cells against the oxidative stress [61]. Contrary to this, rapid induction of heme oxygenase following rhabdomyolysis was found to be associated with a striking reduction in mortality [62]. In another recent study, heme oxygenase was found to mediate an adaptive response to oxidative stress in human skin fibroblasts [63]. In this study, the authors showed that human skin fibroblasts, pre-irradiated with ultraviolet A (UVA) radiation are associated with increased levels of heme oxygenase and sustain less membrane damage during a subsequent exposure to UVA radiation than cells that had not been pre- irradiated. Pretreating cells with heme oxygenase antisense oligo-nucleotide inhibited the irradiation-dependent induction of the heme oxygenase enzyme and abolished the

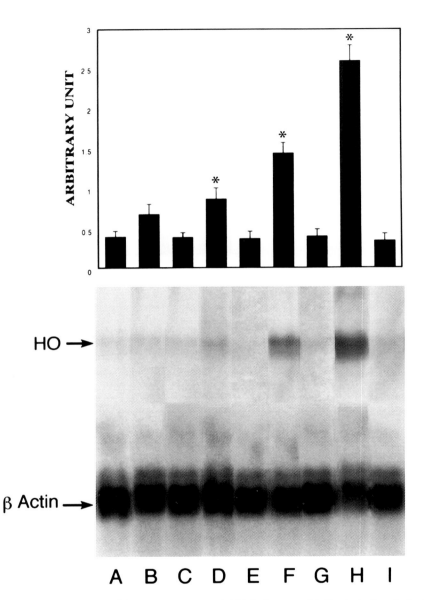

Figure 5 - Northern blot of heme oxygenase mRNA in hearts with 5 min ischemia(isc) and reperfusion(rep). Groups pre-perfused with SOD and catalase for 15 min, control group with buffer. BOTTOM: A:Baseline; B: 5 min isc/15 min rep; C: SOD + Catalase-5 min isc/15 min rep; D: 5 min isc/30 min rep; E: SOD + Catalase - 5 min isc/30 min rep; F: 5 min isc/45 min rep; G: SOD + catalase - 5 min isc/45 min rep; H: 5 min isc/60 min rep; I: SOD + catalase - 5 min isc/60 min rep. TOP: Densitometry(mean ± SEM) for six different experiments for each time point. *p < 0.05 to baseline.

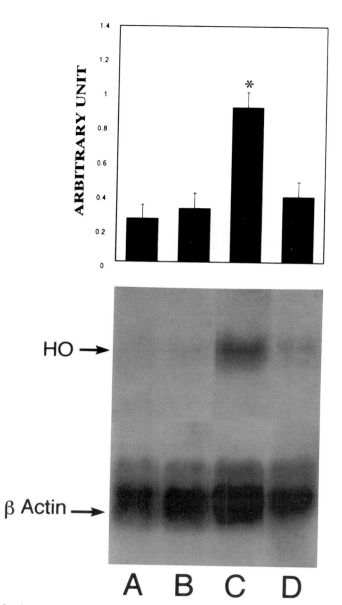

Figure 6 - Northern blot analysis of heme oxygenase mRNA in hearts subjected to perfusion with OH. generating system. (Maulik et al, J. Mol Cell Cardiol, in press). BOTTOM: A: Baseline; B: 15 min perfusion with SOD + catalase; C : 30 min perfusion with OH. generating system; D: 15 min pre-perfusion with SOD + catalase followed by 30 min perfusion with OH. generating system.TOP: Densitometry (mean ± SEM) for six different experiments for each time point. *p < 0.05 to baseline.

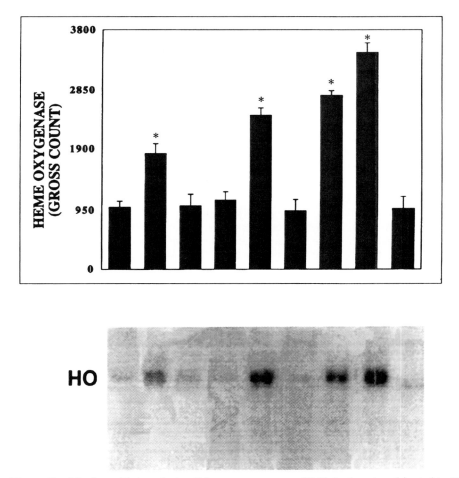

Figure 7 - Northern blot analysis of heme oxygenase mRNA in hearts subjected to 30 min ischemia followed by 30 min of reperfusion and the effects of NO (Maulik et al, Mol Cell Biochem, in press). BOTTOM : Lane 1: Baseline; Lane 2: 15 min perfusion with L-arginine; Lane 3: 15 min perfusion with L-arginine with 650 uM protophorphyrin; Lane 4: 30 min ischemia; Lane 5: 15 min perfusion with L-arginine and protophorphyrin followed by 30 min. ischemia; Lane 6: 15 min perfusion with L-arginine and protoporphyrin followed by 30 min ischemia; Lane 7: 30 min reperfusion after 30 min ischemia; Lane 8: 15 min perfusion with L-arginine followed by 30 min ischemia and 30 min reperfusion; Lane 9: 15 min perfusion with L-arginine and protoporphyrin followed by 30 min ischemia and 30 min reperfusion. TOP: Densitometry (mean ± SEM) of 6 experiments for each time point as shown on blot.
* $p < 0.05$ compared to baseline.

protective effect of pre-irradiation implicating heme oxygenase as the initial inducible mediator of the adaptive process.

At least three plausible mechansims may be put forward to support the beneficial role of heme oxygenase. Firstly, induction of heme oxygenase would increase the cellular capacity to generate biliverdin and bilirubin, potent antioxidants capable of scavenging peroxy radicals and inhibit lipid peroxidation. A recent study has indicated a direct role of bilirubin resulting from the heme oxygenase activation as a physiological protector against oxidative injury [64]. Oxidative stress is likely to potentiate the release of the pro-oxidant heme prosthetic group from the intracellular heme proteins. Heme oxygenase would degrade the heme and replace it with bilirubin. Secondly, induction of heme oxygenase is coupled to the synthesis of ferritin, a proven cytoprotective antioxidant [65]. Thirdly, the process of heme oxygenase activation and bilirubin formation generate CO, a potential chemical messenger that lead to the generation of cGMP [66]. Activation of cGMP is likely to potentiate the activation of signal transduction pathway leading to the generation of diacylglycerol and protein kinase C. A recent study from our laboratory has demonstrated that a precursor of nitric oxide (NO), L-arginine, increased the transcripts of HO-1 mRNA, simultaneously stimulating cGMP content and potentiating CO signaling (66-68) (Figure 7). Protoporphyrin, a heme oxygenase inhibitor, blocked the induction of HO-1 mRNA simultaneously attenuating the NO-mediated improvement in post-ischemic left ventricular functions (Table III).

UBIQUITIN

Ubiquitin is a 76-residue protein which is ubiquiteously present in mammalian cells either in free form or covalently bound through its carboxy terminal Gly residue to other proteins including chromosomal histones, nuclear and cytoplasmic proteins [69]. Ubiquitin has not been detected in bacteria. It has been characterized as an heat shock-induced protein in human, chicken, pig, yeast as well as in other organisms [70 -72]. During the initial periods of heat shock, the protein-ubiquitin conjugation undergoes rapid and pronounced changes presumably due to the deubiquitination of histone H2A and subsequent accumulation of aberrant proteins. After a heat shock, in Trypanosoma cruzi about 100 ubiquitin genes were found to be clustered in a 27kb genomic fragment. [73]. Five of them were fusion genes with a C-terminal extension of their open reading frames by a 52-amino acid residue basic domain. They were transcribed when the temperature was raised from 26oC to 42oC. The altered transcription of ubiquitin gene seems to be essential for restoration of normal activities [74]. Deletion of the heat shock-inducible polyubiquitin gene makes the yeast cells defective in sporulation and hypertensive to stress [75].

It is universally believed that for eukaryotes, initial steps of many intracellular proteolysis consists of covalent conjugation of ubiquitin to short-lived proteins [76]. The coupling of ubiquitin to proteins is catalyzed by ubiquitin-conjugating enzymes

Table III. Effect of NO and Heme Oxygenase Inhibition on the Post-Ischemic Ventricular Recovery

Isolated working rat hearts were made ischemic for 30 min followed by 60 min of reperfusion (control). A separate group of hearts were pre- prefused with 3 mM L-arginine in the presence or absence of 650 mM protoporphyrin for 10 min prior to ischemia. NO induced the expression of HO-1 mRNA which was blocked by protoporphyrin (Mol Cell Biochem, in press) *$p < 0.05$ compared to control; +$p < 0.05$ compared to L-arginine

		REPERFUSION		
		Control	L-arginine	L-arginine+ PP
DP	Baseline	69±1.8	71±3.5	76±2.5
(mm Hg)	I/R	35±1.8	53±4.3*	47±1.4+
dp/dtmax	Baseline	3282±100	3167±223	3044±74
(mm Hg/sec)	I/R	1758±117	2405±125*	2123±78+
Aortic flow	Baseline	43±0.9	43±2.6	44±0.9
(ml/min)	I/R	9.4±1.6	23±1.5*	18±2.0+
Coronary flow	Baseline	25±1.0	26±1.1	24±0.6
(ml/min)	I/R	19±1.6	22±0.8*	19±0.5+

which may function in complexes with ubiquitin ligases [77]. The bonding of ubiquitin with other proteins is reversible, and through the linkage between a-carboxyl group of the ubiquitin and lysine e-amino group of the protein [78]. Ubiquitin is initially activated by an enzyme through an energy-dependent reaction followed by the formation of a thiolester bond with a ubiquitin-conjugating enzyme which subsequently catalyzes isopeptide bond formation with ubiquitin. Ubiquitination of a substrate may result in a substrate-linked multi-ubiquitin chain. In such multi-ubiquitin chains, Lys48 of a ubiquitin moity was believed to be bound with another ubiquitin moiety within a chain [79]. A recent study suggested that ubiquitin-ubiquitin isopeptide bonds in substrate-linked multi-ubiquitin chains involve both Lys48 and Lys29 of ubiquitin [80].

It should be clear from the above discussion that ubiquitin plays an essential role for the degradation of many eukaryotic proteins. While the mechanism of ubiquitination is extremely complex, the role of ubiquitin in the selective protein turnover associated with the stress insult is of great importance. In response to a stress such as heat shock, oxidative stress, or ischemia-reperfusion, the cells undergo rapid changes including both degradation and turnover of proteins. Successful adaptive modification depends on both degradation of selective proteins and induction of the expression of new proteins essential for the survival in the new environment. Ubiquitin seems to be essential for the degradation of the non-essential harmful proteins.

Studies exist in the literature to suport the role of ubiquitin in the myocardial preservation. In a study using ischemic reperfused pig heart, ubiquitin gene was detected in both non-ischemic and ischemic heart tissues [38]. Transcription of the ubiquitin gene was increased during 30 and 120 min of the second reperfusion period. The transient increase of tissue levels of ubiquitin mRNA was associated with temporary formation of new ubiquitin protein conjugates. In the brain, enhanced levels of ubiquitin-protein conjugates were found after five minutes of cerebral ischemia [81]. In a recent study, we have shown a coordinated expression pattern of HO-1 and ubiquitin gene in the same porcine model in which the left anterior descending coronary artery (LAD) was occluded for 10 min and reperfused for 30 min, and after a second occlusion of 10 min, reperfused for up to 210 min [82]. The expression of ubiquitin mRNAs was drammatically enhanced in hearts after second occlusion, with most expression found after 90 min of reperfusion. Several-fold induction of the expression of ubiquitin genes were found in the hearts of pigs fed with coenzyme Q10 for one month (Figure 8). The coenzyme Q10 fed pig hearts were found to be more resistant to ischemia reperfusion injury (Table IV).

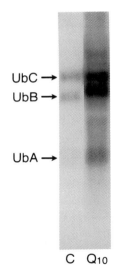

UbC →
UbB →

UbA →

C   Q10

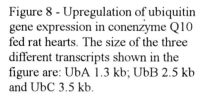

Figure 8 - Upregulation of ubiquitin gene expression in conenzyme Q10 fed rat hearts. The size of the three different transcripts shown in the figure are: UbA 1.3 kb; UbB 2.5 kb and UbC 3.5 kb.

Table IV. Effect of Coenzyme Q10 on the Post-Ischemic Ventricular Recovery
Pigs were fed Coenzyme Q10 (2 mg/kg) for one month. After that pigs were sacrificed, and isolated in situ pig hearts were subjected 60 min of LAD occlusion followed by 60 min of cardioplegic arrest and 60 min of reperfusion. *p < 0.05 compared to control.

		Baseline	60min Reperf.
LVDP	Control	198±35	83±13
(mm Hg)	Q10	211±31	110±7*
LVEDP	Control	24±3	21±2
(mm Hg)	Q10	13±2	16±3*
LVmaxdp/dt	Control	2887±943	630±136
(mm Hg/sec)	Q10	4993±88	823±136*
LVmindp/dt	Control	-1793±746	-434±95
(mm Hg/sec)	Q10	-2986±442	711±170*

SUMMARY

It should be clear from the above discussion that high molecular weight HSP genes are found in both prokaryotes and eukaryotes while small HSP genes such as those encoding ubiquitin and HSP 27 have been identified only in the eukaryotes. The functions of small HSP genes are distinct from those for the high molecular weight HSP genes such as HSP 70, which primarily function as molecular chaperones by facilitating protein folding and maintaining conformation. Contrary to that, the major function of HSP 27 is related to cellular growth and development. In addition HSP 27 seems to be an important component of the signal transduction regulating the adaptive modification of cells under stress. A stressed cell must be able to selectively degrade any abnormal intracellular proteins, and this task is performed by another small HSP, ubiquitin. After stress, many proteins are translocated prior to activation, and ubiquitin facilitates this process. The other small HSP discussed in this chapter, i.e., HSP 32 is also an oxidative stress inducible protein, HO-1. A growing body of evidence suggests its direct role in cellular protection against environmental stress.

It seems, therefore, logical to assume that the induction of small HSP genes such as HSP 32, HSP 27 and ubiquitin, plays an important role in the protection of the cells when challenged by stress. Ischemia/reperfusion is an unique example of a stress that consists of at least two major components, ischemic stress and oxidative stress. Results from many laboratories including our own have demonstrated that the mRNAs encoding the proteins for HSP 32, HSP 27 and ubiquitin are induced in the ischemic/ reperfused hearts. However, except for HSP 32, a direct correlation between the induction of these small HSP genes and myocardial protection from ischemia/ reperfusion injury has not been demonstrated.

The mechanisms of ischemia/reperfusion-induced expression of these HSP genes and their transcription regulation is not known. A heat shock element (HSE) seems to be necessary for most of these expressions. HSEs are also known to regulate the transcription process by binding with the transcription factor (HSF). After stress, HSFs becomes phosphorylated which enhances their ability to enhance transcription. Recently, an antioxidant response element (ARE) has been identified which induces the expression of NQO1 and GST genes in response to environmental stress. The increased activities of these genes are found to play a direct role in cellular protection against diverse stresses including oxidative stress. Such protection results from a two-electron reduction catalyzed by NQO1 that would compete with the reactive oxygen species. It is tempting to speculate that an analogous system is instrumental for the induction of these small HSP genes which confer protection against stresses such as ischemia/reperfusion.

ACKNOWLEDGEMENTS

This study was supported in part by NIH HL 22559, HL 33889, and a Grant-In-Aid from the American Heart Association # 007.

REFERENCES

1.Rebbe NF, Ware J, Betina RM, Modrich P, Stafford DW. Nucleotide sequence of a cDNA for a member of the human 90kDa heat shock protein family. Gene 53 : 235-245, 1987.

2. Brugge JS. Interaction of the Rous sarcoma virus protein pp60src, with the cellular proteins, pp 60 and pp 90. Curr Top Microbiol. Immunol 122: 59-81, 1985

3. Catelli MG, Binart N, Jung-Testas I, Renoir JM, Baulieu EE, Feramisco JR, Welch WJ The common 90 kd protein component of non transformed 8S steroid receptors isaheat schock protein. EMBO J. 4: 3131-3135, 1985.

4. Skowyra D, georgopoulos C, Zycliz M. The E.coli dnaK product, the hsp 70 homolog, can reactivate heat-inactivated RNA polymerase in an ATP hydrolysis-dependent manner. Cell 62: 939-944, 1990.

5. Donnelly TJ, Sievers RE, Visseren FLJ, Welch WJ, Wolfe CL. Heat shock protein induction in rat hearts: a role for improved myocardial salvage after ischemia and reperfusion? Circulation 85: 769-778, 1992.

6. Currie RW, Karmazyn M, Kloc M, Mailer K. Heat shock response is associated with enhanced postischemic ventricular recovery. Circ Res 63: 543-549, 1988.

7. Hutter MM, Sievers RE, Barbosa V, Wolfe CL. Heat shock protein induction in rat hearts. A direct correlation between the amount of heat-shock protein induced and the degree of myocardial protection. Circulation. 89: 355-360, 1994.

8. Liu X, Engelman RM, Moraru II, Rousou JA, Flack JE, Deaton DW, Maulik N, Das DK. Heat shock: A new approach for myocardial preservation in cardiac surgery. Circulation. 86 (suppl II) 358-363, 1992.

9. Plumier, J.C.L., Ross, B.M., Currie, R.W., Angelidis, C.E., Kazlaris, H., Kollias, G., and Pagoulatos, G.N. Transgenic mice expressing the human heat shock protein 70 have improved post-ischemic myocardial recovery. J. Clin Invest. 95: 1854-1860, 1995.

10. Marber, M.S., Mestril, R., Chi, S-H., Sayen, R., Yellon, D.M., and Dillman, W.H. Overexpression of the rat inducible 70-kD heat stress protein in a transgenic mouse increses the resistance of the heart to ischemic injury. J. Clin Invest   95: 1446-1456, 1995.

11. Ingolia TD, Craig EA. Four small Drosophilia heat shock proteins are related to each other and to mammalian a-crystallin. Proc. Natl. Acad. Sci., USA 79: 2360-2364, 1982.

12. Mason PJ, Hall LMC, Gausz J. The expression of heat genes during normal development in Drosophila melanogaster. Molec Gen Genet   194: 73-78, 1984.

13. Glaser RL, Wolfner MF, Lis JT. Spatial and temporal pattern of HSP 26 expression during normal development. EMBO J   5: 747-754, 1986.

14. Pauli D, Tonka CH, Tissieres A, Arrigo AP. Tissue-specific expression of the heat shock protein HSP 27 during Drosophila melanogaster development. J. Cell Biol 111 : 817-828, 1990.

15.   Thomas SR, Lengyel JA. Ecdysteroid-regulated heat-shock gene erxpression during Drosophila melanogaster development. Devl Biol 115: 434-438, 1986.

16. Cohen RS, Meselson M. Separate regulatory elements for the heat-inducible and ovarian expression of the Drosophila HSP 26 gene. Cell 43: 737-746, 1985;   Hoffman EP, Gerring SL, Corces VG. the ovarian, ecdysterone, and heat-shock-responsive promoters of the Drosophila melanogaster HSP 27 gene react very differently to perturbations of DNA sequence. Molec Cell Biol 7: 973-981, 1987.

17. Mayer RJ, Arnold J, Laszlo L, Landon M, Lowe J. Ubiquitin in health and disease. Biochem Biophys Acta. 1089: 141-157, 1991.

18. Ayme A, Tissieres A. Locus 67B of Drosophila melanogaster contains seven, not four, closely related heat shock genes. EMBO J. 4: 2949-2954, 1985),

19. Loomis WF, Wheeler S. Chromatin-associated heat shock proteins in Dictyostelium. Dev Biol   90: 412-418, 1982.

20. Darasch S, Mosser DD, Bols NC, Heikkila JJ. Heat shock gene expression in Xenopus laevis A6 cells in response to heat shock and sodium arsenite. Biochem Cell Biol 66: 862-870, 1988.

21 . Mansfield MA, Key JL. Synthesis of low molecular weight heat shock proteins in plants. Plant Physiol 84: 1007-1017, 1987.

22. Neumann D, Nover L, Parthier B, Rieger R, Scharf KD, Wollgiehn R, zur Nieden U. Heat shock and other stress response systems of plants. Biol Zentralbl 108: 1-156, 1989.

23. Gaestel M, Gross B, Benndorf R, Strauss M, Schunk W-H, Kraft R, Otto A, Boehm H, Stahl J, Drabsch H, Bielka H. Molecular cloning, sequencing and expression in Escherichia coli of the 25-kDa growth-related protein of Ehrlich ascites tumor and its homology to mammalian stress proteins. Eur J. Biochem   179: 209-213, 1989.

24. Hickey E, Brandon SE, Sadis S, Smale G, Weber LA. Molecular cloning of sequences encoding the human heat-shock proteins and their expression during hyperthermia. Gene 43: 147-154, 1986.

25. Zhou M, Lambert H, Landry J. Transient activation of a distinct serine protein kinase is responsible for 27 kDa heat shock protein phosphorylation in mitogen-stimulated and heat-shocked cells. J. Biol Chem 268: 35-43, 1993.

26. Shakoori AR, Oberdorf AM, Owen TA, Weber LA, Hickey E, Stein JL, Lian JB, Stein GS. Expression of heat shock genes during differentiation of mammalian osteoblasts and promyelotic leukomia cells. J. Cell Biochem 48: 277-287, 1992.

27. Spector NL, Samson W, Ryan C, Gribben J, Urban W, welch WJ, Nadler LM. Growth arrest of human B lymphocytes is accompanied by induction of the low molecular weight mammalian heat shock protein (HSP 28). J. Immunol 148: 1668-1673, 1992.

28. Santell L, Bartfel N, Levin E. Identification of a protein transiently phosphorylated by activators of endothelial cell function as the heat shock protein HSP 27. Biochem J. 284: 705-710, 1992.

29. Gaestel M, Schroder W, Benndorf R, Lippmann C, Buchner K, Hucho F, Erdmann VA, Bielka H. Identification of the phosphorylation sites of the murine small heat shock protein HSP 25. J. Biol Chem 266: 14721-14724, 1991.

30. Lavoie J, Hickey E, Weber LA, Landry J. Modulation of actin microfilament dynamics and fluid phase pinocytosis by phosphorylation of heat shock protein 27. J. Biol Chem 268: 24210-24214, 1993.

31. Bitar K, Kaminski M, Hailat N, Cease K, Strahler J. HSP 27 is a mediator of sustained smooth muscle contraction in response to bombesin. Biochem Biophys Res Commun 181: 1192-1200, 1991.

32. Piotrowicz R, Weber LA, Hickey E, Levin EG. Accelerated growth and senescence of arterial endothelial cells expressing the small molecular weight heat-shock protein HSP 27. FASEB J 9: 1079-1084, 1995.

33. Lavoie J, Gingras-Breton G, Tanguay R, Landry J. Induction of chinese hamster HSP 27 gene expression in mouse cells confers resistance to heat shock. J. Biol Chem. 268: 3420-3429, 1993.

34. Mehlen P, Briolay J, Smith L, Diaz-Latoud C, Fabre N; Pauli D, Arrigo A-P. Analysis of the resistance to heat and hydrogen peroxide stress in Cos cells transiently expressing wild type or deletion mutants of the Drosophila 27-kDa heat shock protein. Eur J. Biochem. 215: 277-284, 1993.

35. Shibanuma M, Kuroki T, Nose K. Cell cycle dependent phosphorylation of HSP 28 by TGFb1 and H2O2 in normal mouse osteoblastic cells (MC3T3-E1), but not in their ras-transformants. Biochem Biophys Res Commun 187: 1418-1425, 1992.

36. Nose K, Ohba M, Shibanuma M, Kuroki T. Involvement of hydrogen peroxide in the actions of TGFB1. In: Oxidative stress, Cell activation,m and Viral infection. C. Pasquier, R.Y.Oliver, C. Auclair and L. Packer, eds. Birkhauser Verlag, Basel, Switzerland, pp 21-34.

37. Arata S, Hamaguchi S, Nose K. Effects of the overexpression of the small heat shock protein, HSP 27, on the sensitivity of human fibroblast cells exposed to oxidative stress. J. Cell Physiol 163: 458-465, 1995.

38. Andres J, Sharma HS, Knoll R, Stahl J, Sassen LMA, Verdouw PD, schaper W. Expression of heat shock proteins in the normal and stunned porcine myocardium. Cardiovasc. Res 27: 1421-1429, 1993.

39. Das DK, Engelman RM, Kimura Y. Molecular adaptation of cellular defences following preconditioning of the heart by repeated ischemia. Cardiovasc Res 27: 578-584, 1993.

40. Maulik N, Engelman RM, Wei Z, Lu D, Rousou JA, Das DK. Interleukin-1a preconditioning reduces myocardial ischemia reperfusion injury. Circulation 88 (part II) : 387-394, 1993.

41. Maulik N, Wei Z, Liu X, Engelman RM, Rousou JA, Das DK. Improved postischemic ventricular functional recovery by amphetamine is linked with its ability to induce heat shock. Mol Cell Biochem. 137: 17-24, 1994.

42. Maulik N, Engelman RM, Wei Z, Liu X, Rousou JA, Flack JE, Deaton DW, Das DK. Drug-induced heat-shock preconditioning improves post-ischemic ventricular recovery after cardiopulmonary bypass. Circulation 92 (suppl II): 381-388, 1995.

43. Das DK, Moraru II, Maulik N, Engelman RM. Gene expression during myocardial adaptation to ischemia and reperfusion. Annal NY Acad Sci. 723: 292-307, 1993

44. Zu Y-L, Gilchrist A, Sha'afi RI, Das DK, Huang, C-K. Heat shock, oxidative stress, or phorbol ester stimulate activation of MAPKAP kinase2 and HSP 25 phosphorylation in rat cardiac myocytes. (communicated).

45. Das DK, Maulik N. Moraru II. Gene expression in acute myocardial stress. Induction by hypoxia, ischemia, reperfusion, hyperthermia and oxidative stress. J. Mol Cell Cardiol 27: 181-193, 1995.

46. Ciocca DR, Oesterreich S, Chamness GC, McGuire WL, Fuqua SAW. Biological and clinical implications of HSP 27, J Natl Cancer Inst 85: 1558-1570, 1993.

47. Tenhunen R, Marver HS, Schmid R. Microsomal heme oxygenase. J. Biol Chem 244: 6388- 6394, 1969.

48. Keyse SM, Tyrrell RM. Heme oxygenase is the major 32 KDa stress protein induced in human skin fibroblasts by UVA radiation, hydrogen peroxide and sodium arsenite. Proc Natl Acad Sci 86 : 99-103, 1989.

49. Keyse SM, Applegate LA, Tromvoukis Y, Tyrrell RM. Oxidant stress leads to transcriptional activation of the human heme oxygenase gene in cultured skin fibroblast. Mol Cell Biol 10: 4967-4969, 1990.

50. McCoubery WK, Ewing JF, Maines MD. Human heme oxygenase: Characterization and expression of a full length cDNA and evidence suggesting the two HO-2 transcripts differ by choice of polyadenylation signal. Arch. Biochem Biophys 295: 13-20, 1992.

51. Maines MD, Mayer RD, Ewing JF , McCoubrey WK. Induction of kidney heme oxygenase -1 (HSP 32) mRNA and protein by ischemia/reperfusion : Possible role of heme as both promoter of tissue damage and regulator of HSP 32. J. Pharmacol Exp Therapeu 264 : 457-462, 1993.

52. Vile GF, Tyrrell RM. Oxidative stress resulting from ultraviolet A irradiation of human skin fibroblasts leads to a heme oxygenase-dependent increase in ferritin. J. Biol Chem 268 : 14678-14681, 1993.

53. Knowlton AA, Brecher P, Apstein CS. Rapid expression of heat shock Protein in the rabbit after brief cardiac ischemia. J. Clin Invest 87: 139-147, 1991.

54. Tacchini L, Schiaffonati L, Pappalardo C ,Gatti S,.Bernelli-Zazzera A. Expression of HSP 70, immediate-early response and heme oxygenase genes in ischemic-reperfused rat liver. Lab Invest 68: 465-471, 1993.

55. Raju VS, Maines MD. Coordinated expression and mechenism of induction of HSP32 (heme oxygenase 1) mRNA by hyperthermia in rat organs .Biochemica Biophysica Acta 1217: 273-280,1994.

56. Shibahara S, Muller RM, Taguchi H. Transcriptional control of the rat heme oxygenase by heat shock. J. Biol Chem. 262: 12889-12892, 1987.

57. Lavrovsky Y, Schwartzman ML, Levere RD, Kappas A, Abraham NG. Identification of binding sites for transcription factors NF-kappa B and AP-2 in the promoter region of the human heme oxygenase 1 gene. Proc. Natl. Acad. Sci., USA. 91: 5989-5991, 1994.

58. Ewing JF, Raju VS, Maines MD . Induction of heart heme oxygenase-1 (HSP 32) by hyperthermia: Possible role in stress-mediated elevation of cyclic 3':5'-guanosine monophosphate. J. Pharmacol Exp Therapeu. 271: 408-414, 1994.

59. Balla J, Nath KA, Balla G, Juckett MB, Jacob HS, Vercellotti GM. Endothelial cell heme oxygenase and ferritin induction in rat lung by hemoglobin in vivo. Am J. Physiol 268: L321-L327, 1995.

60. Maulik N, Sharma HS, Das DK. Induction of heme oxygenase gene expression during reperfusion of ischemic myocardium. J. Mol Cell Cardiol 28:1261-1270,1996.

61. Nutter LM, Sierra EE, Ngo NG. Heme oxygenase does not protect human cells against oxidant stress. J Lab Clin Med 123, 506-14, 1994.

62. Nath KA, Balla G, Vercellotti GM, Balla J,Jacob HS, Levitt MD, Rosenberg ME. Induction of heme oxygenase is a rapid, protective response in rhabdomyolysis in the rat. J. Clin Invest. 90: 267-270, 1992.

63. Vile GF, Basu-Modak S, Waltner C, Tyrrell RM. Heme oxygenase 1 mediates an adaptive response to oxidative stress in human skin fibroblasts. Proc. Natl. Acad. Sci., USA 91: 2607-2610, 1994.

64. Llesuy SF, Tomar ML. Heme oxygenase and oxidative stress. Evidence of involvement of bilirubin as physiological protector against oxidative damage. Biochim Biophys Acta : 1223 : 9-14, 1994.

65. Balla G, Jacob HS, Balla J, Rosenberg M, Nath K, Apple F, Eaton JW, Vercellotti GM. Ferritin: a cytoprotective antioxidant strategem of endothelium. J. Biol Chem 267 : 18148-18152, 1992.

66. Maulik N, Engelman DT, Watanabe M, Engelman RM, Das DK. Nitric oxide - a retrograde messenger for carbon monoxide signaling in ischemic heart. Mol Cell Biochem. 157: 75-86, 1996.

67. Maulik N, Engelman D, Watanabe M, Engelman RM, Rousou JA, Flack J, Deaton D, Das DK. Nitric oxide/cabon monoxide : A free radical dependent molecular switch for myocardial preservation during ischemic arrest. Circulation (in press).

68. Maulik N, Engelman DT, Watanabe M, Engelman RM ,Maulik G, Cordis GA, Das DK. Nitric oxide signaling in ischemic heart. Cardiovasc Res 30: 593-601, 1995.

69. Finley D, Varshavsky A. The ubiquitin system : functions and mechanisms.Trends Biochem Sci 10 : 343-346, 1985.

70. Baker ZT, Board PG. The human ubiquitin gene family structure of a gene andpseudogenes from the UbB subfamily. Nucl. Acids Res 15: 443-463, 1987.

71. Ozkaynak E, Finley D, Solomon MJ, Varshavsky A. the yeast ubiquitin genes: A family of natural gene fusions. EMBO J. 6: 1429-1439,1987.

72. Bond U, Schlesinger MJ. Ubiquitin is a heat shock protein in chicken embryo fibroblasts. Mol Cell Biol 15: 949-956, 1985.

73. Swindle J, Ajioka J, Eisen H, Sanwal B, Jacquemot C, Browder Z, Buck G. the genomic organization and transcription of the ubiquitin genes of Trypanosoma cruzi. EMBO J. 7: 1121-1127, 1988.

74. Parag HA, Raboy B, Kulka RG. Effect of heat shock on protein degradation in mammalian cells: Involvement of ubiquitin system. EMBO J. 6:55-63, 1987.

75. Finlay D, Ciechanover A, Varshavsky A. Thermolability of ubiquitin-activating enzyme from the mammalian cell cycle mutant ts85. Cell 37: 43-55, 1984.

76. Altschul SF, Gish W, Miller W, Myers EW, Lipman DJ. Basic local alignment search tool. J. Mol Biol 215: 403-410, 1990.

77. Ciechanover A. The ubiquitin proteasome proteolytic pathway .Cell 79: 13-21, 1994.

78. Hochstrasser M. Ubiquitin, proteosomes, and the regulation of intracellular protein degradation. Curr Opin. Cell Biol 1 7: 215-223, 1995.

79. The Molecular Biology of the Yeast Saccharomyces (Broach JR, Pringle JR, Jones EW eds.) vol 2, pp 539-581. Cold Spring Harbor Laboratory Press, Cold Spring Harbor, NY.

80. Johnson ES, Ma PCM, Ota IM, Varshavsky A. A proteolytic pathway that recognizes ubiquitin as a degrading signal. J. Biol Chem. 270: 17442-17456, 1995.

81. Hayashi T, Takeda K, Matsuda M. Post-transient ischemia increase in ubiquitin conjugates in the early reperfusion. NeuroReport 3: 519-520, 1992.

82. Sharma HS, Maulik N, Gho BCG, Das DK, Verdouw PD. Coordinated expression of heme oxygenase-1 and ubiquitin in the porcine heart subjected to ischemia and reperfusion. J. Mol Cell Biochem 157: 111-116, 1996.

10

THE INFLUENCE OF HEAT SHOCK PROTEINS IN ATHEROGENESIS

Georg Schett[1,2], Bernhard Metzler[1], Albert Amberger[1],
Dorothea Michaelis[1], Maria Romen[2], Qingbo Xu[1] and Georg Wick[1,2]

[1]Institute for Biomedical Aging Research, Austrian Academy of Sciences, Innsbruck, and [2]Institute for General and Experimental Pathology, University of Innsbruck, Medical School, Innsbruck, Austria.

Correspondence to: Dr. Georg Wick, Institute for Biomedical Aging Research, Austrian Academy of Sciences, Rennweg 10, A-6020 Innsbruck, Austria. Tel. +43-512-583 9190 Fax. +43-512-583 9198

INTRODUCTION

Atherosclerosis is the most prevalent human vascular disorder, affects the great majority of Western populations, and is a leading cause of death. Almost every adult has atherosclerotic lesions in his/her vascular tree, but the severity and clinical manifestations show a high degree of variance between individuals. Since atherosclerosis is multifactorial, chronic and slowly progressive, onset and clinical manifestations are separated by large time periods, making it difficult to pinpoint the influence of a putative atherogenic agent on disease progression. Consequently, classical risk factors for atherosclerosis do not necessarily conform to etiologic factors, but can also modulate pre-existing disease.

Two often overlooked features of atherosclerosis complicate the identification of a single risk factor, such as elevated serum cholesterol levels, as the causal agent. First, one of the hallmarks of atherosclerosis is early onset, which contradicts the general belief that long term exposure to deleterious factors, such as high serum cholesterol levels, initiates vessel wall alterations. Fatty streaks, cushion-like, whitish intimal areas commonly considered predecessors of atherosclerotic plaques, appear as early as ten years of age and often increase rapidly before age twenty (Stary, 1989). Second, atherosclerosis is an arterial, not a venous disease and has a focal character even within the arterial tree, preferentially affecting areas subjected to high hemodynamic stress.

Therefore, a putative agent causing atherosclerosis must be both ubiquitous and present at young ages, explaining the overall prevalence of disease even in young people. On the other hand, it must affect specific predilection sites, explaining the characteristic disease localization.

The arterial intima, which is successively altered and rebuilt during the pathogenic process, is the primary target of atherosclerosis. Proliferation and accumulation of smooth muscle cells and lipid-laden macrophages ("foam cells"), as well as lipid influx and extracellular matrix accumulation are classical histological signs of fully developed atherosclerotic lesions. Cell death due to necrosis and/or apoptosis and degenerative features, like exulcerations and calcifications, are commonly seen in advanced lesions. Two basic concepts have emerged over the past few decades from extensive investigations into the development of atherosclerotic lesions. One, called the *"response to injury"*-hypothesis, focus on compromised arterial endothelial integrity as the initial step of disease, and incriminates chemical (hypercholestolemia, smoking, toxins), mechanical (blood pressure) and microbial (viruses) stressors as initiating agents (Ross, 1993). It further postulates that endothelial damage leads to production and secretion of growth and chemotactic factors by injured cells, followed by adhesion, transmigration and accumulation of mononuclear cells in the intimal layer (Libby and Hansson, 1991; Ross, 1993). As a consequence of lipid uptake by intimal macrophages, fatty streaks can develop and growth factor-induced migration and proliferation of smooth muscle cells from the media finally result in formation of atherosclerotic plaques.

The *"modified lipoprotein"*-theory identifies modifications of plasma low density lipoproteins (LDL) as a primary pathogenic factor in atherogenesis (Steinberg and Witztum, 1990). Indeed oxidation of LDL can change its biological characteristics so it becomes chemotactic for monocytes. This theory stresses that fatty streaks originate from modified LDL deposition in the arterial intima, which then attracts monocytes and, after scavenger receptor mediated uptake, accumulates in the cytoplasm, resulting in foam cell formation. Thereafter, progression to atherosclerotic plaques according to the above described mechanisms may occur.

IMMUNOLOGIC PHENOMENA IN ATHEROSCLEROSIS

Immunopathologic mechanisms have long been neglected or considered only anecdotally in atherosclerosis research. However, since classical theories of atherosclerosis have failed to satisfactorily explain pathogenesis, especially in its initial stages, and growing evidence indicates the presence of a variety of immune mechanisms within atherosclerotic lesions, immune and inflammatory processes warrant further attention (Emerson and Robertson, 1988, Hansson et al., 1989, Libby and Hansson, 1991). As a consequence, several questions have arisen regarding the nature and function of T cells and antibodies, respectively, present in atherosclerotic lesions which is/are the putative antigen(s) responsible for inducing immunocompetent cells and/or antibodies, and why do they accumulate in the vessel wall? What is the function of the immune system in atherogenesis, and are the immune reactions of primary or secondary nature? In this context, it is also critical to know whether the immune response aggravates the atherosclerotic process or plays a protective role, and if humoral and/or cellular mechanisms are essentially involved. Another key question is whether immunopathologic mechanisms can explain the fact that atherosclerosis, as a single defined pathologic state, is "caused" by various risk factors such as hypercholesterolemia, smoking, blood pressure or diabetes, which at first glance have no common denominator.

Immunodominant antigens in atherosclerotic lesions are of major scientific interest, but have not yet been clearly identified. Several candidate antigens have been suggested, a few of which have been shown to play some role in T cell and antibody accumulation within lesions. Thus, oxidized LDL (oxLDL) is present in atherosclerotic lesions, and antibodies as well as T cells reacting with this antigen have been demonstrated in the diseased intima. However, since only a small portion of total T cells and antibodies in the intima exhibit this specificity, additional important antigen(s) must be present. Furthermore, those antigens should be of major interest in promoting the early inflammatory stages of atherosclerosis and may represent the basis of the disease. Basically, three different mechanisms are considered to generate antigenic determinants that may be important in atherosclerotic lesions: 1) cell necrosis can lead to the exposure of cryptic antigens, otherwise not accessible to the immune system (Schattner and Rager-Zisman, 1990); 2) physical, chemical or infection-mediated denaturation of vessel wall proteins may be followed by the formation of "altered self" antigens, and, 3) antigenic mimicry of exogenous, e.g. microbial antigens with possible partial homologies to self antigens may entail cross-reactive immune reactions (Cohen, 1990). Theoretically as detailed later in this article, all three mechanisms may trigger the induction of autoimmunity to hsp: hsp60 as a predominantly intracellular antigen can be released after cell death, its expression can be altered by a variety of different stimuli, and it is a major immunogenic and highly conserved antigen of many microbes. The association of atherosclerotic lesions in chickens infected with Marek's disease virus (MDV), and herpes virus and cytomegalovirus, as well as certain strains of *Chlamydia pneumoniae* in humans, exemplifies the possible involvement of microbial antigens (Valtonen, 1991; Yamashiroya et al., 1988). Immunohistochemical assessment of early and late atherosclerotic lesions proved the occurrence of both humoral and cellular immune processes in the diseased vascular intima (Xu et al., 1990). Granular immunoglobulin deposition and accumulation of immune complexes were found in the atherosclerotic intima and represent early changes in the course of disease. In parallel, activation of the complement cascade has been demonstrated by the presence of the terminal lytic complex C_{5-9} as a typical feature of atherosclerotic lesions (Hollander et al., 1979). Complement components are co-localized with macrophages expressing high levels of complement receptors for C3b (CR1) and C3bi (CR3) (Seifert and Hansson, 1989). In contrast to the scarcity of B lymphocytes in all stages of atherosclerotic lesions, which makes *in situ* production of (auto)antibodies unlikely, considerable amounts of T lymphocytes can be observed in the atherosclerotic intima (Xu et al., 1993). Sequential immunohistochemical investigations of the cellular composition of normal intima, transition zone (between normal intima and fatty streak), fatty streak and atherosclerotic plaque, proved that infiltration of arterial intima by T lymphocytes, together with monocytes, is the earliest detectable change in the formation of atherosclerotic lesions. As a matter of fact, the number of T lymphocytes in the

185

transition zone exceeds that of macrophages. The more advanced the lesions become, the more heterogenous the cellular infiltration, with an increasing number of macrophages, foam cells and smooth muscle cells (Xu et al., 1992). The majority (up to 70%) of early intimal T cells are of the CD4+ helper phenotype, the remainder are CD8+. However, not all T cells in early atherosclerotic changes bear the a/b-T cell receptor (TCR); approximately 10 % of infiltrating lymphocytes are of the g/d-TCR phenotype, indicating an up to ten-fold enrichment of these cells compared to peripheral blood (only 1% g/d-TCR positive) (Kleindienst et al., 1993). Whatever attracts these cells, heat shock proteins (hsp) may be good candidate antigens since only the hsp-reactive TCR-Vd1-subset, not the Vg9/d2 TCR-subset characteristic of circulating g/d-T cells (Jindal et al., 1989; Kaufmann, 1990), is increased . Since both atherosclerotic lesions and normal intima at sites of major hemodynamic stress contain considerable quantities of these cells, an initial atherogenic function cannot be ruled out. On the other hand, these cells could screen the blood for potentially harmful antigenic material, a possibility raised upon the discovery of small T cell accumulations in the intima of healthy arteries in children, which led us to postulate the existence of a so-called "vascular-associated lymphoid tissue (VALT)" similar to the mucosa-associated lymphoid tissue (MALT) (Wick et al., 1992).

T cells infiltrating early atherosclerotic lesions are in an activated state, expressing HLA-DR and interleukin 2 -receptors, but sensitization of these cells seems to occur outside the intima, e.g. in the regional lymph nodes, since aberrant expression of MHC-class II molecules on endothelium has never been observed without an underlying, mononuclear infiltration providing a source for g-interferon (Xu et al., 1990). Concerning TCR-gene usage, Southern blot analyses demonstrated a completely heterogenous distribution in lymphocytes of advanced lesions, but whether polyclonality is also true for lymphocytes populating early lesions or fatty streaks remains to be determined(Stemme et al., 1991).

In addition to the presence of antibodies and T lymphocytes, it should be noted that a number of growth factors and cytokines responsible for various inflammatory and immunologic reactions are also produced by intimal cells within atherosclerotic lesions (Libby and Hansson, 1991; Ross, 1993). Some of these are essential for cell growth, differentiation and migration, the best example of which is the platelet-derived growth factor (PDGF), which represents a main mediator of smooth muscle cell proliferation and their migration from the vascular media into the intima.

ATHEROSCLEROSIS- AN AUTOIMMUNE DISEASE INDUCED BY HEAT SHOCK PROTEIN 65/60?

Our research on the possible role of stress proteins in atherogenesis is based on the postulates for identification of autoimmune diseases by Milgrom and Witebsky (1962) and our own previous work on spontaneous experimentally-induced autoimmune disease in animal models. Several years ago while searching for putative immunodominant and atherogenic antigens inside atherosclerotic lesions, we defined that mycobacterial hsp65 was capable of inducing arteriosclerotic lesions in rabbits.

Extensive immunization experiments in rabbits using total proteins from human or rabbit atherosclerotic lesions emulsified in complete Freunds adjuvant (CFA) revealed disease only in rabbits immunized with CFA regardless of the additional antigens used (Xu et al., 1992). Since one of the major components of CFA, containing heat-killed *Mycobacterium tuberculosis*, is hsp65, we hypothesized that hsp65 was a possible atherogenic agent, and proved this by induction of arteriosclerotic lesions in rabbits immunized with recombinant hsp65, and the failure to induce disease using adjuvants devoid of hsp65 (e.g. Ribi or lipopeptide). These immunization-induced lesions consisted of lymphoid cells and, similar to classical human lesions, smooth muscle cells and macrophage infiltration, but deposition of foam cells and extracellular lipid was lacking. Additional cholesterol feeding led to the development of more severe lesions, that corresponded exactly to advanced human atherosclerotic plaques, including the presence of foam cells. Until now, the induction of atherosclerotic lesions has not been observed with any other antigen except hsp65. Furthermore, it was possible to show that atherosclerotic lesions induced by immunization of normocholesterolemic rabbits with hsp65 can regress, in contrast to those in hypercholesterolemic animals (Xu et al., 1996).

This animal model of hsp65-induced atherosclerosis exhibited two major characteristics deemed essential for understanding atherogenesis. First, a potentially pathogenic immune reaction with T cells and antibodies specific for hsp65 was induced. Second, lesions developed only in areas of major hemodynamic stress, such as the aortic arch and branching sites of large vessels, indicating focally-increased susceptibility to hsp-induced atherogenic damage (Kleindienst et al., 1993; Xu et al., 1993). These two central aspects of the "immunology of atherosclerosis" constitute two major lines of research in our laboratory: a possible pathogenic immune and autoimmune reaction to hsp in atherosclerosis, and the stress-response of the target organ structures, such as endothelial cells, which may predispose for lesion development.

As mentioned previously, both cellular and humoral immune reactions seem to play a part in atherogenesis (Wick et al., 1995). On the cellular side of the immune system, functional studies of T cells in human atherosclerosis are relatively cumbersome, due to problems with the availability of very early atherosclerotic lesions and autologous feeder cells for cultivation and therefore knowledge about their specificity and possible hsp65-reactivity is rare. However, since hsp65 is a major antigen for g/d-Tcells, the presence of unexpectedly high numbers of T cells bearing the g/d-TCR in early atherosclerotic lesions points to the recognition of intimal hsp65/60 as a cellular antigen (Xu et al., 1993). Furthermore, we demonstrated in our rabbit model an accumulation of hsp65-reactive lymphocytes among plaque-infiltrating lymphocytes. Whether this holds true in early atherosclerotic lesions of humans remains to be shown. However, since the mammalian hsp65 homologue hsp60 is abundantly present in atherosclerotic lesions and is known to effectively trigger T cell responses, the presence of hsp65/60-specific T cells in the intima of atherosclerotic lesions should be further investigated.

Since hsp65 is not only an immunodominant antigen for T cells, but can also induce a strong humoral immune response, our interest also extends to anti-hsp65/60 antibodies. It should be noted that low amounts of anti-hsp65 antibodies and T cells are present in almost every healthy human. A large epidemiologic study of 879 randomly-selected, clinically-healthy inhabitants of Bruneck, a small town in Northern Italy just across the

Tyrolean border ("Bruneck-Study"), revealed an association between anti-hsp65 antibodies and sonographically-demonstrable but clinically inapparent carotid atherosclerosis (Xu et al., 1993). Significantly elevated serum antibody titers against hsp65 coincided with the presence of atherosclerotic plaques in the carotid arteries. Since this correlation was highly significant and demonstrated to be independent from other classical risk factors, such as hypercholesterolemia, smoking, hypertension and diabetes, these antibodies may constitute an independent risk factor and be of diagnostic value. Recent unpublished studies proved a similar elevation of anti-hsp65 antibodies in coronary heart disease.

Due to high interspecies sequence homology within the hsp60 family, anti-hsp65/60 antibodies not only recognize mycobacterial hsp65 but also cross-react with the analogous component of *E. coli* -groEL and, most important, with human hsp60 (Kaufmann, 1990). We hypothesized that anti-hsp65/60 antibodies, in addition to their proven diagnostic value, may also act as pathogenic autoantibodies, recognizing or even destroying stressed cells of the vessel wall. This was corroborated by immunohistochemical studies demonstrating positive staining of endothelial cells as well as lesion macrophages and smooth muscle cells by anti-hsp65/60 high titer antisera (Xu et al., 1993). For a detailed analysis of binding specificity and functional activity of hsp-antibodies, we purified specific antibodies from human high titer sera from the Bruneck-Study by affinity chromatography over hsp65 columns and used this preparation to analyze epitope specificity and cytotoxicity to endothelial cells and macrophages.

A systematic binding analysis of anti-hsp65/60 Ab to both soluble and plastic pin-bound (Geysen et al., 1987; Hajeer et al., 1992) hsp65 overlapping peptides revealed strong antibody binding to three distinct short linear sequences. Two epitopes were located at the N-terminal part of hsp65 (amino acid residues 97-109 and 179-187), and a third was defined within its C-terminal portion (amino acid residues 504-512) (Metzler et al., 1996). Since mycobacterial hsp65 and *E.coli* groEL display a high degree of sequence homology, it was possible to study the localization and conformation of these three epitopes relative to the known three-dimensional structure of *E. coli*-groEL, as mentioned above. This approach was especially prompted by the fact that anti-hsp65/60 serum antibodies exhibit a high cross-reactivity to *E. coli*-groEL. Sequence I (aa 97-109) and sequence III (504-512), located distantly from each other on the 540 amino acid hsp65 sequence, are closely related areas on the corresponding tertiary groEL structure. Both sequences are within the equatorial domain of groEL and form two side-by-side a-helices oriented towards the outside of the heptamer ring structure (Braig et al., 1994). In contrast, sequence II (179-187) is located within the small intermediate domain of groEL.

In vivo, chaperonins of the hsp60 family form heptamers, which implies the necessity of a panel of contact-forming amino acids. All but four of these 35 contact-forming sites are located distantly from the three described sequences of serum antibody binding. While sequence III is not included in any intersubunit bound, sequence I comprises two such domains, but both are located at the C-terminal end of the respective sequence (Lys105 and Ala109), which led us to postulate the accessibility of both sequences within the heptameric ring structure of hsp60. In contrast, two inter-subunit bounds (Thr181, Leu183) are located exactly in the middle of sequence II (aa 179-187) where they probably interfere with antibody binding. The existence of antibodies against sequence II, however, suggests their accessibility for the humoral immune system. We hypothesize that degradation of the heptameric ring structure in connection with prokaryotic or eukaryotic cell death or physiological turnover of hsp molecules leads to increased accessibility of sequence II and immunogenic recognition of this cryptic epitope.

During the last few years, a number of major and minor T cell epitopes has been identified on hsp65, rendering it highly immunogenic for the cellular immune system. Thus, our sequence II is identical with the major T cell epitope thought to play a role in human rheumatoid arthritis and adjuvant arthritis in rats (van Eden et al., 1988). In addition, sequence I has been described as a hsp65- T cell epitope associated with the appearance of recurrent oral ulcers (Hasan et al., 1995). Sharing of identical epitopes in T- and B cell recognition is known in various autoimmune diseases. In addition to its role as a humoral and cellular hsp65-epitope, sequence II shows homology with a peptide of toxic shock syndrome toxin-1 (TSST-1) (Ramesh et al., 1994).

We hypothesize that hsp60-epitopes constituted by these three defined sequences may act as autoantigens in the pathogenesis of atherosclerosis. Further studies stressing the definition of additional conformational hsp65-epitopes are ongoing, and should clarify the role of each sequence in the anti-vascular autoimmune reaction as well as other autoimmune diseases, such as systemic scleroderma, lupus erythematosus and rheumotoid arthritis.

Based on the observation that anti-hsp65/60 antisera recognize a 60kD band in extracts from stressed, but not unstressed, endothelial cells on Western blots, we also studied their possible functional role on endothelial cells. Using laser confocal microscope scanning, surface binding of human affinity-purified hsp65 Ab to heat-stressed, but not unstressed, human endothelial cells was detected, indicating the presence of this mitochondrial hsp60, or at least certain parts of it, on the surface of stressed cells. Furthermore, when complement or peripheral blood mononuclear cells were present as effectors, surface binding was accompanied by cytotoxicity towards stressed, but not unstressed cells. Complement-mediated cytotoxicity and antibody-dependent cellular cytotoxicity (ADCC) were only observed in the presence of anti-hsp65/60 Ab, not with anti-hsp65/60 Ab-free preparations (Schett et al., 1995) *(Figure 1)*. Considering the high induction of hsp60-expression of endothelial cells at sites of major hemodynamic stress, e.g. the carotid bifurcation, anti-hsp65/60 Ab may selectively damage the endothelium at sites especially prone for atherosclerosis. Alternatively, endothelial hsp60 expression may be induced by an underlying preexisting mononuclear cell infiltration that produces proinflammatory cytokines, such as IL-1 and TNF-alpha.

Macrophages are known to be among the earliest cells infiltrating arterial intima and are essential in atherogenesis. Thus we addressed the question whether anti-hsp65/60 Abs also have the potential to induce macrophage damage. Several different factors, including mechanical and chemical stressors, may be involved in the induction of hsp60.

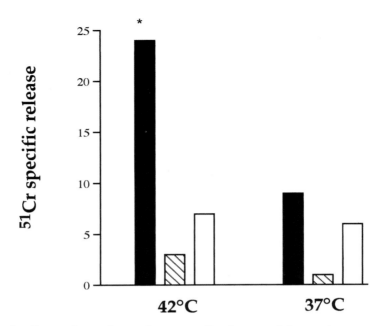

Figure 1- Comparison of complement-mediated cytotoxicity on heat-stressed and unstressed endothelial cells. Confluent endothelial cells in 96-well plates were incubated at 42°C for 30 min. followed by 90 min. at 37°C, or kept without treatment throughout. After three washes with medium 199, 5 uCi ^{51}Cr in 100 ul of medium 199 containing 10% FCS was added to each well, and the cells incubated at 37°C for 1.5 h. After two further washes, antibodies (solid bar, affinity purified anti-hsp65 antibodies; hatched bar, unbound Ig fraction; open bar, mouse mAb anti-CD3) in 100 ul of the medium were added and incubated at 37°C for 7 h in the presence of guinea pig serum as a source of complement. After incubation, supernatant radioactivity was determined in a gamma counter. The experiments were performed in triplicates. * P < 0.01 vs. untreated cells.

Oxidative stress by altered lipoproteins seems to play an important role, since oxLDL is abundant in human serum and atherosclerotic lesions, and is a potent activator of monocytic stress protein synthesis both by free radical production and its phagocytosis, which also induces hsp. Hypoxia, which is considered a powerful inducer of hsp, might be increasingly important in the core region, particularly when the lesion thickens and nutrition becomes critical. Third, cytokine production is a common and early feature of all cells participating in atherogenesis, and TNFa and IL-1 also trigger hsp induction in addition to a variety of other proinflammatory changes. Fourth, differentiation of blood monocytes to tissue macrophages after their transmigration to the intima is likely accompanied by hsp induction. In agreement with the results obtained with endothelial cells, anti-hsp65/60 Abs also react with the surface of stressed macrophages and could lyse them via complement-mediated cytotoxicity and ADCC. Regardless of the main effector mechanism, cytotoxicity of anti-hsp65/60 antibodies could lead to severe cell damage or even death, especially at macrophage-rich and highly stressed areas of the atherosclerotic lesion. This, in part, might entail the progression and perpetuation of the atherogenic process and explain phenomena such as formation of the necrotic core and plaque rupture, which are known to coincide with abundant monocytic infiltration.

The development of autoimmune disease depends on a combination of target organ susceptibility and the presence of an autoimmune repertoire, i.e. autoreactive T cells or autoantibodies (Wick et al., 1986; Wick et al., 1987; Wick et al., 1992). While the immunologic repertoire in autoimmune diseases has been intensively investigated, primary changes of the target organ/ structure facilitating immunpathologic damage have not. A"well-balanced" combination of autoimmune repertoire and target organ susceptibility, can initiate and promote autoimmune disease, which neither can do alone. In the case of stress protein-induced autoimmunity, the nature of the target organ is crucial, since almost every individual bears at least low levels of autoreactive hsp-specific T cells and/or autoantibodies, of which only a minor portion develops disease. In addition, despite the presence of a similar immunologic repertoire, disease type (e.g. atherosclerosis or arthritis) and localization (e.g. arteries or joints) may vary widely among individuals. We hypothesize that shear stress and oxLDL are factors that essentially modify arteries, rendering them susceptible to immunologic attack and/or lowering the threshold to the effect of other vasoactive stressors. The expression of hsp in the arterial wall is regulated by a variety of factors, the most important of which are mechanical injury by high blood pressure, oxLDL and cytokines. Immunohistochemical studies revealed that normal endothelium, and the intima of healthy arterial and venous vessels exhibited only low amounts of hsp60. However, coincidental with an atherosclerotic alteration and, to a lesser extent at sites of major hemodynamic stress hsp60 expression is highly induced in both endothelium and intimal cells *(Figure 2)*. Endothelial cells overlying transition zones, fatty streaks and atherosclerotic plaques, are all hsp60-positive, and shear stress seems to be the most important stress factor contributing to this process. Macrophages and lymphocytes infiltrating arterial intima are among the first cells positively stained for hsp60, a feature that is shared by smooth muscle cells in later stages of atherosclerotic lesions. Potential factors, that might induce hsp60 production by intimal cells have been discussed above.

As one approach to investigate the role of target organ susceptibility, we cultivated human arterial and venous endothelial cells and compared their responses to typical cardiovascular stress factors. Adhesion molecule expression of these two cell types showed different expression patterns in response to stress. For example, *E. coli* lipopolysaccharide or cytokines, such as tumor necrosis factor a (TNFa) or IL-1, showed a long-lasting upregulation of vascular cell adhesion molecule-1 (VCAM-1) in arterial, but not venous, endothelial cells. In addition, oxLDL lead to long-term induction of intercellular adhesion molecule-1 (ICAM-1), VCAM-1 and endothelial leucocyte adhesion molecule-1 (ELAM-1) in arterial endothelial cells, but had no significant effect on venous endothelial cells (Amberger et al., 1996). This effect of oxLDL is dependent

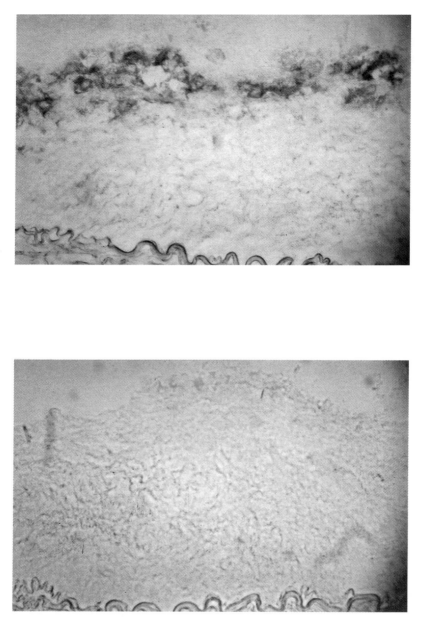

Figure 2- Detection of hsp60 in atherosclerotic lesions. Cryostat sections from the aortic arch of rabbits immunized with hsp65 and fed a 0.2% cholesterol diet for 14 weeks labeled with monoclonal antibody ML-30 against hsp65/60 and visualized with the APAAP system (top panel). Note the presence of positive staining of the endothelium and the intima of the atherosclerotic lesions. Lower panel is a negative control treated with normal mouse IgG. Lumen of the aorta at top in each photomicrograph. X400.

on the presence of preexisting mRNA for adhesion molecules induced by serum depletion or cytokines. It remains to be clarified if differential regulation is also true for hsp60 expression in arterial and venous endothelial cells, and how shear stress alters the threshold for expression of adhesion molecules and heat shock proteins induced by other stress factors. Such experiments may provide clues as to why people suffer from "arteriosclerosis" but not from "venosclerosis", and the reasons for hsp60 expression within atherosclerotic lesions. Furthermore, they may explain why restenosis occurs in veins used in coronary bypass operations. Since almost all individuals display basal levels of autoreactive T cells and antibodies against hsp60, genetically-determined differences in target organ structures could be a prime factor in rendering certain areas of the vascular tree susceptible to autoimmune attacks. Thus, differential responses of endothelial cells to changes in blood pressure and to oxLDL may be crucial in facilitating or impeding autoimmune damage.

The data presented form the basis of a new *immunologic hypothesis of atherogenesis* (Wick et al., 1995), postulating that the first stages of atherosclerotic lesions result from an immune reaction against hsp60 followed by formation of foam cells in the presence of additional risk factors, such as high serum cholesterol levels. The inflammatory reaction to hsp60 and hsp60 expression itself is a response to injury initiated by several stress-factors known to be risk factors for atherosclerosis, such as hypertension, smoking, viral infection or chemically- modified LDL. Mechanical shear stress may lower the threshold for other risk factors, leading to the hsp60 expression and induction of lesions in arteries, but not in veins. Whether cellular or humoral components of the immune system are responsible for initiating that reaction, and whether sensitization to hsp60/65 is a consequence of bacterial infection or of *bona fide* autoimmunity, remains to be clarified.

ACKNOWLEDGEMENTS

This work was supported by grants to G.W. form the Austrian Science Fund (projects 8925 and 10677), the Sandoz Foundation for Geronotological Research, the Austrian National Bank and the State of Tyrol to G.W. Dr. J. Willeit (Clinic of Neurology, Innsbruck), Dr. B. Hochleitner and Dr. C. Trieb (Clinic of Surgery, Innsbruck) we thank for excellent clinical collaboration. Dr. R. Van der Zee (Inst. for Infectious Diseases, Utrecht, Netherlands), Dr. Satish Jindal (PerSeptive Biosystems, Framinham, MA), Dr. M. Singh (GBF, Braunschweig, Germany), Dr. L. Mizzen (Stressgen Biotechn., Victoria, Canada), Dr. R.S. Gupta (McMaster Univerity, Hamilton, Canada), Dr. T. Ottenhoff (Dep. of Immunohematology, Leiden, Netherlands), Dr. R. Bernstein (Dep. of Rheumatology, Manchester, UK) and Dr. G. Jürgens (Inst. of Biochemistry, Graz, Austria) for production hsp65 and 60 as well as peptides, cDNA probes and LDL preparations. We also thank T. Öttl, A. Mair and G. Dobler for excellent technical assistance.

REFERENCES

Braig K, Otwinowski Z, Hegde R, Boisvert D.C, Joachimiak A, Horwich A.L, Sigler P. (1994) The crystal structure of the bacterial chaperonin GroEL at 2.8Å. Nature 371:578-586.

Cohen R. I. (1990) A heat shock protein, molecular mimicry and autoimmunity. Israel J. Med. Sci. 26:673-676.

Emeson E, RobertsonA. L.Jr. (1988) T lymphocytes in aortic and coronary intimas: Their potential role in atherogenesis. Am J Pathol. 130:369-376.

Geysen H.M, Rodda S.J, MasonT.J, Tribbick G, and Schoofs P.G. (1987) Strategies for epitope analysis using peptide synthesis. J Immunol Methods 102:259-274.

Hajeer A.H, Worthington J, Morgan K, and Bernstein R.M. (1992) Monoklonal Antibody epitopes of mycobacterial 65-kD heat shock protein defined by epitope scanning. Clin. Exp. Immunol. 89:115-119.

Hansson G. K, JonassonL, SeifertP. S, and Stemme S. (1989) Immune mechanisms in atherosclerosis. Arteriosclerosis. 9:567-578.

Hasan A, Childerston e A, Pervin K, Shinnick T, Mizushima Y, van der Zee R, Vaughan R, and Lehner T. (1995) Recognition of a unique peptide epitope of the mycobacterial and human heat shock protein 65-60 antigen by T cells of patients with recurrent oral ulcers. Clin. Exp. Immunol. 99: 392-397.

Hollander W, Colombo M. A, Kirkpatrick B, and Paddock J. (1979) Soluble proteins in the human atherosclerotic plaque. Atherosclerosis 34:391-405.

Jindal S, Dudani A.K, Singh B, Harley C.C, and Gupta R.S. (1989) Primary structure of a human mitochondrial protein homologous to the bacterial and plant chaperonins and to the 65-kilodalton mycobacterial antigen. Mol. Cell Biol. 9: 2279-2283.

Jones D. B, CoulsonA. F. W, and Duff G. W. (1993) Sequence homologies between hsp60 and autoantigens. Immunol. Today 14:115-118.

Kaufmann S.H.E. (1990) Heat shock proteins and immune response. Immunol Today 11:129-136.

Kleindienst R, Xu Q, Willeit J, Waldenberger F, Weimann S, and Wick G. (1993) Immunology of atherosclerosis: Demonstration of heat shock protein 60 expression and T-lymphocytes bearing a/b or g/d receptor in human atherosclerotic lesions. Am J Pathol. 142:1927-1937.

Libby P, and Hansson G. K. (1991) Involvement of the immune system in human atherogenesis: current knowledge and unanswered questions. Lab. Invest. 64:5-15.

Metzler B, Schett G, Kleindienst R, Xu Q, van der Zee R, Ottenhoff T, Hajeer A, Bernstein R, and Wick G. (1996) Epitope specificity of anti-heat shock protein 65/60 serum antibodies in atherosclerosis. (submittd).

Milgrom W, Witebsky E. (1962) Autoantibodies and autoimmune disease. JAMA 181: 706-717.

Ramesh N, Parronchi P, Ahern D, Romanagni S, and Geha R. (1994) A toxic shock syndrom toxin-1 peptide that shows homology to amino acids 180-193 of mycobacterial heat shock protein 65 is presented as conventional antigen. Immunol. Invest 23:381-391.

Ross R. (1993) The pathogenesis of atherosclerosis: a perspective for the 1990s. Nature. 362:801-809.

Schattner A, and Rager-Zisman B. (1990) Virus-induced autoimmunity. Rev. Infect. Dis. 12:204-222.

Schett G, Xu Q, Amberger A, van der Zee R, Recheis H, Willeit J, and Wick G. (1995) Autoantibodies against heat shock protein 65 mediate endothelial cytotoxicity. J. Clin. Invest. 96:2569-2577.

Seifert P. S, and Hansson G. K. (1989) Complement receptors and regulatory proteins in human atherosclerotic lesions. Arteriosclerosis 9:802-811.

Stary H. C. (1989) Evolution and progression of atherosclerotic lesions in coronary arteries of children and young adults. Arteriosclerosis Suppl. I, 9:19-32.

Steinberg D, and WitztumJ. L. (1990) Lipoproteins and atherogenesis: current concepts. J. Am. Med. Assoc. 264:3047-3052.

Stemme S, Rymo L, and Hansson G. K. (1991) Polyclonal origin of T lymphocytes in human atherosclerotic plaques. Lab. Invest. 65:654-660.

Valtonen V.V. (1991) Infection as a risk factor for infarction and atherosclerosis. Ann. Med. 23:539-543.

van Eden W, Thole J. E. R, van der Zee R , Noordzij A,. van Embden J. D. A, Hensen E. J, and CohenI. R. (1988) Cloning of the mycobacterial epitope recognized by T lymphocytes in adjuvant arthritis. Nature 331:171- 173.

Wick G, and Xu Q. (1991) Heat shock protein 65 as an antigen in atherogenesis.(abstr.) Arterioscler. Throm. 11:1526a.

Wick G, Hala K, Wolf H, Ziemiecki A, Sundick R.S, Stöffler-Meilicke M, DeBaets M (1986) The role of Genetically-Determined Primary Alterations of the Target organ in the Developement of Spontaneous Autoimmune Thyreoiditis in Obese Strain (OS) Chickens. Immunol Reviews 94:113-136.

Wick G, Kleindienst R, Dietrich H , and Xu Q. (1992) Is atherosclerosis an autoimmune disease. Trends Food Sci. Technol. 3:114-119.

Wick G, Krömer G, Neu N, Fässler R, Ziemiecki A, Müller R.G, Ginzel M, Beladi I, Kühr T, and Hala K. (1987) The multi-factorial pathogenesis of autoimmune disease. Immunol. Lett. 16:249-258.

Wick G, Schett G, Amberger A, Kleindienst R, and Xu Q. (1995) Is atherosclerosis an immunologically mediated disease? Immunol Today 16: 7-33.

Xu Q, Dietrich H, Steiner H. J, Gown A.M, Schoel B, Mikuz G, Kaufmann S.H.E, and Wick G. (1992) Induction of arteriosclerosis in normocholesterolemic rabbits by immunization with heat shock protein65. Arterioscler .Thromb. 12:789-799.

Xu Q, Kleindienst R, Schett G, Waitz W, Jindal S, Gupta R.S, Dietrich H, and Wick G. (1996) Regression of arteriosclerotic lesions induced by immunization with heat shock protein 65-containing material in normocholesterolemic, but not hypercholesterolemicrabbits. Atherosclerosis (in press).

Xu Q, Kleindienst R, Waitz W, Dietrich H, and Wick G. (1993) Increased expression of heat shock protein 65 coincides with a population of infiltrating T lymphocytes in atherosclerotic lesions of rabbits specifically responding to heat shock protein 65. J. Clin. Invest. 91:2693-2702.

Xu Q, Luef G, Weimann S, Gupta R.S, Wolf H, and Wick G. (1993) Staining of endothelial cells and macrophages in atherosclerotic lesions with human heat-shock protein reactive antisera Arterioslcer. Thromb. 13:1763-1769.

Xu Q, Oberhuber G, Gruschwitz M, and Wick G. (1990) Immunology of atherosclerosis: cellular composition and major histocompatibility complex class II antigen expression in aortic intima, fatty streaks, and atherosclerotic plaques in young and aged human specime. Clin Immunol. Immunopathol. 56:344-359.

Xu Q, Willeit J, Marosi M, Kleindienst R, Oberhollenzer F, Kiechl S, Stulnig T, Luef G and Wick G. (1993) Association of serum antibodies to heat- shock protein 65 with carotid atherosclerosis. Lancet. 341:255-259.

Yamashiroya H. M, Ghosh L, Yang R, and RobertsonA. L. Jr. (1988) Herpesviridae in coronary vessels and aorta of young trauma victims. Am. J. Pathol. 130:71-79.

11

THE STRESS RESPONSE IN HYPOXIC-ISCHEMIC BRAIN:
CORRELATION OF TISSUE CULTURE FINDINGS WITH IN VIVO
MODELS

Robert N. Nishimura, M.D.
Chief of Molecular Neurobiology Laboratory
Veterans Affairs Hospital and UCLA
Department of Neurology 111N-1
16111 Plummer St.
Sepulveda, CA 91343

Barney E. Dwyer, Ph.D.
Chief of Molecular Neurobiology Laboratory
Veterans Affairs Hospital and Dartmouth Medical School
Department of Medicine (Neurology)
Research Service 151
White River Junction, VT 05009

INTRODUCTION

A great deal of interest has been directed to the pathogenesis of brain injury after stroke in human disease. In the United States approximately 175,000 fatalities and many more disabled are directly attributed to stroke every year (Adams and Victor, 1993). Many metabolic and biochemical processes occur during and after the cessation of blood flow to specific areas of the brain which might directly affect the clinical outcome. In recent years studies in animal models have identified and described the heat shock or stress response in hypoxic-ischemic brain. This chapter summarizes the main findings of the stress response and HSP 70 in the brain after hypoxia-ischemia and then correlates those findings with work performed in cell culture models. Included is a discussion of the regulation of HSP 70, associated signal transduction pathways, cellular proteins and metabolites. Finally a brief discussion of future directions using new experimental models of stress proteins is presented.

Much attention has centered around the induction of the highly inducible member of the 70 kDa heat shock protein family, HSP 70, in hypoxia-ischemia. This protein is also known commonly as HSP 68, HSP 72, and HSP 70i. HSP 70 is distinguished from HSC 70, the abundant constitutive member of the HSP 70 family.

STRESS PROTEINS IN HYPOXIC-ISCHEMIC BRAIN INJURY

Since the description of HSP 70 induction in rat brain after heat shock and ischemia (Currie and White, 1981) numerous studies have described the induction of HSP 70 in various models of hypoxia-ischemia. Those include studies of global and focal ischemia with the expression of HSP 70 and other HSPs which have become characteristic of the mammalian heat stress response (Nowak, 1985; Dienel et al, 1986; Jacewicz et al, 1986; Kiessling et al, 1986). Since the original observations the studies performed are too numerous to critique individually. We will attempt to use selected studies to describe and illustrate the role of HSP 70 in the pathophysiology of neuronal damage in hypoxia-ischemia.

Neonatal Hypoxia-Ischemia

Early and persistent inhibition of protein synthesis is a characteristic of hypoxia-ischemia in brain (Dwyer et al, 1987). In the presence of protein synthesis inhibition, synthesis of HSP 70 was observed in unilateral common carotid ligation followed by several hours of hypoxia (8% oxygen), in ipsilateral (side of ligation) but not contralateral hippocampus during recovery of three hours duration (Dwyer et al, 1989). Synthesis was noted by radiolabeled HSP 70 and confirmed by western blot analysis using a polyclonal antibody developed against human HSP 70 . However, HSP 70 was not detected in those same experimental tissues when probed with the monoclonal antibody, C-92, also developed against human HSP70. Immunocytochemical staining using the C-92 antibody demonstrated HSP 70 staining of the ipsilateral cerebral cortex one hour after hypoxia and the CA3 region of the hippocampus by 12 hours after hypoxia in the same model (Ferriero et al, 1990). More severe injury resulted in more intense immunostaining of the cerebral cortex and the CA1 region of the hippocampus. Two important points can be made from those studies. First HSP 70 was found in areas of histologically injured neurons. Secondly HSP 70 was induced by one hour in the hippocampus, an area in adult animals where HSP 70 was not immunostained until approximately 12 hours. Further studies using this model in developing older animals showed increased expression of c-fos mRNA after two hours of recovery in multiple areas of the ipsilateral hemisphere after hypoxia while HSP 70 mRNA was not expressed until 24 hours and then predominantly in the hippocampus (Blumenfeld et al, 1992). Those investigators also showed induction of c-fos mRNA in 15 and 23 day old rats primarily in the entorhinal cortex and the dentate gyrus of the hippocampus. In contrast only a minority of rats at both ages showed scattered expression of HSP 70 mRNA in the ipsilateral hemisphere. Twenty four hours of recovery showed c-fos mRNA was nearly normalized in the ipsilateral hemisphere while HSP 70 mRNA was increased in the same areas in the 7, 15 and 23 day old rats. Another study of immediate early gene expression using the unilateral carotid ligation model showed c-fos and c-jun mRNA induced in the ipsilateral cortex, hippocampus and striatum. HSP 70 mRNA was also induced in most of those areas but was frequently absent from areas where c-fos and c-jun was expressed in the 7 day old animals (Munell et al, 1994). Also in that model, ATP levels were severely decreased in the whole ipsilateral hemisphere immediately after hypoxia but by two hours of recovery only the cortex showed consistently decreased ATP levels (Kobayashi and Welsh, 1995). That correlated with increased HSP 70 mRNA. In contrast white matter showed recovery of ATP levels but also showed marked induction of HSP 70 mRNA. By 24 hours no correlation of ATP levels with HSP 70 mRNA could be found, but neuronal necrosis was correlated with decreased ATP levels.

In the developing gerbil, a 20 minute transient global ischemia induced HSP 70 mRNA and protein in the hippocampus in postnatal animals aged 15, 21, and 30 days four days after the ischemia (Soriano et al, 1994a). Postnatal 7 day old animals showed no histological injury to the hippocampal neurons or induction of HSP 70 mRNA or protein. Postnatal 15 day old animals showed HSP 70 immunoreactivity in the dentate gyrus and granular and molecular layers of the hippocampus. HSP 70 immunoreactivity of the CA1 pyramidal cell layer was noted in 21 day and 30 day old and adult animals, and in the CA3 pyramidal cell layer in the 30 day old and adult animals. Histological cell necrosis was observed in CA3 in 15 postnatal day and older animals. CA1 cells were necrotic in 30 day and adult animals. The correlation of induction of HSP 70 in affected areas was age dependent but little correlation was made with the areas of HSP 70 induction and histological cell survival.

Collectively, those studies indicated that in the developing rat brain the ability to synthesize HSP 70 after hypoxia-ischemia changed in older animals, implying that the mechanism of induction in the developing animals was different than the neonatal animals. However, while the mechanism of induction may differ during development, the susceptibility of the brain to injury also changes. It was possible that neurons in younger animals were not injured to the same degree from a similar insult resulting in the differences noted. The mechanism for that change in rate of HSP 70 synthesis was unresolved but may be important since the delay in synthesis of HSP 70 may indicate an increased susceptibility to injury secondary to hypoxia-ischemia. The relationship of immediate early gene expression and the induction of HSP 70 was not clear. The proto-oncogene expression of c-fos and c-jun did not appear to be directly related to the synthesis of HSP 70. Rather their expression probably represented a general signal of cellular injury. The persistence or return to normal of the expression of c-fos indicated the extent of injury and not a signal for HSP 70 synthesis. Finally the acute marked decrease of ATP levels in the hypoxic-ischemic brain seemed to correlate well with the subsequent induction of HSP 70. Persistence of decreased ATP levels probably indicated irreversible neuronal injury and the return of ATP levels to normal permitted the resumption of protein synthesis and HSP 70 synthesis. However, the association of HSP 70 synthesis with neuronal survival did not imply that HSP 70 was central to the survival of neurons in that type of injury. In fact in the young gerbil ischemic model, HSP 70 synthesis was not correlated with neuronal survival.

Global Ischemia

Expression of HSP 70 in adult models of global ischemia was first identified in gerbils (Nowak, 1985) and rats (Dienel et al, 1986) after 24 hours of recovery from global ischemia. Increased and prolonged HSP 70 mRNA was isolated from gerbil brain 24 hours after global ischemia but peaked 6 hours after ischemia (Nowak et al, 1990; Abe et al, 1991). Transcription of HSP 70 mRNA was localized to neurons after brief global ischemia using in situ hybridization techniques (Kawagoe et al, 1992b; Nowak, 1991). The latter study showed that neurons in the hippocampus, striatum and ischemic cortex readily induced HSP 70 mRNA but more than three hours after the brief ischemia in gerbils. With more severe ischemia increased neuronal localization of HSP 70 mRNA was evident in ischemic areas and involved more neurons. Similar findings were noted in rat but with a more prolonged ischemia (Kawagoe et al, 1993b). The induction of HSC 70 mRNA also followed the induction of HSP70 in the gerbil brain after graded global ischemia (Aoki et al, 1993; Kawagoe et al, 1992c) and rat brain (Kawagoe et al, 1992b). More severe ischemia resulted in induction of HSC 70 mRNA in CA1, neocortex, and thalamus. However, the induction decreased with time after ischemia. Those findings pointed out the issue of differences in thresholds between neurons and glial cells of the brain. The mechanisms responsible for the induction of HSP 70 are not fully understood in neurons. The lack of induction in glial cells was also a striking finding. That finding implied a difference in the mechanisms of transcription in neurons versus glial cells. The delay in the induction of HSP 70 mRNA predicted that HSP 70 synthesis was also delayed in those models.

Immunocytochemical localization of HSP 70 in gerbil and rat models of global ischemia showed similar results. A study in gerbil brain observed the chronological appearance of HSP 70 by immunocytochemistry in different brain regions (Vass et al, 1988). HSP 70 was first noted in the dentate gyrus of the hippocampus by 4 hours but not prominently until 16 hours after ischemia. By 24 hours prominent staining was noted in the dentate gyrus and beginning to appear in the CA1 and CA3 regions of the hippocampus. Only prominent staining was noted in the CA3 region. By 48 hours after ischemia the CA3 region was intensely stained for HSP 70 while the dentate and CA1 regions were beginning to lose immunoreactivity. Staining of the striatum and cerebral cortex began with few detectable immunostained neurons 12 hours after ischemia and increased in the number of cells and intensity of staining 24 and 48 hours after ischemia.

The cerebral cortex remained intensely stained 96 hours after ischemia. In the rat more prominent staining of the CA1 neurons of the hippocampus was noted after mild ischemia (Chopp et al, 1991; Simon et al, 1991). In more prolonged and severe ischemia HSP 70 immunostaining expanded beyond the hippocampus to other neuronal populations (Simon et al, 1991; Kirino et al, 1991). Milder conditions of ischemia resulted in increased expression of HSP 70 in the CA1 and hilar neurons in rat and gerbil (Simon, 1991; Kirino et al, 1991). Interventions to prevent injury resulted in decreased HSP 70 expression in ischemic injury (Nowak, 1989; Nowak, 1991). As expected, with very severe ischemia immunostaining of non-neuronal cells including glia and endothelial cells was noted (Gonzalez et al, 1991). From those studies it was apparent that survival of neurons in the ischemic brain was correlated with synthesis of HSP 70. However, the synthesis of the protein was not an indicator of cellular survival. Rat CA1 neurons subjected to 10 minutes of ischemia resulted in severe damage and cell death despite the robust synthesis of HSP 70 in those cells (Chopp et al, 1991; Simon et al, 1991). Those findings were in contrast to the gerbil model of global ischemia where 10 minutes of ischemia resulted in barely detectable HSP 70 in CA1 neurons (Vass et al, 1988; Kirino et al, 1991). Since generalized protein synthesis inhibition is well known in neurons after ischemia (Dienel et al, 1980; Kirino and Sano, 1984; Thilmann et al, 1986; Widmann et al, 1991; Hu and Wieloch, 1993) the findings in the gerbil were not unexpected, but did not explain the findings in the rat model. Also, in the gerbil model other regions adjacent to CA1 induced significant HSP 70.

The explanation for the differences in induction of HSP 70 in different rodent models may be secondary to species differences but may also represent altered mechanisms of induction in the rat versus gerbil CA1 neurons. It was also possible that HSP 70 in the gerbil CA1 did not stain because the epitope was occupied by adjacent or reactive protein complexes or peptides. That may have been the case in cultured neurons (Marini et al, 1990). Of more clinical importance was the fact that all studies showed significant lag time from the time of insult to the appearance of HSP 70. If the fate of cells was determined within minutes of the primary ischemic injury then HSP 70 was synthesized too late to be protective. In that case HSP 70 represented an epiphenomenon in ischemia and may have had no direct effect on the outcome. HSP 70 then represented a marker of cell injury (Gonzalez et al 1989). However, that result did not preclude HSP from occupying a protective function in neurons after injury since it was not present in neurons at the time of injury. Also since the stress response involved the induction of many more stress proteins it did not exclude their role in the protection of neurons from ischemic injury.

Several points were partially or fully supported in the rat model of global ischemia. The first finding was that HSP 70 synthesis was delayed or absent in many regions of the ischemic brain. That implied that the threshold for HSP 70 synthesis was different in various regions of the brain and also in selected neurons. Those differences remain unexplained. The delay in synthesis may have been the result of a global decrease in protein synthesis which is a hallmark of ischemic injury (Dienel et al, 1980; Kirino and Sano, 1984; Thilmann et al, 1986; Widmann et al, 1991; Hu and Wieloch, 1993). However, a final explanation may involve differences in mechanisms of HSP 70 induction in neurons since glial cells and endothelial cells in the ischemic brain did not

201

significantly synthesize HSP 70. Recent work showed bipolar cells tentatively identified as type 2 astrocytes and microglia were HSP 70 immunoreactive after global ischemia (Gaspary et al, 1995). Despite those findings neuronal HSP 70 still provided the majority of immunoreactivity in most studies. As mentioned previously, it was possible that the immunoreactivity was decreased in glial cells because of protein-protein interactions between HSP 70 and glial proteins which resulted in false negative staining. Finally if glial cells were not actively involved in the stress response by induction of HSP 70 synthesis then it may represent an altered mechanism of induction in those cells. In gerbil hippocampus a 10 minute ischemia caused an increase in HSP 70 in hilar neurons but much later in glial fibrillary acidic protein positive astrocytes in the same region (Araki et al, 1994). The cellular signal transduction pathways for the stress response was unclear but may be different in glial cells compared with neurons.

Though the majority of work centered around the induction of HSP 70 in ischemia, the stress response as it applied to ischemia involved other less studied stress proteins. The induction of HSC 70 mRNA after ischemia mirrored the induction of HSP 70 mRNA in global ischemia in the gerbil (Abe et al, 1991; Sato et al, 1992; Aoki et al, 1993c) but was not corroborated with immunoblot evidence of an increase in expression of HSC 70. Other stress protein families were studied in the setting of hypoxia-ischemia. HSP 90 alpha heat shock protein mRNA was induced in gerbils after 10 minutes of transient global ischemia (Kawagoe, et al, 1993a). In situ hybridization showed that HSP 90 alpha mRNA was induced after ischemia and peaked 8 hours into recovery. In CA1 hippocampal cells HSP 90 mRNA was continuously induced for 24 hours and diminished by 48 hours after recovery. The findings supported a generalized stress response in CA1 neurons after global ischemia. The family of HSP 70 genes is expanding. Using subtractive hybridization of cDNA libraries constructed from gerbil ischemic brain a DNA sequence having 91.3 % homology with human HSP 70 was isolated (Abe et al, 1993b). Besides the stress proteins, expression of other mRNAs and proteins were described after ischemic injury. They included cytoskeletal proteins (Saito et al, 1995), ornithine decarboxylase (Dienel et al, 1985; Muller et al, 1991), superoxide dismutase (Matsuyama et al, 1993), and growth factors (Lindvall et al, 1992).

Since HSP 70 mRNA was not predictive of neuronal survival, other investigators have looked at other neuronal specific markers such as microtubule-associated proteins (MAP 2b and 2c) to predict survival (Saito et al, 1995). MAPs are expressed developmentally in the nervous system and were hypothesized to be expressed in those injured neurons as a regenerative response. MAP 2c mRNA was expressed in neurons destined to survive as a late postischemic response. The authors, however, admitted that a transient expression of MAP 2c may have been present in neurons destined to die. In contrast, HSP 70 mRNA was expressed in brain regions where neurons were destined to survive or die after ischemia. The persistence of HSP 70 mRNA expression correlated with increased postischemic cell injury.

In rat four-vessel occlusion model of ischemia, induction of tau, a microtubule associated protein, was noted within two hours after ischemia in those hippocampal neurons which eventually demonstrated HSP 70 immunostaining (Geddes et al, 1994). In contrast, MAP 2 showed less correlation with HSP 70 induction and was not a predictor of neuronal death. Because HSP 70 induction was noted after tau induction the latter was an early indicator of ischemic cell injury. Examination of another cell marker, parvalbumin, showed that survival of parvalbumin-immunoreactive neurons in the gerbil hippocampus and cortex after ischemia did not depend on HSP 70 induction (Ferrer et al, 1995).

In an attempt to establish mechanisms of induction of HSP70, proto-oncogenes were studied. Induction of immediate early genes c-jun and jun B was rapid and transient in the hippocampal dentate gyrus while c-fos remained at an upregulated state for many hours (Woodburn et al, 1993). HSP 70 mRNA was induced in dentate early and CA1, CA3 and cerebral cortex at 24 hours after ischemia. Co-expression of c-fos and HSP 70 mRNA after 2 and 5 minutes of ischemia was studied by in-situ hybridization in gerbil hippocampus (Ikeda et al, 1994). Immunocytochemical studies of gerbil brain after 15 minutes of ischemia revealed c-fos induction in CA3 and CA4 followed by c-jun in CA3 and later still HSP 70 (Takemoto et al, 1995). Selected cortical regions also showed a similar induction pattern. Notably CA1 did not show induction of c-fos, c-jun or HSP 70. With 5 minutes of ischemia induction of c-fos and c-jun was more rapidly induced in the brain except for the hippocampus. Again HSP 70 was not immunodetected until 24 hours after ischemia. It was another study which showed a delay in HSP 70 synthesis after ischemia. It also showed that proto-oncogene immunostaining might predict subsequent HSP 70 synthesis in surviving neurons. However, in a recent study, K+ channel openers prevented global ischemia induced expression of c-fos, c-jun, HSP 70 and APP (Heurteaux et al, 1993). Coincident with those findings was that neuronal cell death in CA1 was abolished. Those results seemed to undermine the importance of HSP 70 in cell survival. However, since cell injury was abolished then HSP 70 induction was not expected.

Ubiquitin is a small heat stress protein which is involved in the degradation of denatured proteins. These proteins become complexed with ubiquitin and targeted for degradation through cytoplasmic proteasomes. After 7.5 minutes of sublethal ischemia in gerbils, ubiquitin-protein complexes were found in hippocampal pyramidal cells and for prolonged periods in CA1 neurons (Hayashi et al, 1991). Those complexes were Triton X-100 insoluble following 20 minutes of ischemia and increased especially in the mitochondria (Hayashi et al, 1992; Hayashi et al, 1993). The persistence of those complexes indicated the degree of intracellular damage to the CA1 neurons. As a result of those complexes free ubiquitin was depleted in the CA1 neurons (Morimoto et al, 1996). Ubiquitin depletion whether due to failure to convert conjugated ubiquitin to free ubiquitin or failure of new synthesis would have impaired the ability of the neurons to reverse injury.

HSP 32 or heme oxygenase is the rate-limiting enzyme in heme catabolism. It catalyzes heme to bilirubin and releases carbon monoxide and ferrous iron in the process (Maines, 1993). The induction of the enzyme was noted in heavy metal toxicity and oxidative stress (Keyse and Tyrrell, 1989; Taketani et al, 1989; Zhang and Liu, 1992). After transient global ischemia the inducible form of heme oxygenase (HO-1) was increased in the ischemic hemisphere and reached a maximum after 12 hours of reperfusion. In situ hybridization showed wide distribution in both neurons and glial-like cells in the cerebral cortex, hippocampus and thalamus (Takeda et al, 1994). With more prolonged global ischemia followed by reperfusion, HO-1 mRNA was found in the cerebral cortex>striatum>hippocampus (Paschen et al, 1994). Zinc protoporphyrin pretreatment prior to transient MCA occlusion reduced infarct size after 22 hours of reperfusion (Kadoya et al, 1995). Zinc protoporphyrin was noted to be an IL-1 antagonist and therefore implicated in the ischemic injury. However, zinc protoporphyrin is also a potent heme oxygenase inhibitor. Another interpretation of the results was that HO-1 and the constitutive heme oxygenase (HO-2) found in neurons were inhibited (Panizzon et al, 1996). That would have resulted in decreased heme degradation, but also less ferrous iron and carbon monoxide. Iron released theoretically would increase free radical formation through the Fenton reaction and lead to oxidative cell injury. However, the antioxidant effect of the heme degradation product, bilirubin, and the guanylyl cyclase regulatory properties of carbon monoxide might easily justify the induction of HO-1 during acute stress to protect the cells from injury. Whether HO-1 is beneficial or harmful during ischemic injury remains to be determined in animal models.

HSP 60, a mitochondrial heat stress protein showed increased expression during the immediate reperfusion period in the gerbil global ischemia model (Abe et al, 1993a). CA1 neurons showed increased expression of HSP 60 mRNA up to 24 hours after ischemia. In contrast HSP 70 and HSC 70 mRNAs were peaking at 24 hours and persisted past 48 hours. That occurred while mitochondrial encoded mRNA for cytochrome oxidase decreased, a sign of mitochondrial DNA damage. Those findings implicated energy failure in the pathophysiology of CA1 hippocampal ischemic damage.

The interaction of HSP 70 with tubulin, a neural protein, was described (Sanchez et al, 1994). In-vitro experiments showed binding of tubulin to carboxyterminal residues 431-444 which were also associated with other microtubule-associated proteins. The significance of that binding was unknown. In transient global ischemia in the gerbil alpha-tubulin mRNA was expressed in regions of cells destined to survive while HSP 70 was induced in regions where survival and cell death occurred (Kumar et al, 1993).

Association of HSP70 was made with beta/A4 amyloid protein precursor (APP) after transient graded global ischemia in gerbil (Tomimoto et al, 1994). After ischemia for three minutes and reperfusion for 48 hours a few neurons in CA1 and layer V/VI of the frontoparietal cortex positively immunostained for APP. After more severe ischemia and 24 hours of reperfusion densely stained neurons were noted in the subiculum and CA3 or the hippocampus and layers III and V/VI of the frontoparietal cortex. In penumbral neurons, those surrounding regions of infarction, co-localization of APP and HSP 70 was noted. APP is thought to have a significant role in neuronal death in Alzheimer's disease and perhaps HSP 70-APP interactions modulate the toxicity of APP.

Studies of HSP 70 induction in human stroke victims are sparse. However, in autopsy cases of long-term stroke survival , HSP 70 expression was noted in CA2, CA3, and CA4 together with gliosis (Kitamura, 1994). Few conclusions can be made on the available human data but the prolonged expression of HSP 70 may have indicated continued subclinical injury or repair of the injured brain.

Focal Cerebral Ischemia

Though the underlying pathophysiological processes are probably not substantially different in focal cerebral ischemia compared with global cerebral ischemia, there are certain histological features which more closely mimic the human condition of cerebral stroke. The focality of the ischemic area also enables the observer to examine and compare normal brain with ischemic brain in the same animal. Also in the global ischemia models, the hippocampus demonstrates more neuronal cell death than cortical neurons. That observation is reversed in the focal ischemia models. The majority of literature described the evolution of infarction relative to the synthesis of HSP 70 in transient focal ischemia in rat brain. Since the suggestion that HSP 70 was a marker of neuronal injury (Gonzalez et al, 1989) many studies confirmed that HSP 70 was present in neurons in areas of infarction. The pattern of infarction involved islands of infarcted tissue among relatively normal areas of brain. HSP 70 was present in neurons within the infarct and in astrocytes in the periphery of the infarct (Sharp et al, 1991). In experiments involving graded duration of focal ischemia for up to 2 hours, no HSP 70 staining was noted in astrocytes (Li et al, 1992). Those investigators found that HSP 70 immunostaining was most intense after 30 minutes of focal ischemia followed by 48 hours of reperfusion. Thirty to 60 minutes of ischemia was the limit of neuronal viability before histological cell death occurred in the damaged area. Longer duration of ischemia was accompanied by a smaller area of HSP 70 positive cortex and more microglial and endothelial cell HSP 70 positive cells. Microglial cells were reported to become HSP 70 positive at one hour after 60 minutes of middle cerebral artery (MCA) occlusion only (Soriano et al, 1994b). Those results clearly indicated a hierarchy of induction in the various cell types in the brain.

After one hour of permanent occlusion of the (MCA), tissue levels of HSP 70 mRNA within the vascular territory increased for the next 24 hours while c-fos mRNA increased in the whole ischemic cortex by 15 minutes and extended up to 3 hours (Welsh et al, 1992). That suggested to those investigators that spreading depression was responsible for the c-fos elevation. In another model both carotids were occluded in combination with permanent MCA occlusion (Welsh et al, 1992). After one hour of combined ischemia and no carotid reperfusion, HSP 70 mRNA was expressed only in the area surrounding the MCA vascular territory. With reperfusion for 2 hours, HSP 70 mRNA became intensely expressed in most of the hemisphere (including the MCA territory) with the combined vascular insults. By 24 hours, HSP 70 mRNA was only evident within the MCA territory. Those results indicated that HSP 70 mRNA was a marker of the ultimately injured cortex and that the induction of HSP 70 mRNA required oxidative metabolism. After permanent occlusion of the MCA and ligation of the ipsilateral common and external carotid arteries, HSP 70 mRNA was induced within 4 hours and persisted for 24 hours within a small area of infarcted MCA territory (Kinouchi et al, 1993a). Some neurons in areas considered to be in the ischemic penumbra were intensely stained for HSP 70. The findings were very similar to those of the transient focal ischemia greater that 90 minutes duration (Li et al, 1992; Kinouchi et al, 1993b).

The latter authors, however, found staining after 60-90 minutes of ischemia and reperfusion in endothelial cells greater than glial cells and neurons.

In situ hybridization studies of oncogenes and other HSPs are not appreciably different than those results seen in global ischemia. In the MCA and ipsilateral ligation model of ischemia, oncogenes c-fos and jun B mRNAs were induced throughout the affected hemisphere within 1 hour of MCA occlusion and by 4 hours induction was increased further in the thalamus and caudate-putamen (Kinouchi et al, 1994). By 24 hours all structures were returning to baseline induction. Interestingly c-jun mRNA was not induced early in the affected hemisphere but later in selected penumbral areas. HSP 70 mRNA correlated with the induction of c-fos and jun B induction. HSC 70 mRNA was studied in the MCA occlusion model and increased in the infarcted cortex at 3, 8 and 24 hours after occlusion and returned to normal by 7 days. HSC 70 protein was not studied (Kawagoe et al, 1992b). Immunohistochemistry localized HSP 27 to microglia in the center of the infarct by 4 hours and by 24 hours staining included reactive astrocytes throughout the affected hemisphere (Kato et al, 1995). Those authors also found HSP 27 in reactive glial in the unaffected hemisphere. It was unclear from that study whether HSP 27 immunoreactivity was associated with new HSP 27 synthesis. It was possible that the epitope was hidden from antibody staining since no staining was noted in control brain and HSP 27 is thought to represent a constitutively expressed HSP. Also no western blot data was presented to show the specificity of the antibody. An earlier study involving multiple HSP mRNAs showed that HSP 27 mRNA was not substantially induced until 8 hours after ischemia (Higashi et al, 1994). In that same study HSP 47 mRNA, a collagen binding protein, was induced after 4 hours of ischemia and increased until 48 hours after ischemia while 78 kDa glucose regulated protein, grp 78, mRNA remained elevated but relatively stable during the same period. HSP 90 was unchanged compared with the untreated animals. In separate studies a new member of the HSP 70 family has been recently cloned and described in focal ischemia, grp 75, or 75 kDa glucose regulated protein (Massa et al, 1995). After ischemia grp75 mRNA was upregulated in neurons of the ischemic forebrain, hippocampus, and basal ganglia. It was suggested that grp 75 represented a marker of metabolic compromise after ischemia.

HSP 70 was also associated with p53, a product of the p53 tumor suppressor gene (Chopp, et al, 1992). After two hours of middle cerebral artery occlusion and 12 hours of recovery, p53 immunostaining was associated with histological neuronal necrosis while HSP 70 was associated with histologically intact neurons. Those investigators suggested that HSP 70 somehow regulated the synthesis of p53. However, since the study was not over several days the presence of HSP 70 may have only marked those neurons which survived for 12 hours and were also destined to die later. A second study showed that p53 was present in regions of brain which were destined to sustain severe neuronal necrosis up to 96 hours of recovery (Li et al, 1994). That association suggested that HSP 70 was a marker of neuronal survival in other brain areas.

Most of the previous studies in the focal ischemia models in the rat centered attention on HSP 70. However, as in the global ischemia models, the appearance of HSP 70 in the ischemic area was very late. If we conclude that after 30 minutes of ischemia HSP 70 induction would not help neuronal survival then the presence of HSP 70 in those affected neurons would primarily represent a marker for neuronal injury. Most of the reviewed studies showed that neurons which synthesized HSP 70 were likely to survive the focal ischemia. Likewise, neurons that did not induce HSP 70 in the area of injury were more likely to die. A conclusion that HSP 70 protected cells from cell death could not be made from those studies. Since HSP 70 induction was late and the fate of the neuron in question was determined much earlier, then it was probable that survival at least in the early period after ischemia was determined by other factors. How HSP 70 might promote the survival and recovery of neurons from ischemia remains unknown.

STRESS PROTEINS IN PRECONDITIONING

The development of tolerance to various stresses is of interest to biologists and now neurobiologists since it integrates the heat shock response and specifically HSP 70. Tolerance was produced by subjecting the targeted cells, tissue or organs to a mild stress then subjecting the tissue to a more severe similar or new stress. It was thought that the mild conditioning stress induced tolerance through the induction of heat shock proteins, specifically HSP 70.

Reports of ischemic tolerance in the brain in vivo, paralleled the development of tolerance in other tissues such as the heart. Hyperthermia in rats for 15 minutes duration at 41.5°C, 24 hours prior to global cerebral ischemia produced striking protection in the dorsal-lateral striatum, inferior frontal cortex, and parasagital cortex in animals examined 7 days after the ischemia (Chopp et al, 1989). Less protection was noted in the subiculum and hippocampus. Similar preheat treatment of 42-42.5° C for 15 minutes 18 hours prior to a brief 5 minute global ischemia resulted in significant neuronal protection in the CA1 region of the hippocampus (Kitagawa et al, 1991a). However, pretreatment 3, 6, 24 or 50 hours prior to ischemia resulted in lack of significant protection. Double pretreatments at 36 and 18 hours prior to ischemia also resulted in protection in CA1 similar to the single 18 hour pretreatment animals. The pretreatments in both studies were capable of producing HSP 70 and it was implied that HSP 70 and/or the general heat shock response was responsible for the protection noted. It is important to note that absolute protection was not achieved by conditioning in those experiments.

Ischemic preconditioning in vivo and subsequent ischemic tolerance was studied in rat and gerbil. In the rat, 3 minutes of conditioning forebrain ischemia resulted in protection of CA1 neurons from 6 minutes and possibly 8 minutes of global ischemia 3 days after the conditioning stress in animals which survived 7 days after the second ischemic insult (Liu et al, 1992). Preconditioning did not protect neurons from a second 10 minute global ischemia. The authors also showed that 3 minutes of ischemia resulted in HSP 70 immunoreactivity. Similar results of tolerance were found by others in variants of the rat global ischemia model (Liu et al, 1993; Nishi et al, 1993). A conditioning stress 24 hours before a second MCA occlusion resulted in protection in the cortex of ischemic animals (Simon et al, 1993). Other investigators showed that the induction of tolerance was not due to changes in cerebral perfusion (Matsushima and Hakim, 1995), arterial pH, paO_2, or glucose during the experiment (Glazier et al, 1994). In the gerbil a similar paradigm of 2 or 5 minute conditioning global ischemia 2 days prior to a second 5 or

10 minute global ischemia resulted in neuronal protection in the hippocampus, cerebral cortex, striatum and thalamus of animals surviving 7 days of recovery after the second ischemia (Kitagawa et al, 1991b; Kirino et al, 1991). HSP 70 was induced by 2 minutes of ischemia. The authors also showed that protection was not afforded by only 1 minute of conditioning ischemia which also did not induce HSP 70 synthesis as shown by western blot analysis. Immunohistochemical staining of ischemia sensitive CA1 neurons after three 2 minute ischemic insults administered at one hour intervals resulted in no HSP 70 staining 24 and 48 hours later (Kato et al, 1993). Those neurons were destined to die from the insult. Ischemia resistant CA3 neurons treated the same way were slightly stained for HSP 70 but survived the insults. Preconditioning hippocampus accelerated subsequent HSP 70 mRNA transcription and HSP 70 immunoreactivity in CA1 neurons in gerbil after the second ischemic insult (Aoki et al, 1993b). The result was greater neuronal survival in CA1. It was concluded form those studies that HSP 70 induction was strongly associated with ischemic tolerance. The timing of the conditioning stress was also crucial to the development of tolerance. Those results also showed that different thresholds of tolerance were present in different neuronal populations and that repeated sublethal insults could result in significant neuronal death.

In supporting studies of the role of HSP 70 in tolerance, quercetin and anti-HSP 70 antibody were infused into the lateral ventricles of preconditioned gerbils (Nakata et al, 1993). That resulted in a marked inhibition of ischemic tolerance. Quercetin was used as an inhibitor of HSP 70 synthesis but since its mode of action is by inhibiting heat shock transcription factor 1 (Nagai et al, 1995), its effects were less specific and involved other stress proteins not studied in that report. The mechanism for the uptake of anti-HSP 70 antibody into neurons was not shown in that study but was unlikely because of its molecular size. Because of the shortcomings of that study, the role of HSP 70 in the development of ischemic tolerance was uncertain. HSP 70 was not a prerequisite for ischemic tolerance in the gerbil CA1 neurons (Abe and Nowak, 1994). By elevating the temperature to 39.5°C during the conditioning stress and comparing those animals with normothermic conditioning stress, the investigators noted that after a second ischemic insult 2 days after the conditioning stress both normothermic and hyperthermic CA1 neurons survived. However, only 50% of normothermic animals induced HSP 70 mRNA compared with all of the hyperthermic group. Accelerated synthesis of HSC 70 was also noted in the same experimental conditions and mirrored the expression of HSP 70 in the same neuronal populations (Aoki et al, 1993a). That was unlike HSP 27 which was induced by preconditioning but was noted in different cellular populations from those staining for HSP 70. HSP 27 was primarily induced in glial cells (Kato et al, 1994b). In separate studies, the amount of HSP 70 induced by preconditioning in dorsal root ganglion cells was more important than the type of preconditioning stress when neurons were exposed to a severe ischemic insult (Amin et al, 1995). Induction of oxidative stress also induced ischemic tolerance in gerbils which supported the hypothesis that multiple types of conditioning stress could induce tolerance to ischemia (Ohtsuki et al, 1992). All of the mentioned studies did not show that HSP 70 induction was necessary for the development of ischemic tolerance.

The mechanism of induced ischemic tolerance is not well understood but may involve

N-methyl-D-aspartate receptor activation, since MK-801, an antagonist of the receptor inhibited the induction of tolerance in previously mentioned gerbil models (Kato et al, 1992). Interestingly a protein synthesis inhibitor, anisomycin, which reduced HSP 70 synthesis did not inhibit tolerance in that study. That latter finding seemed to partially dispel the thought that tolerance was secondary to the recovery of protein synthesis after ischemic injury (Furuta et al, 1993). In contrast early recovery of protein synthesis, as measured by radiolabeled valine, following ischemia was induced by ischemic tolerance in the gerbil hippocampus (Nakagomi et al, 1993). More recently it was shown that adenosine was essential for the development of ischemic brain tolerance (Heurteaux et al, 1995). Adenosine liberated during the conditioning stress stimulated extracellular adenosine A1 receptors in brain which in turn resulted in opening ATP-sensitive K+ channels. Those results indicated that HSP 70 was not essential for the development of tolerance. Further support for those findings included evidence that spreading depression induced by application of KCl to the cerebral cortex resulted in ischemic tolerance (Kobayashi et al, 1995). In both of those models it would have been interesting if the presence of HSP 70 increased ischemic tolerance. The explanation for ischemic tolerance becomes more complicated since repeated stresses reduced expression of c-fos in rat brain. Those cellular processes which turn on or off via the c-fos proto-oncogene are not fully understood and may be of importance in regulating ischemic tolerance. Inhibitors of protein kinase C reduced development of thermotolerance (Kim et al, 1993) and may likely do the same in ischemic tolerance. PKC inhibitors also inhibited ischemic conditioning in the heart (Speechly-Dick et al, 1994).

The explanations for development of ischemic tolerance in neurons did not include what the effect was on other cell types such as glial cells, microglia and endothelial cells. Since all of those cells produce growth factors and cytokines, it was possible that they also contributed to the survival of neurons after severe stress and also conditioning stress. Histological involvement of astrocytes and microglia in the development of ischemic tolerance of CA1 was supported by observing reactive astrocytes and reactive microglia in CA1 after the conditioning stress (Kato et al, 1994a).

DEFINING THE ROLE OF STRESS PROTEINS IN NEURO-PROTECTION: USE OF CULTURED NEURONS AND GLIAL CELLS

The preceding sections revealed convincing evidence for the heat shock phenomenon or stress response in rodent hypoxia-ischemia. Despite the association of neuronal survival and HSP 70 and perhaps other HSPs, the definitive role of HSP 70 in neuronal protection was still unanswered. That was a product of the complexity of the pathophysiology of hypoxia-ischemia and also the evolving signalling pathways resulting in cell death. HSP 70 is likely to emerge as only a part of the entire story of cell death. This section will discuss data primarily from cell culture studies that showed that HSP 70 was necessary for survival from heat shock and possibly from other types of stress. The regulation of HSP 70 will also be discussed in neural cells. We will also suggest models which might answer the questions raised by the previous sections in this chapter.

There were numerous cell culture studies which showed the association of HSP 70 with thermotolerance. There numbers were too great to review here but several monographs are available for those who wish to review the recent literature (Morimoto et al, 1994; Mayer and Brown, 1994). Two significant mammalian cell culture studies showed the necessity of HSP 70 in thermotolerance. In the first Chinese hamster ovary cells were transfected with multiple copies of the heat shock gene promoter minus the HSP 70 coding region (Johnston and Kucey, 1988). The rationale for that was that activated heat shock transcription factor 1 (HSF1) would become activated after heat shock and bound to the transfected heat shock promoter, effectively titering out the available HSF1 for the native cellular heat shock promoters. The result was a striking inhibition of HSP 70 gene translation and transcription and resultant cell death after heat shock. That study showed that HSP 70 was primarily decreased after heat shock but other heat shock genes were largely unaffected. That result was puzzling since all heat shock genes are activated by heat and why HSP 70 alone was decreased remains unanswered. The second study used monoclonal antibodies specific to HSP 70 and HSC 70, that were microinjected into rat fibroblasts and then the cells were heat treated (Riabowol et al, 1988). The result was that HSP 70 and HSC 70 were synthesized but the newly synthesized and constitutive HSC 70 were unable to translocate into the nucleus after the heat stress, being bound by the injected antibodies. That resulted in fibroblast cell death. One conclusion was that HSP 70 synthesis was not adequate to protect the cell unless the protein was able to also translocate into the nucleus with HSC 70. It would have been interesting if heat stress were administered prior to microinjection of the antibodies. Since the translocation of HSP 70 and HSC 70 occurs soon after the heat stress, we would predict that the microinjection of the antibodies would have less or no detrimental effect on cell survival.

In the nervous system only one study showed the necessity of HSP 70 during stress. Microinjection of a mouse monoclonal antibody with specificity to HSP 70 and HSC 70 into cultured cerebral neurons was reported to lead to thermosensitivity (Khan and Sotelo, 1989). Despite the scant data it supported the previous reports that HSP 70 and likely HSC 70 were important in cellular thermoprotection.

Most of the early in-vitro work in the nervous system which implicated HSP 70 as a neuroprotective protein was by indirect observation and association. A basic design of experiments was to induce HSP 70 by heat shock in cultured neurons then subject those same neurons to a second stress. The second stress was either another severe heat stress or excitotoxin such as glutamate (Lowenstein et al, 1991; Rordorf et al, 1991). In both of those studies cerebellar granule cells (Lowenstein et al, 1991) and cortical neurons in mixed cortical cell cultures (Rordorf et al, 1991) were protected from glutamate toxicity by the conditioning stress. Nonspecific protein synthesis inhibitors inhibited the protective effect of the conditioning stress (Rordorf et al, 1991). That finding implied that the synthesis of protein and likely HSP 70 was responsible for the protection. However, the major question remained unanswered: Did HSP 70 protect neurons from neurotoxicity due to a variety of sources or was it a more general stress response? Since the prestress induced HSP 70 and many other proteins and HSPs the conclusion that HSP 70 was protective was unclear. HSP 70 as a marker of injury or recovery was just as likely. Another question was related to the presence of HSP 70 in the neurons prior to the second stress. The interval between stresses ranged from 14 to 24 hours in those studies. What was the basis for the selection of the timing interval between the preheat stress and the second stress? It was clear from non-nervous system and nervous system studies in vitro that the time interval between the conditioning stress and subsequent stress was very important. It implied that a certain level of HSP 70 correlate with protection and perhaps a certain subcellular location was also required as well. Those questions remain unanswered. A possible answer was that the neurons were recovering from heat stress and that the appearance and disappearance of HSP 70 presented a window where many cellular protective processes were operating and contributing to neuronal protection. Another possibility was that HSP 70 had a direct effect on cellular survival by "protecting" essential cytoplasmic proteins and removing denatured peptides and proteins caused by the stress. HSP 70 and HSC 70 interacted with newly synthesized polypeptide chains after stress (Beckmann et al, 1990). However, during stress that interaction was not transient as in normal growth conditions which implied that normal protein folding reactions were disrupted. In neurons after stress many cellular proteins specific to neurons might be affected and the ability of HSP 70, HSC 70 and probably other HSPs to chaperone and protect those proteins from inactivation were crucial for neuronal survival. Virtually no information is available which demonstrates direct interaction of HSP 70 and neuronal specific proteins.

One of the first studies in vivo which demonstrated an association of HSP 70 with cellular protection in the nervous system was performed in the rat retina (Barbe et al, 1988). In that study the rats were first preheat stressed then allowed to recover and then subjected to an intense retina damaging light source. In the pretreated animals significant and optimal protection of the photoreceptor cells was afforded by heat shock 18 hours prior to the light stress. That correlated with the highest levels of HSP 70 in the retina when measured by western blot analysis. Other findings included the lack of protection if the interval between stresses was increased to 50 hours or decreased to less than 10 hours. In addition to an elevation of HSP 70, HSC 70 and HSP 110 were increased by the prestress. Again the association of HSP 70 and photoreceptor cell survival was implied but unproven. That in vivo study emphasized that other processes and perhaps HSPs were acting to help produce retinal tolerance to light since the window of protection was not necessarily only during the optimal levels of HSP 70 production.

To resolve the dilemma of unspecified cellular responses confounding whether HSP 70 was involved in cellular survival, different strategies were developed. The first was to develop cell lines which constitutively overexpressed HSP 70 so that a prestress was not needed to induce HSP 70. Since the other HSPs were not increased and other cellular responses related to heat shock or stress were not induced then any effect on cellular survival during many types of stress, were related to the presence of HSP 70. When the HSP 70 human gene was stably transfected into cells lines several investigators reported that those cell lines acquired thermoresistance (Angelidis et al, 1991; Li et al, 1991; Li et al 1992). Transfection of the gene and expression of HSP 70 also protected a tumor necrosis factor-alpha (TNF) sensitive cell line from toxicity by 1000 fold (Jaattela et al, 1992). In related experiments expression of an antisense HSP 70 RNA in a clone increased their sensitivity to TNF. The mechanism for protection from the cytotoxic cytokine was unresolved but the resistant clones showed no difference in TNF binding to its receptor.

In neural cells the transfection of the HSP 70 gene into primary rat dorsal root ganglion cells (Uney et al, 1993; Mailhos et al, 1994) and a neuronal cell line (Mailhos et al, 1994) protected those cells from heat stress. Stable transfection of HSP 90 also protected neurons from heat stress (Mailhos et al, 1994). However, neurons and the cell lines were not protected with NGF deprivation which induced apoptosis in transfected and nontransfected cells (Mailhos et al, 1994). Those same investigators reported that heat shock delayed and protected neurons from apoptosis (Mailhos et al, 1993). The apparent discrepancy was likely related to the many other effects which heat shock induces which were not induced by the presence of HSP 70 alone. Methodological questions regarding the morphology of the DRG neurons and other unspecified cell types made it unclear as to the degree of purity of those cultures for assessment of cell death (Uney et al, 1993). Those authors also believed that unspecified glial cells were also sensitive to heat shock though in our experience rat cortical astrocytes and oligodendrocytes are quite resistant to heat stress even above 45°C (unpublished observations). Both of those studies raised the question of what the mode of cell killing was after heat shock in neurons. Was it apoptosis? It was also reported that the constitutive synthesis of HSP 70 did not protect neurons from other types of cell injury. That implied that other HSPs or factors were responsible for protection from other types of stress. The overexpression of HSP 90 and subsequent conferring of thermoresistance in neurons (Mailhos et al, 1994) indicated that other HSPs might be active in the process of thermoprotection. In rat-1 cells the overexpression of HSP 70 modulated HSF1 phosphorylation and subsequent binding to the heat shock element of the promoter, a possible explanation of improved thermotolerance of those cells (Kim et al, 1995). However, the overexpression of HSP 27 in human fibroblasts did not confer resistance to oxidative stress induced by H_2O_2 (Arata et al, 1995). Those same transfected cells were thermoresistant.

The in vitro HSP 70 gene transfection studies have become more relevant with the recent introduction of two strains of HSP 70 transgenic mice (Marber et al, 1995; Plumier et al, 1995). Each transgene was under the control of the beta-actin promoter. Expression of human HSP 70 (Plumier et al, 1995) and rat HSP 70 (Marber et al, 1995) conferred myocardial resistance to ischemic injury and improved post-ischemic recovery. We studied the rat HSP 70 transgenic mouse and found that those mice appeared and acted normally during an observation period greater than 10 months. Western blot analysis of transgenic brain regions showed transgenic rat HSP 70 in cortex, basal ganglia, thalamus, hippocampus, brainstem and cerebellum (unpublished observations). In addition we have found that those mice expressed the transgene immunohistochemically in neurons of all areas studied. One notable exception to immunostaining was the cerebellar granule cell type. Astroglia and oligodendroglia did not appear to express large amounts of the transgenic HSP 70. Cellular morphology and cerebral architecture appeared normal by standard hematoxylin and eosin staining. Future experiments are planned to test whether the presence of HSP 70 will protect neurons from transient ischemia.

Besides testing the central hypothesis of whether HSP 70 will protect cells, cell culture helped to explore the mechanisms of induction of HSP 70 under conditions which mimicked hypoxia-ischemia or other injuries. Related to that aim, cell culture provided models to study the regulation of the heat shock response and transcription factors which control transcription of the HSPs. It is well known that HSP 70 induction is primarily controlled by the transcription factor denoted as heat shock transcription factor 1 (HSF1). This factor has been extensively characterized in mammalian cells (Wu et al, 1994; Morimoto et al, 1994b). HSF1 is constitutively synthesized and present within cells as an unphosphorylated monomer. After heat shock and likely other stresses, HSF1 becomes trimerized and phosphorylated. That step in the activation of the heat shock genes remains to be fully characterized. Some clues to that activation pathway came from the inhibition of HSP70 synthesis by staurosporine, a multiple protein kinase inhibitor (Erdos and Lee, 1994). Their work implied that phosphorylation was required in the induction pathway or of HSF1 before expression of HSP 70 could occur. Nitric oxide, a cellular second messenger, may be involved in the induction of HSP 70. Heat shock of rats increased nitric oxide production in many tissues including brain (Malyshev et al, 1995). The production of nitric oxide was inhibited when the animals were treated with N-nitro-L-arginine, a nitric oxide synthase inhibitor, and the synthesis and accumulation of HSP 70 was decreased in many tissues. Brain was not measured. In rat cortical neuronal cultures another nitric oxide synthase inhibitor, aminoguanidine, applied 24 hours prior to heat stress decreased HSP 70 synthesis (Nishimura and Dwyer, unpublished observations). That effect was not seen in cultured rat cortical astrocytes. The role of nitric oxide production in the pathogenesis of neuronal cell death is controversial (Choi, 1993). The relationship of nitric oxide to HSP 70 synthesis warrants further investigation in hypoxia-ischemia. In other studies calcium was necessary for HSF1 activation and protein kinase was necessary for HSP 70 transcription (Price and Calderwood, 1991). Stress-activated protein kinases activated c-jun (Sanchez et al, 1994). Their role in the activation of stress protein transcription was not studied.

In regards to ischemia, it was demonstrated that HSF1 was activated within 30 minutes of reperfusion in the gerbil hippocampus after transient ischemia and remained activated for at least 3 hours after reperfusion (Nowak and Abe, 1994). That prolonged activation partially explained the delayed synthesis of HSP 70 in regions of the brain after ischemic injury. Those studies were verified and extended to other regions of ischemic cortex (Higashi et al, 1995). Another mammalian heat shock transcription factor 2 (HSF2) was also characterized in the ischemic cortex but its role in the acute activation of HSP 70 was unlikely since HSF2 activation was not demonstrated by gel shift mobility assay (Higashi et al, 1995).

Conditions which mimicked the extracellular and intracellular environment created by ischemia were studied in cell culture. Glial cultures induced HSP 70 after heat shock (Nishimura et al, 1988b). Using purified astrocytes HSP 70 was induced by conditions important in the pathophysiology of ischemia such as oxidative stress created by exposure to hydrogen peroxide (Nishimura et al, 1988a), hypoxia (Copin et al, 1995) and acidosis (Nishimura et al, 1989). However, the mechanisms of induction were not studied. The mechanism of induction of HSP 70 in acidosis was clarified when it was

213

shown that HSF1 was activated and trimerized and bound to the heat shock promoter sequence (Zimarino et al, 1990).

Clues to the mechanism of activation of HSF1 after ischemic injury come from recent studies of the activation of HSF1 after heat shock. In vivo work showed that the heat shocked animal activated HSF1 in a time frame and pattern similar to that induced by ishemia (Higashi et al, 1995). Rat neuronal cultures showed immediate but prolonged activation of HSF1 after heat shock when compared with astrocytes (Nishimura and Dwyer, 1996). That correlated with the delayed synthesis of HSP 70 over a 24 hour period when compared with astrocytes. Immunocytochemical localization revealed that a significant number of smaller non-process bearing neurons never showed HSP 70 staining. Neurons also showed localization of HSF1 in the cytoplasm and nucleus while astrocytes showed only nuclear localization before, during and after heat shock. HSF2 was present in astrocytes and showed no phosphorylation. However, HSF2 was absent in neurons by western blot analysis. Those findings showed distinct regulatory differences between cortical neurons and astrocytes related to HSP 70 synthesis. Those findings were in sharp contrast to the regulation of HSP 70 synthesis in cultured hippocampal neurons (Marcuccilli et al, 1996). In that study HSP 70 was not induced in primary rat hippocampal neurons after one hour of 42°C heat stress when analyzed up to 24 hours later and compared with cultured astrocytes treated in comparable conditions. Further, HSF1 was absent from hippocampal neurons as analyzed by gel shift mobility assay. HSF2 was present in hippocampal neurons when compared with astrocytes which contained both HSF1 and HSF2. Both studies pointed out differences between astrocytes and two types of neurons. The heterogeneity of neurons was also evident in that some populations expressed different heat shock transcription factors which resulted in different responses to the same stress. It remains to be proven whether differences in transcription factor expression result in selective neuronal vulnerability to ischemia. One hypothesis that could be studied is whether the presence of both HSF1 and HSF2 in neuronal cells will result in increased survival and resistance to a variety of stresses since increased amounts of HSF1 or HSF2 might result in increased expression of a number of HSPs and swifter synthesis of all HSPs. That was in fact the case in rat-1 cells which were transfected with human HSF1 genes and subsequently constitutively expressed increased HSF1 without increasing HSP 70 (Nussenzweig et al, 1994). The transfected cells induced HSP 70 and thermotolerance more rapidly than nontransfected cells but also show decreased duration of HSF1 activation (Shen et al, 1994). HSP 27 and HSP 90 expression were unmodified in unstressed cells.

If HSP 70 is found to protect cells from ischemic damage it would be helpful to have mechanisms to induce HSP 70 without the often deleterious effects of heat or ischemia as a conditioning stress. Recent studies provided clues to the mechanisms of induction of HSP 70. Two conditions activated HSF1 and promoted binding of activated HSF1 to the heat shock promoter; acidosis (Zimarino et al, 1990) and exposure of cells to salicylate (Jurivich et al, 1992). Both conditions were tested in astrocyte cultures and resulted in HSP 70 induction when 1,10 phenanthroline was added in both conditions (Nishimura and Dwyer, 1995). The proposed mechanism was that 1,10 phenanthroline found its way into the nuclear DNA and intercalated, causing transcription of HSP 70 mRNA, but only if HSF1 was already activated. Those experiments showed that the induction of HSP 70 was at least a two step process and that HSP 70 could be chemically induced without heat stress. Those findings need verification in an in vivo model.

Cell culture provided the opportunity to discover conditions which induced other specific HSPs. That was the case in cultured rat astrocytes which induced HSP 32, heme oxygenase 1 (HO1), after oxidative stress caused by exposure of the astrocytes to H_2O_2 (Nishimura et al, 1988a; Dwyer et al, 1992; Dwyer et al, 1995). Brief exposure of cells to H_2O_2 led to induction of HO1 with little induction of HSP 70 in astrocytes. Cultured rat cortical neurons showed little induction of HO1 and no induction of HSP 70 in the same conditions. The mechanism of induction of HO1 was undefined. HO1 activity could lead to the release of free metal ions such as ferrous ion which can directly produce free radical hydroxyl ions through the Fenton reaction. Since oxidative injury may be a major cause of injury in hypoxia-ischemia, heme oxygenase could provide clues to the final pathway of ischemia-induced injury. Recent studies in hippocampal slices showed the protective effect of metalloporphyrins in whole slice hypoxia (Panizzon et al, 1996). It was inferred that heme oxygenase activity was inhibited by the metalloporphyrins. If heme oxygenase activity was detrimental to neuronal survival then the use of metalloporphyrins may become useful as a treatment in hypoxia-ischemia as was shown in the treatment of neonatal hyperbilirubinemia in humans (Kappas et al, 1988; Valaes et al, 1994).

FUTURE DIRECTIONS

The future will bring new models which will increase our knowledge of HSPs in the response to hypoxic ischemic injury. These might take the form of specific knockouts of HSPs (if not lethal) or mutated proteins to decrease the effectiveness of the native proteins. Future studies will involve the overexpression of HSPs in neuronal cells and the antisense knockout of specific HSPs. Each of those models will also provide the opportunity to study the role of other HSPs or factors such as growth factors and cytokines in the pathogenesis of hypoxic-ischemic injury.

The transgenic mouse which overexpresses HSP 70 provides an in vivo model to test the role of HSP 70 in neuronal injury. If results of studies in the transgenic ischemic heart model are as encouraging for the role of HSP 70 in reducing ischemic injury to the brain then the study of regulation and function of HSP 70 and other stress proteins such as heme oxygenase will likely bring new therapeutic strategies for stroke. Another transgenic mouse model which overexpresses Cu-Zn-superoxide dismutase showed prolonged expression of HSP 70 mRNA and neuronal survival after transient focal ischemia (Kamii et al, 1994). That model and others to be developed will demonstrate the influence and interactions of various neuroprotective proteins with HSP 70. Finally, despite the major interest in HSP 70 in ischemic brain injury it is the authors' opinion that many new and exciting findings will be made regarding the functions of HSPs and that many new HSPs remain to be discovered together with other HSP-associated proteins. The finding that HSF1 was localized to over 150 sites within the *Drosophila* chromosomes (Westwood et al, 1991) makes our current understanding of the HSPs only the "tip of the iceberg" of what remains to be learned.

SUMMARY

The induction of stress proteins including HSP 70 is characteristic of the ischemic brain. However, it is apparent from the neonatal, adult-global, and adult-focal ischemic models that HSP 70 expression is not directly correlated with neuronal survival. The expression of HSP 70 in neurons was noted in those areas of brain which were selectively more vulnerable to injury such as various regions of the hippocampus and cerebral cortex. Increased severity of injury resulted in differential expression of HSP 70 in glial cells and endothelial cells. Expression of other HSPs were also studied in neurons and glia in ischemia. Regulation of the expression is still largely unknown except that the transcription factor, HSF1, was found upregulated in ischemia. Oncogene expression has not been directly correlated with HSP 70 expression. Whether HSP 70 or other stress proteins contribute to neuronal survival in animal models remains unanswered.

The phenomenon of acquired tolerance has been extended to animal models of brain ischemia. Mild conditioning thermal and ischemic stress reduced brain damage in several models of ischemic brain injury. Again, although stress protein synthesis was coincident with conditioning, a conclusive role for HSP 70 or other stress protein in ameliorating ischemic neuronal injury *in vivo* remains unresolved.

HSP 70 is inducible in cultured primary glial cells of rat brain under conditions of hyperthermia, acidosis, and oxidative stress, conditions relevant to ischemic brain injury. Neuronal induction of HSP 70 was less robust and delayed in culture. The striking induction of HSP 70 in ischemic brain compared with the weak induction in tissue culture may reflect the severity of injury and other inducers in *in vivo* models.
HSP 70 expression by transfection studies of primary dorsal root ganglion cells showed that HSP 70 protected neurons from heat stress but not from NGF deprivation induced apoptosis. Those studies have not conclusively shown that HSP 70 can protect central nervous system neurons from ischemic stress.

The regulation of HSP 70 induction appears to involve the activation of HSF1 and not HSF2 in brain cells. Culture studies have shown that HSF2 is not present in primary cortical neurons while HSF 1 is not present in primary hippocampal neurons. Those differences may help to explain the differential expression and selective vulnerability of neurons to hypoxic-ischemic injury.

HSP 70 can now be pharmacologically regulated with various chemical treatments and conditions and raises the possibility that clinically relevant strategies can be devised to elevate the expression of HSP 70 in targeted tissues such as brain.

ACKNOWLEDGEMENTS

This work was supported by VHA Medical Research funds at the Veterans Health

Administration Medical Center, Sepulveda, California; Veterans Health Administration Medical Center and ROC, White River Junction, Vermont and the UCLA, Department of Neurology, Los Angeles, California. Additional support was provided by the American Heart Association, Los Angeles Chapter, and the United Cerebral Palsy Research Foundation. We would like to thank Dr. Shi-Yi Lu, Su-Ting Fu, Ruth Cole, Linda Esmaili, Iman Abdalla, Raissa Marasigan-Hill, Bill Gardner, and Shauna McClure for providing technical expertise in our work. We would also like to thank Dr.'s William Welch, UCSF; Richard I. Morimoto, Northwestern University; and Ruben Mestril and Wolfgang Dillman, UCSD for their contributions to our work.

REFERENCES

Abe, H. and Nowak, T.S.Jr., Stress protein induction is not required to express ischemic tolerance in the gerbil, *Soc. Neurosci. Abs.* 20:1036, 1994.

Abe, K., Kawagoe, J., Aoki, M., and Kogure, K., Changes of mitochondrial DNA and heat shock protein gene expressions in gerbil hippocampus after transient forebrain ischemia, *J. Cerebral Blood Flow Metab.* 13:773-780, 1993a.

Abe. K., Sato, S., Kawagoe, J., Lee T.H., and Kogure, K., Isolation and expression of an ischaemia-induced gene from gerbil cerebral cortex by subtractive hybridization, *Neurological Res.* 15:23-28, 1993b.

Abe, K., Tanzi, R.E., and Kogure, K., Induction of HSP70 mRNA after transient ischaemia in gerbil brain, *Neurosci. Lett.,* 125:166-168, 1991.

Adams, R.D., and Victor, M., Cerebrovascular diseases, In: *Principles of Neurology*, Adams, R.D., and Victor, M. (eds), 5th ed., pp. 669, McGraw-Hill, New York, 1993.

Angelidis, C.E., Lazaridis, I., and Pagoulatos, G.N., Constitutive expression of heat-shock protein 70 in mammalian cells confers thermoresistance, *Eur. J. Biochem.* 199:35-39, 1991.

Aoki, M., Abe, K., Kawagoe, J., Nakamura, S., and Kogure, K., Acceleration of HSP 70 and HSC 70 heat shock gene expression following transient ischemia in the preconditioned gerbil hippocampus, *J. Cerebral Blood Flow Metab.* 13:781-788, 1993a.

Aoki, M., Abe, K., Kawagoe, J., Nakamura, S., and Kogure, K., The preconditioned hippocampus accelerates HSP 70 heat shock gene expression following transient ischemia in the gerbil, *Neurosci. Lett.* 155:7-10, 1993b.

Aoki, M, Abe, K., Kawagoe, J., Sato, S., Nakamura, S., and Kogure, K, Temporal profile of the induction of heat shock protein 70 and heat shock cognate protein 70 mRNAs after transient ischemia in gerbil brain, *Brain Res.* 601:185-192, 1993c.

Amin, V., Cumming, D.V.E., Coffin, R.S., and Latchman, D.S., The degree of protection provided to neuronal cells by a pre-conditioning stress correlates with the amount of heat shock protein 70 it induces and not with the similarity of the subsequent stress, *Neurosci. Lett.* 200:85-88, 1995.

Araki, T., Kato, H., Liu, XE, Kogure, K., and Itoyama, Y., Induction of heat shock protein 70 and glial fibrillary acidic protein in the postischemic gerbil hippocampus, *Metab. Brain Dis.* 9:369-375, 1994.

Arata, S., Hamaguchi, S., and Nose, K., Effects of the overexpression of the small heat shock protein, HSP 27, on the sensitivity of human fibroblast cells exposed to oxidative stress, *J. Cell. Physiol.* 163:458-465, 1995.

Barbe, M.F., Tytell, M., Gower, D.J., and Welch, W.J., Hyperthermia protects against light damage in the rat retina, *Science* 241:1817-1820, 1988.

Beckmann, R.P., Mizzen, L.A., and Welch, W.J., Interactions of HSP 70 with newly synthesized proteins: implications for protein folding and assembly, *Science* 248:850-854, 1990.

Blumenfeld, KS., Welsh, RA., Harris, V.A., and Pensenson, M A., Regional expression of c-fos and heat shock protein-70 mRNA following hypoxia-ischemia in immature rat brain, *J. Cerebral Blood Fl. and Metab.* 12:987-995, 1992.

Chopp, M., Chen, H., Ho, K.-L., Dereski, M.O., Brown, E., Hetzel, F.W., and Welch, K.M.A., Transient hyperthermia protects against subsequent forebrain ischemic cell damage in the rat, *Neurology* 39:1396-1398, 1989.

Chopp, M., Li, Y., Dereski, ML., Levine, S.R, Yoshida, Y. and Garcia, J.H., Neuronal Injury and Expression of 72-kDa Heat-Shock Protein After Forebrain Ischemia in the Rat, *Acta Neuropath.* 83:66-71, 1991

Chopp, M, Li, Y., Zhang, Z.G., and Freytag, S.O., p53 expression in brain after middle cerebral artery occlusion in the rat, *Biochem. Biophvs. Res. Commun.* 182:1201-1207, 1992.

Currie, R.W., and White, F.P., Trauma-induced protein in rat tissues: a physiological role for a "heat shock" protein?, *Science* 214:72-73, 1981.

Dienel, G.A., Pulsinelli, W.A., and Duffy, T.E., Regional protein synthesis in rat brain following acute hemispheric ischemia, *J. Neurochem.* 35:1216-1226, 1980.

Dienel, G.A., Cruz, N.F., and Rosenfeld, S.J., Temporal profiles of proteins responsive to transient ischemia, *J. Neurochem.* 44:600-610, 1985.

Dienel, G.A., Kiessling, M., Jacewicz, M., and Pulsinelli, W.A., Synthesis of heat shock proteins in rat brain cortex after transient ischemia, *J. Cerebral Blood Flow Metab.* 6:505-510, 1986.

Dwyer, B.E., Nishimura, R.N., Powell, C.L., and Mailheau, S.L., Focal protein synthesis inhibition in a model of neonatal hypoxic-ischemic brain injury, *Exp. Neurol.* 95:277-289, 1987.

Dwyer, B.E., Nishimura, RN., and Brown, I.R, Synthesis of the major inducible heat shock protein in rat hippocampus after neonatal hypoxia-ischemia, *Exp. Neuro.* 104:28-31, 1989.

Dwyer, B.E., Nishimura, R.N., de Vellis, J., and Yoshida, T., Heme oxygenase is a heat shock protein and PEST protein in rat astroglial cells, *Glia* 5:300-305, 1992.

Dwyer, B.E., Nishimura, R.N., Lu, H.-Y., Differential expression of heme oxygenase-1 in cultured cortical neurons and astrocytes determined by the aid of a new heme oxygenase antibody. Response to oxidative stress, *Mol. Brain Res.* 30:37-47, 1995.

Erdos, G., and Lee, Y.J., Effect of staurosporine on the transcription of HSP 70 heat shock gene HT-29 cells, *Biochem. Biophys. Res. Commun.* 202:476-483, 1994.

Ferrer, I., Soriano, M.A., Vidal, A., and Planas, A.M., Survival of parvalbumin-immunoreactive neurons in the gerbil hippocampus following transient forebrain ischemia does not depend on HSP-70 protein induction, *Brain Res.* 692:41-46, 1995.

Ferriero, D.M, Soberano, H.Z., Simon, RP. and Sharp, F.R, Hypoxia-ischemia induces heat shock proteinlike (HSP 72) immunoreactivity in neonatal rat brain, *Dev. Brain Res.* 53:145-150, 1990.

Furata, S. Ohta, S., Hatakeyama, T., Nakamura, K., and Sakaki, S., Recovery of protein synthesis in tolerance-induced hippocampal CA1 neurons after transient forebrain ischemia, *Acta Neuropathol.* 86:329-336, 1993.

Gaspary, H., Graham, S.H., Sagar, S.M., and Sharp, F.R., HSP 70 heat shock protein induction following global ischemia in the rat, *Mol. Brain Res.* 34:327-332, 1995.

Geddes, J.W., Schwab, C., Craddock, S., Wilson, J.L., and Pettigrew, L.C., Alterations in tau immunostaining in the rat hippocampus following transient cerebral ischemia, *J. Cerebral Blood Flow Metab.* 14:554-564, 1994.

Glazier, S.S., O'Rourke, D.M., Graham, D.I., and Welsh, F.A., Induction of ischemic tolerance following brief focal ischemia in rat brain, *J. Cerebral Blood Flow Metab.* 14:545-553, 1994.

Gonzalez, M.F., Lowenstein, D., Femyak, S., Hisanaga, K., Simon, R., and Sharp F.R., Induction of heat shock protein 72-like immunoreactivity in the hippocampal formation following transient global ischemia, *Brain Res. Bull.* 26:241-250, 1991.

Gonzalez, M.F., Shiraishi, K., Hisanaga, K., Sagar, S.M., Mandabach, M., and Sharp, F.R., Heat shock proteins as markers of neural injury, *Mol. Brain Res.*6:93-100, 1989.

Hayashi, T., Takada, K., and Matsuda, M., Changes in ubiquitin and ubiquitin-protein conjugates in the CA1 neurons after transient sublethal ischemia, *Mol. Chem. Neuropathol.* 15:75-82, 1991.

Hayashi, T., Takada, K., and Matsuda, M., Subcellular distribution of ubiquitin-protein conjugates in the hippocampus following transient ischemia, *J. Neurosci. Res.* 31:561-564, 1992.

Hayashi, T., Tanaka, J., Kamikubo, T., Takada, K., and Matsuda, M., Increase in ubiquitin conjugates dependent on ischemic damage, *Brain Res.* 620:171-173, 1993.

Heurteaux, C., Bertaina V., Wldmann, C., and Lazdunski, M., K+ channel openers prevent global ischemia induced expression of c-fos, c-jun, heat shock protein, and amyloid beta-protein precursor genes and neuronal death in rat hippocampus, *Proc. Natl. Acad. Sci. (USA)* 90:9431-9435, 1993.

Heurteaux, C., Lauritzen, I., Widmann, C., and Lazdunski, M., Essential role of adenosine, adenosine A1 receptors, and ATP-sensitive K+ channels in cerebral ischemic preconditioning, *Proc. Natl. Acad. Sci. (USA)* 92:4666-4670, 1995.

Higashi, T., Takechi, H., Uemura, Y., Kikuchi, H., and Nagata, K., Differential induction of mRNA species encoding several classes of stress proteins following focal cerebral ischemia in rats, *Brain Res.* 650:239-248, 1994.

Higashi, T., Nakai, A., Uemura, Y., Kikuchi, H., and Nagata, K., Activation of heat shock factor 1 in rat brain during cerebral ischemia or after heat shock, *Mol. Brain Res.* 34:262-270, 1995.

Hu, B.R., and Wieloch, T., Stress-induced inhibition of protein synthesis initiation: modulation of initiation factor 2 and guanine nucleotide exchange factor activities following transient cerebral ischemia in the rat, *J. Neurosci.* 13:1830-1838, 1993.

Ikeda, J., Nakajima, T., Osborne, O.C., Mies, G., and Nowak T.S. Jr., Coexpression of c-fos and hsp70 mRNAs in gerbil brain after ischemia: induction threshold, distribution and time course evaluated by in situ hybridization, *Mol. Brain Res.* 26:249-258, 1994.

Jaattela, M., Wissing, D., Bauer, P.A., and Li, G.C., Major heat shock protein hsp70 protects tumor cells from tumor necrosis factor cytotoxicity, *EMBO J.* 11:3507-3512, 1992.

Jacewicz, M., Kiessling, M., and Pulsinelli, W.A., Selective gene expression in focal cerebral ischemia, *J. Cerebral Blood Flow Metab.* 6:263-272, 1986.

Jurivich, D.A., Sistonen, L., Kroes, R.A., and Morimoto, R.I., Effect of sodium salicylate on the human heat shock response, *Science* 255:1243-1245, 1992.

219

Kadoya, C., Domino, E.F., Yang, G.-Y, Stern, J.D., and Betz, A.L., Preischemic but not postischemic zinc protoporphyrin treatment reduced infarct size and edema accumulation after temporary focal cerebral ischemia in rats, *Stroke* 26:1035-1038, 1995.

Kamii, H., Kinouchi, H., Sharp, F.R., Koistinaho, J., Epstein, C.J., and Chan, P.H., Prolonged expression of hsp70 mRNA following transient focal ischemia in transgenic mice overexpressing Cu-Zn-superoxide dismutase, *J. Cerebral Blood Flow Metab.* 14:478-486, 1994.

Kappas, A., Drummond, G.S., Manola, T., Petmezaki, S., and Valaes, T., Sn-protoporphyrin use in the management of hyperbilirubinemia in term new-borns with direct Coombs-positive ABO incompatibility, *Pediatrics* 81:485-497, 1988.

Kato, H., Liu, Y., Araki, T., and Kogure, K., MK-801, but not anisomycin, inhibits the induction of tolerance to ischemia in the gerbil hippocampus, *Neurosci. Lett.* 139:118-121, 1992.

Kato, H., Kogure, K., Araki, T., and Itoyama, Y., Astroglial and microglial reactions in the gerbil hippocampus with induced ischemic tolerance, *Brain Res.* 664:69-76, 1994a.

Kato, H., Liu, Y., Kogure, K., and Kato, K., Induction of 27-kDa heat shock protein following cerebral ischemia in a rat model of ischemic tolerance, *Brain Res.* 634:235-244, 1994b.

Kato, H., Liu, X.-H., Nakata, N., and Kogure, K., Immunohistochemical visualization of heat shock protein-70 in the gerbil hippocampus following repeated brief cerebral ischemia, *Brain Res.* 615:240-244, 1993.

Kato, H., Kogure, K., Liu, X.-H., Araki, T., Kato, K., and Itoyama, Y., Immunohistochemical localization of the low molecular weight stress protein HSP 27 following focal cerebral ischemia in the rat, *Brain Res.* 679:1-7, 1995.

Kawagoe, J., Abe, K., Sato, S., Nagano I., Nakamura S., and Kogure K., Distributions of heat shock protein (HSP) 70 and heat shock cognate protein (HSC) 70 mRNAs after transient focal ischemia in rat brain, *Brain Res.* 587: 195-202, 1992a.

Kawagoe, J., Abe, K., Sato, S., Naganao, I., Nakamura, S., and Kogure, K., Distributions of heat shock protein-70 mRNAs and heat shock cognate protein-70 mRNAs after transient global ischemia in gerbil brain, *J. Cerebral Blood Flow Metab.* 12:794-801, 1992b.

Kawagoe, J., Abe, K., and Kogure, K., Different thresholds of HSP 70 and HSC 70 heat shock mRNA induction in post-ischemic gerbil brain, *Brain Res.* 599:197-203, 1992c.

Kawagoe, J., Abe, K, Aoki, M, and Kogure K., Induction of HSP 90 alpha heat shock mRNA after transient global ischemia in gerbil hippocampus, *Brain Res.* 62:121-125, 1993a.

Kawagoe, J., Abe, K., and Kogure, K., Regional difference of HSP 70 and HSC70 heat shock mRNA inductions in rat hippocampus after transient global ischemia, *Neurosci. Lett.* 153: 165-168, 1993b.

Keyse, S.M., and Tyrrell, R.M., Heme oxygenase is the major 32-kDa stress protein induced in human skin fibroblasts by UVA radiation, hydrogen peroxide, and sodium arsenite, *Proc. Natl. Acad. Sci. (USA)* 86:99-103, 1989.

Khan, N.A., and Sotelo, J., Heat shock stress is deleterious to CNS cultured neurons microinjected with anti-HSP 70 antibodies, *Biol. Cell* 65:199-202, 1989.

Kiessling, M., Dienel, G.A., Jacewicz, M., and Pulsinelli, W.A., Protein synthesis in postischemic rat brain: a two-dimensional electrophoresis analysis, *J. Cerebral Blood Flow Metab.* 6:642-649.1986.

Kim, D., Ouyang, H., and Li, G.C., Heat shock protein hsp70 accelerates the recovery of heat-shocked mammalian cells through its modulation of heat shock transcription factor HSF1, *Proc. Natl. Acad. Sci. (USA)* 92:2126-2130, 1995.

Kim, S.H., Kim, J.H., Erdos, G., and Lee, Y..J., Effect of staurosporine on suppression of heat shock gene expression and thermotolerance development in HT-29 cells, *Biochem. Biophys. Res. Commun.* 193:759-763, 1993.

Kinouchi, H., Sharp, F.R., Koistinaho, J., Hicks, K., Kamii, H., and Chan, P.H., Induction of heat shock hsp 70 mRNA and hsp 70 kDa protein in neurons in the 'penumbra' following focal cerebral ischemia in the rat, *Brain Res.* 619:334-338, 1993a.

Kinouchi, H., Sharp, F.R., Hill, M.P., Koistinaho, J., Sagar, S.M., and Chan, P.H., Induction of 70-kDa heat shock protein and hsp 70 mRNA following transient focal cerebral ischemia in the rat, *J. Cerebral Blood Flow Metab.* 13:105-115, 1993b.

Kinouchi, H., Sharp, F.R., Chan, P.H., Koistinaho, J., Sagar, S.M., and Yoshimoto, T., Induction of c-fos, junB, c-jun, and hsp70 mRNA in cortex, thalamus, basal ganglia, and hippocampus following middle cerebral artery occlusion, *J. Cerebral Blood Flow Metab.* 14:808-817, 1994.

Kirino, T., Tsujita, Y., and Tamura, A., Induced tolerance to ischemia in gerbil hippocampal neurons, *J. Cerebral Blood Flow Metab.* 11:299-307, 1991.

Kitagawa, K., Matsumoto, M., Tagaya, M., Kuwabara, K., Hata, R., Handa, N., Fukunaga, R., Kimura, K., and Kamada, T., Hyperthermia-induced neuronal protection against ischemic injury in gerbils, *J. Cerebral Blood Flow Metab* 11:449-452, 1991a.

Kitagawa, K., Matsumoto, M., Kuwabara, K., Tagaya, M., Ohtsuki, T., Hata, R., Ueda, H., Handa, N., Kimura, K., and Kamada, T., 'Ischemic tolerance' phenomenon detected in various brain regions, *Brain Res.* 561:203-211, 1991b.

Kitamura, O., Immunohistochemical investigation of hypoxic-ischemic brain damage in forensic autopsy cases, *Int. J. Legal Med.* 107:69-76, 1994.

Kobayashi, S., and Welsh, F.A., Regional alterations of ATP and heat-shock protein-72 mRNA following hypoxia-ischemia in neonatal rat brain, *J. Cerebral Blood Flow Metab.* 15: 1047-1056, 1995.

Kobayashi, S., Harris, V.A., and Welsh, F.A., Spreading depression induced tolerance of cortical neurons to ischemia in rat brain, *J. Cerebral Blood Flow Metab.* 15:721-727, 1995.

Kumar,K.,Savithiry,S., and Madhukar, B.V., Comparison of alpha-tubulin mRNA and heat shock protein 70 mRNA in gerbil brain following 10 minutes of ischemia, *Mol. Brain Res.* 20:130-136, 1993.

Li, G.C., Li, L., Liu, Y.-K., Mak, J.Y., Chen, L., and Lee, W.M., Thermal response of rat fibroblasts stably transfected with the human 70-kDa heat shock protein-encoding gene, *Proc. Natl. Acad. Sci. (USA)* 88:1681-1685, 1991.

Li, Y., Chopp, M., Garcia, J.H., Yoshida, Y., Zhang, Z.G., and Levine, S.R., Distribution of the 72-kd heat-shock protein as a function of transient focal cerebral ischemia in rats, *Stroke* 23:1292-1298, 1992.

Li, Y., Chopp, M., Zhang, Z.G., Zalonga, C., Niewenhuis, L., and Gautam, S., p53-immunoreactive protein and p53 mRNA expression after transient middle cerebral artery occlusion in rats, *Stroke* 25:849-856, 1994.

Lindvall, O., Ernfors, P., Bengzon, J., Kokaia, Z., Smith, M.-L., Siesjo, B.K., and Persson, H., Differential regulation of mRNAs for nerve growth factor, brain-derived neurotrophic factor, and neurotrophin 3 in the adult rat brain, following cerebral ischaemia and hypoglycemic coma, *Proc. Natl. Acad. Sci. (USA)* 89:648-652, 1992.

Liu, Y., Kato, H., Nakata, N., and Kogure, K., Protection of rat hippocampus against ischemic neuronal damage by pretreatment with sublethal ischemia, *Brain Res.* 586:121-124, 1992.

Liu, Y., Kato, H., Nakata, N., and Kogure, K., Temporal profile of heat shock protein 70 synthesis in ischemic tolerance induced by preconditioning ischemia in rat hippocampus, *Neurosci.* 56:921-927, 1993.

Lowenstein, D.H., Chan, P.H., and Miles, M.F., The stress protein response in cultured neurons: characterization and evidence for a protective role in excitotoxicity, *Neuron* 7:1053-1060, 1991.

Mailhos, C., Howard, M.K., and Latchman, D.S., Heat shock protects neuronal cells from programmed cell death by apoptosis, *Neurosci.* 55:621-627, 1993.

Mailhos, C., Howard, M.K., and Latchman, D.S., Heat shock proteins hsp 90 and hsp 70 protect neuronal cels from thermal stress but not from programmed cell death, *J. Neurochem.* 63:1787-1795, 1994.

Maines, M.D., Carbon monoxide: An emerging regulator of cGMP in the brain, *Mol. Cell Neurosci.*, 4:389-397, 1993.

Malyshev, I.Y., Manukhina, E.B., Mikoyan, V.D., Kubrina, L.N., and Vanin, A.F., Nitric oxide is involved in heat-induced HSP70 accumulation, *FEBS Lett.* 370:159-162, 1995.

Marber, M.S., Mestril, R., Chi, S.-H., Sayen, R., Yellon, D., and Dillman, W.H., Overexpression of the rat inducible 70-kD heat stress protein in a transgenic mouse increases the resistance of the heart to ischemic injury, *J. Clin. Invest.* 95:1446-1456, 1995.

Marini, A.M., Kozuka, M., Lipsky, R.L., and Nowak, T.S. Jr., 70-kilodalton heat shock protein induction in cerebellar astrocytes and cerebellar granule cells in vitro: comparison with immunocytochemical localization after hyperthermia in vivo, *J. Neurochem.* 54:1509-1516, 1990.

Massa, S.M., Longo, F.M., Zuo, J., Wang, S., Chen, J., and Sharp, F.R., Cloning of rat grp75, an hsp70-family member, and its expression in normal and ischemic brain, *J. Neurosci. Res.* 40:807-819, 1995.

Matsushima, K. and Hakim, A.M., Transient forebrain ischemia protects against subsequent focal cerebral ischemia without changing cerebral perfusion, *Stroke* 26:1047-1052, 1995.

Matsuyama, T., Michishita, H., Nakamura, H., Tsuchiyama, M., Shimizu, S., Watanabe, K., and Sugita, M., Induction of copper-zinc superoxide dismutase in gerbil hippocampus after ischaemia, *J. Cerebral Blood Flow Metab.* 13:135-144, 1993

Mayer, J., and Brown, I. (eds), *Heat Shock Proteins in the Nervous System*, Academic Press, New York, 1994.

Morimoto, Richard I., Tissieres, Alfred, and Georgopoulos, C. (eds) *The Biology of Heat Shock Proteins and Molecular Chaperones*, Cold Spring Harbor Laboratory Press, Cold Spring Harbor, 1994.

Morimoto, R.I., Jurivich, D.A., Kroeger, P.E., Mathur, S.K., Murphy, S.P., Nakai, A., Sarge, K., Abravaya, K., and Sistonen, L.T., Regulation of heat shock gene transcriptioon by a family of heat shock factors, In *The Biology of Heat Shock Proteins and Molecular Chaperones*, Morimoto, R.I., Tissieres, A., and Georgopoulos, C. (eds), pp. 417-455, Cold Spring Harbor Laboratory Press, Cold Spring Harbor, 1994b.

Morimoto, T., Ide, T., Ihara, Y., Tamura, A., and Kirino, T., Transient ischemia depletes free ubiquitin in the gerbil hippocampus CA1 neurons, *Am. J. Path.* 148:249-257, 1996.

Muller, M., Cleef, M., Rohn, G., Bonnekoh, P., Pajunen, A.E.I., Bernstein, H.-G. and Paschen, W., Ornithine decarboxylase in reversible cerebral ischaemia: An immunohistochemical study, *Acta Neuropathol.* 83:39-45, 1991.

Munell, F., Burke, R.E., Bandele, A., and Gubits, R.M, Localization of c-fos, c-jun, and hsp 70 mRNA expression in brain after neonatal hypoxia-ischemia, *Dev. Brain Res.*77: 111-121, 1994.

Nakagomi, T., Kirino, T., Kanemitsu, H., Tsujita, Y., and Tamura, A., Early recovery of protein synthesis following ischemia in hippocampal neurons with induced tolerance in the gerbil, *Acta Neuropathol.* 86:10-15, 1993.

222

Nakata, N., Kato, H., and Kogure, K., Inhibition of ischaemic tolerance in the gerbil hippocampus by quercetin and anti-heat shock protein-70 antibody, *NeuroReport* 4:695-698, 1993.

Nishi, S., Taki, W., Uemura, Y. Higashi, T., Kikuchi, H., Kudoh, K., Satoh, M., and Nagata, K., Ischemic tolerance due to the induction of HSP 70 in a rat ischemic recirculation model, *Brain Res.* 615:281-288, 1993.

Nishimura, R.N., Dwyer, B.E., Cole, R., and de Vellis, J., Induction of the 68/72 kDa heat shock protein during hydrogen peroxide toxicity, In: *NATO ASI Series, Cellular and Molecular Aspects of Neural Development and Regeneration*, Gorio, A., de Vellis, J., Haber, B., Perez-Polo, J.R. (eds.), Vol H22, pp. 227-231, Springer-Verlag, New York, 1988a.

Nishimura, R.N., Dwyer, B.E., Cole, R., de Vellis, J., Liotta, K., The induction of the major heat stress protein in purified rat glial cells, *J. Neurosci. Res.* 20:12-18, 1988b.

Nishimura, R.N., Dwyer, B.E., Cole, R., de Vellis, J., and Liotta, Induction of heat-shock like response after rapid changes of extracellular pH in cultured rat astrocytes, *Exp. Cell Res.* 180:276-280, 1989.

Nishimura, R.N., Dwyer, B.E., Clegg, K., Cole, R., and de Vellis, J., Comparison of the heat shock response in cultured cortical neurons and astrocytes, *Mol. Brain Res.* 9:39-45, 1991.

Nishimura, R.N., and Dwyer, B.E., Pharmacological induction of heat shock protein 68 synthesis in cultured rat astrocytes, *J. Biol. Chem.* 270:29967-29970, 1995.

Nishimura, R.N., and Dwyer, B.E., Evidence for different mechanisms of induction of HSP 70i: a comparison of cultured rat cortical neurons with astrocytes, *Mol. Brain Res.* in press, 1996.

Nowak, T.S. Jr., Synthesis of a stress protein following transient ischemia in the gerbil., *J. Neurochem.* 45:1635-1641, 1985.

Nowak, T.S., Jr., MK-801 prevents 70-kDa stress protein-induction in gerbil brain after ischemia: The heat shock response as a marker for excitotoxic pathology, In *Pharmacology of Cerebral Ischaemia 1988: Proceedings of the Second International Symposium on the Pharmacology of Cerebral Ischaemia* , Krieglstein, J. (ed), pp.229-234, Boca Raton, CRC Press, 1989.

Nowak, T.S. Jr., Localization of 70 kDa stress protein mRNA induction in gerbil brain after ischemia, *J. Cerebral Blood Flow Metab.* 11:432-439, 1991.

Nowak, T.S. Jr., and Abe, H., Postischemic stress response iin brain, In *The Biology of Heat Shock Proteins and Molecular Chaperones*, Morimoto, R.I., Tissieres, A., and Georgopoulos, C. (eds), pp. 553-575, Cold Spring Harbor Laboratory Press, Cold Spring Harbor, 1994.

Nussenzweig, A., Burgman, P. Shen, G., and Li, G.C., Rat-1 cells transfected with human HSF1 are thermal resistant but do not express HSP70 in the absence of stress, *Biology of Heat Shock Proteins and Molecular Chaperones Abs,* pp234, Cold Spring Harbor Laboratory Press, Cold Spring Harbor, 1994.

Ohtsuki, T., Matsumoto, M., Kuwabara, K., Kitagawa, K., Suzuki, K., Taniguchi, N., and Kamada, T., Influence of oxidative stress on induced tolerance to ischemia in gerbil hippocampal neurons, *Brain Res.* 599:246-252, 1992.

Panizzon, K.L., Dwyer, B.E., Nishimura, R.N., Wallis, R.A., Neuroprotection against CA1 injury with metalloporphyrins, *Neuroreport* , in press, 1996.

Paschen, W., Uto, A., Djuricic, B., and Schmitt, J., Heme oxygenase expression after reversible ischemia of rat brain, *Neurosci. Lett.* 180:5-8, 1994.

Plumier, J.-C. L., Ross, B.M., Currie, R.W., Angelidis, C.E., Kazlaris, H., Kollias, G., and Pagoulatos, G.N., Transgenic mice expressing the human heat shock protein 70 have improved post-ischemic myocardial recovery, *J. Clin. Invest.* 95:1854-1860, 1995

223

Price, B.D., and Calderwood, S.K., Ca^{2+} is essential for multistep activation of the heat shock factor in permeabilzed cells, *Mol. Cell. Biol.* 11:3365-3368, 1991.

Riabowol, K.T., Mizzen, L.A., and Welch, W.J., Heat shock is lethal to fibroblasts microinjected with antibodies against HSP-70, *Science* 242:433-436, 1988.

Rordorf, G., Koroshetz, W..J., and Bonventre, J.V., Heat shock protects cultured neurons from glutamate toxicity, *Neuron* 7:1043-1051, 1991.

Saito,N., Kawai, K.,and Nowak, T.S.Jr., Reexpression of developmentally regulated MAP2c mRNA after ischemia: colocalization with hsp 72 mRNA in vulnerable neurons, *J. Cerebral Blood Flow Metab.* 15:205-- 215, 1995.

Sanchez, C., Padilla R., Paciucci, R., Zabala J.C., and Avila, J., Binding of heat-shock protein 70 (hsp 70) to tubulin, *Arch. Biochem. Biophys.* 310:428-432, 1994.

Sanchez, I., Hughes, R.T., Mayer, B.J., Yee, I., Woodgett, J.T., Avruch, J., Kyriakis, J.M., and Zon, L.I., Role of SAPK/ERK kinase-1 in the stress-activated pathway regulating transcription factor c-jun, *Nature* 372:794-798, 1994.

Sato, S., Abe, K., Kawagoe, J., Aoki, M., and Kogure, K., Isolation of complementary DNAs for heat shock protein (HSP) 70 and heat shock cognate protein (HSC) 70 genes and their expressions in post-ischaemic gerbil brain, *Neurol. Res.* 14:375-380, 1992.

Shen, G., Li, L., Yang, S.-H., Wu, C., and Li, G.C., Altered heat shock response in rat-1 cells stably and constitutively expressing the human heat shock factor HSF1, *Biology of Heat Shock Proteins and Molecular Chaperones Abs*, pp 276, Cold Spring Harbor Laboratory Press, Cold Spring Harbor, 1994.

Simon, R.P., Niiro, M., and Gwinn, R., Prior ischemic stress protects against experimental stroke, *Neurosci. Lett.* 163:135-137, 1993.

Simon, R.P., Cho, H., Gwinn, R., and Lowenstein, D.H., The Temporal Profile of 72-KDA Heat-Shock Protein Expression Following Global Ischemia, *J. Neurosci.* 11:881-889, 1991.

Soriano, M.A., Tortosa A., Planas, A.M., Rodriguez-Farre, E., and Ferrer, I., Induction of HSP 70 mRNA and HSP 70 protein in the hippocampus of the developing gerbil following transient forebrain ischemia, *Brain Res.* 653:191-198, 1994a.

Soriano, M.A., Planas, A.M., Rodriquez-Farre, E., and Ferrer, I., Early 72-kDa heat shock protein induction in microglial cells following focal ischemia in the rat brain, *Neurosci. Lett.* 182:205-207, 1994b.

Speechly-Dick, M.E., Mocanu, M.M., and Yellon, D.M., Protein kinase C: its role in ischemic preconditioning in the rat, *Circ. Res.* 75:586-590, 1994.

Takeda, A., Onodera, H., Sugimoto, A., Itoyama, Y., Kogure, K., and Shibahara, S., Increased expression of heme oxygenase mRNA in rat brain following transient forebrain ischemia, *Brain Res.* 666:120-124, 1994.

Takemoto, O., Tomimoto, H., and Yanagihara, T., Induction of c-fos and c-jun gene products and heat shock protein after brief and prolonged cerebral ischemia in gerbils, *Stroke* 26: 1639-1648, 1995.

Taketani, S., Kohno, H., Yoshinaga, T., and Tokunaga, R., The human 32-kDa stress protein induced by exposure to arsenite and cadmium ions is heme oxygenase, *FEBS Lett.* 245:173-176, 1989.

Thilmann, R., Xie, Y., Kleihues, P., and Kiessling, M., Persistent inhibition of protein synthesis precedes delayed neuronal death in post-ischemic gerbil hippocampus, *Acta Neuropathol.* 71, 88-93, 1986.

Tomimoto, H., Wakita, H., Akiguchi, I., Nakamura, S., and Kimura, J., Temporal profiles of accumulation of amyloid beta/A4 protein precursor in the gerbil after graded ischemic stress, *J. Cerebral Blood Flow Metab.*

224

14:565-573. 1994.

Uemoto, S., Noguchi, K., Kawai, Y., and Senba, E., Repeated stress reduces the subsequent stress-induced expression of fos in rat brain, *Neurosci. Lett.* 167:101-104, 1994.

Uney, J..B., Kew, J.N.C., Staley, K., Tyers, P., and Sofroniew, M.V., Transfection-mediated expression of human HSP 70i protects rat dorsal root ganglion neurones and glia from severe heat stress, *FEBS Lett.* 334:313-316, 1993.

Valaes, T., Petmezaki, S., Henschke, C., Drummond, G.S., and Kappas, A., Control of jaundice in preterm newborns by an inhibitor of billirubin production: studies with tin-mesoporphyrin, *Pediatrics* 93:1-11, 1994.

Vass, K., Welch, W.J., and Nowak, T.S.Jr., Localization of 70-kDa stress protein induction in gerbil brain after ischemia, *Acta Neuropathol.* 77:128-135, 1988.

Welsh, F.A., Moyer, D.J., and Harris, V.A., Regional expression of heat shock protein-70 mRNA and c-fos mRNA following focal ischemia in rat brain, *J. Cerebral Blood Flow Metab.* 12:204-212, 1992.

Westwood, J.T., Clos, J., and Wu, C., Stress-induced oligomerization and chromosomal relocalization of heat-shock factor, *Nature* 353:822-827, 1991.

Widmann, R., Kuroiwa, T., Bonnekoh, P., and Hossmann, K.-A., [^{14}C] Leucine incorporation into brain proteins in gerbils after transient ischaemia: Relationship to selective vulnerability of hippocampus, *J. Neurochem.* 56:789-796, 1991.

Woodburn, V.L., Hayward N.J., Poat J.A., Woodruff, G.N., and Hughes, J., The effect of dizocilpine and enadoline on immediate early gene expression in the gerbil global ischaemia model, *Neuropharm.*32: 1047-1059, 1993.

Wu, C., Clos, J., Giorgi, G., Haroun R.I., Kim, S.-J., Rabindran, S.K., Westwood, J.T., Wisniewski, J., and Yim, G., Structure and regulation of heat shock transcription factor, In *The Biology of Heat Shock Proteins and Molecular Chaperones*, Morimoto, R.I., Tissieres, A., and Georgopoulos, C. (eds), pp. 395-416, Cold Spring Harbor Laboratory Press, Cold Spring Harbor, 1994.

Zhang, H., and Liu, A.Y.-C., Tributyltin is a potent inducer of the heat shock response in human diploid fibroblasts, *J. Cell. Physiol.* 153:460-466, 1992.

Zimarino, V., Wilson, S., and Wu, C., Antibody-mediated activation of *Drosophila* heat shock factor in vitro, *Science* 249:546-549, 1990.

225

INDEX